Gynecological Laparoscopic Surgery: An Evidence-Based Approach

Gynecological Laparoscopic Surgery: An Evidence-Based Approach

Edited by Florence McClure

AMERICAN
MEDICAL PUBLISHERS
www.americanmedicalpublishers.com

American Medical Publishers,
41 Flatbush Avenue,
1st Floor, New York,
NY 11217, USA

Visit us on the World Wide Web at:
www.americanmedicalpublishers.com

ISBN: 978-1-63927-493-2

Cataloging-in-Publication Data

Gynecological laparoscopic surgery : an evidence-based approach / edited by Florence McClure.
p. cm.
Includes bibliographical references and index.
ISBN 978-1-63927-493-2
1. Laparoscopic surgery. 2. Generative organs, Female--Endoscopic surgery.
3. Generative organs, Female--Surgery. 4. Evidence-based medicine.
I. McClure, Florence.

RG104.7 .G96 2022
618.105 9--dc23

Table of Contents

Preface

In past decades, laparoscopic surgery has emerged as a gynecological surgical procedure with applications in diagnosis and tubal ligations, as well as for the treatment of multiple gynecological conditions. Laparoscopy is widely used for the treatment of endometriosis, removal of ectopic pregnancy, ovarian cystectomy and hysterectomy, as well as the removal of fibroids, ovarian cysts, lymph nodes and uterus. It is also used for correcting pelvic organ prolapse and the cancers of the uterus, ovary and cervix. Compared to laparotomy, laparoscopy is safer, less expensive and has shorter recovery time. This book is compiled in such a manner, that it will provide an in-depth knowledge about the theory and practice of gynecological laparoscopic surgery. The topics included herein are of utmost significance and bound to provide incredible insights to readers. In this book, using case studies and examples, constant effort has been made to make the understanding of the difficult concepts as easy and informative as possible, for the readers.

This book has been the outcome of endless efforts put in by authors and researchers on various issues and topics within the field. The book is a comprehensive collection of significant researches that are addressed in a variety of chapters. It will surely enhance the knowledge of the field among readers across the globe.

It gives us an immense pleasure to thank our researchers and authors for their efforts to submit their piece of writing before the deadlines. Finally in the end, I would like to thank my family and colleagues who have been a great source of inspiration and support.

Editor

1

Non-technical factors influence laparoscopic simulator performance among OBGYN residents

Liv Ahlborg · Leif Hedman · Carsten Rasmussen · Li Felländer-Tsai · Lars Enochsson

Abstract In addition to technical skills, nontechnical factors appear to influence surgical results. This study aims to analyze how visuospatial ability, self-efficacy, and flow are associated with simulated laparoscopic performance of residents in obstetrics and gynecology (OBGYN). In this cohort study, 28 residents in obstetrics and gynecology were tested for visuospatial ability and self-efficacy prior to simulator training. All participants subsequently conducted a basic set of tasks in the simulator. Self-efficacy, once again, and flow were assessed after training. Nineteen of the subjects then completed a 2-day course with identical simulator tasks, although now to a predefined credential level. Visuospatial ability correlated with simulator performance in the technically most advanced simulator task in the basic set ("total time," $r=-0.40$, $p=0.039$). Flow correlated with: "right instrument pathway"($r=-0.40$, $p=0.004$) in that same task and with the 2-day overall training results ($r=-0.56$, $p=0.017$). Self-efficacy correlated with the 2-day result ($r=-0.56$, $p=0.013$) and significantly improved after training ($p=0.011$). When constructing a curriculum for OBGYN residents, visuospatial abilities and non-technical factors like flow and self-efficacy should be considered.

L. Ahlborg · L. Hedman · L. Felländer-Tsai · L. Enochsson
Center for Advanced Medical Simulation and Training (CAMST),
Karolinska University Hospital,
Stockholm, Sweden

L. Ahlborg · L. Felländer-Tsai · L. Enochsson
Department of Clinical Science,
Intervention And Technology (CLINTEC),
Karolinska Institutet at Karolinska University Hospital,
Stockholm, Sweden

L. Ahlborg (✉)
Division of Obstetrics and Gynecology, Södertälje Hospital,
152 86 Södertälje, Sweden
e-mail: liv.karlsson-ahlborg@ki.se

L. Hedman
Department of Psychology, Umeå University,
Umeå, Sweden

L. Enochsson
Divisions of Surgery, Karolinska University Hospital,
Stockholm, Sweden

L. Felländer-Tsai
Divisions of Orthopaedics, Karolinska University Hospital,
Stockholm, Sweden

C. Rasmussen
Divisions of Obstetrics and Gynecology,
Karolinska University Hospital,
Stockholm, Sweden

Keywords Gynecological laparoscopy · Simulator training · Nontechnical skills

Background

The lack of structured training programs for residents performing surgery is jeopardizing patient safety [1–3]. Simulators are becoming important training tools in preparing for various real-life scenarios. For example, computerized simulations appear to be beneficial for enhancing the technical performance among surgery and obstetrics and gynecology (OBGYN) residents [4–6].

In addition to technical skills, nontechnical factors appear to be important when constructing a surgical curriculum. Previous studies have reported behavior-rating systems for surgeons based on skills, such as situation awareness, decision making, communication, and leadership. Such systems appear to be beneficial for safe surgical practice [7–10].

Our research group has focused on trying to identify nontechnical factors that might influence the learning process during image-guided simulator training. Visuospatial ability, commonly defined as the capacity to generate "a mental representation of a two- or three-dimensional structure and then assessing its properties or performing a transformation of the representation" [11] appears to influence operative performance. We have previously reported that visuospatial abilities correlate with simulated laparoscopic performances among surgical novices and for consultants in OBGYN [12–14]. Since simulator training appears to improve surgical performance, testing residents for visuospatial abilities could improve the design of individual training programs.

Another important feature of the learning process is self-efficacy, i.e., one's belief in one's ability to succeed in specific situations [15]. For example, Maschuw et al. [16] reported that low self-efficacy correlates with poor simulator performance among surgical residents. Flow, i.e., "to move or run smoothly with unbroken continuity and concentration and complete absorption in what one does" [17], is another factor that appears to be of importance for task performance. A recent study shows that repeated team training of cardiopulmonary resuscitation in a virtual world increase concentration, as well as self-efficacy in medical students [18]. Assessments of self-efficacy and flow might therefore be useful for evaluating a training program's or an instrument's effectiveness and feasibility.

The aim of the present study was to explore visuospatial ability, self-efficacy, and flow in OBGYN residents in relation to laparoscopic simulator performance, in preparation for constructing a gynecological curriculum.

Methods

The study group consisted of 28 OBGYN residents from 21 different hospitals in Sweden. Exclusion criteria were more than ten independently performed laparoscopic tubal occlusions or attendance at a simulator course prior to the study. The study intended to investigate the abilities among laparoscopic novices with no prior laparoscopic simulator training.

The study was conducted at the Center for Advanced Medical Simulation and Training (CAMST), at Karolinska University Hospital, Stockholm, Sweden, during a week in 2009. The regional Research Ethics Committee of Stockholm approved the study.

Visuospatial ability

In order to test for visuospatial ability, all participants first completed the redrawn Vandenberg and Kuse Mental rotations test, version A (MRT-A) [19]. The test consists of 24 items each containing a target figure to the left with four stimulus figures to the immediate right of the target figure. The task for the test subject is to mentally rotate the stimulus figures around the vertical axis. Participants had to identify both of two correct alternatives in order to get a score of "1." Thus the maximum score was 24. Each participant was given the items organized into two subsets consisting of 12 items each. Three minutes were given to complete each subset. There was a 1-min break between each part. Instructions, procedures, and scoring were identical to those of Peters and collaborators [19].

Simulator performance

For laparoscopic gynecological simulation, we used the LapSimGyn® VR (virtual reality) (Surgical Science AB, Gothenburg, Sweden) simulator, which is an advanced laparoscopic simulator with proven construct validity [20–22]. The system consists of software that runs on a Xeon-1.8 GHz processor using the Microsoft Windows® XP (Microsoft Corporation, Redmond, WA, USA) operating system. The computer is equipped with 256 MB internal RAM, a NVIDIA Quadro2 EX graphics card (NVIDIA Corporation, Santa Clara, CA, USA), a 15-inch monitor, and a virtual laparoscopic interface manufactured by Immersion, Inc. (San Jose, CA, USA).

All participants did one set of basic procedures to get familiar with the simulator and then one to two more sets to complete the basic simulator training.

Additionally, 19 of the subjects completed a 2-day course, which consisted of the same set of tasks. The subjects trained until they reached a predefined credential level in the simulator [4]. The simulator tasks performed were "cutting," "clip applying," "lifting and grasping," "tubal occlusion," and "salpingectomy." The most demanding task in this set was "lifting and grasping," and it was therefore selected in subsequent analyses. This skill, as well as the other in the set, has previously been reported to discriminate between novices and experts, i.e., to demonstrate construct validity [21]. In this task, you need to move a small needle with great precision and use a short distance (instrument path length), a small angle (instrument angular path length), and speed (total time) to reach the credential level.

The simulator parameters analyzed in the task "lifting and grasping" were "total time" (seconds), left and right "instrument angular path length" (degrees), and "instrument path length" (meters). The performance during the 2-day training course was measured by the number of trials until reaching the credential level in the task "lifting and grasping" and the sum of trials of all tasks until reaching credential level.

Self-efficacy

Individual self-efficacy is a capability in which cognitive, social, emotional, and behavioral skills must be organized and effectively orchestrated to serve several different purposes. Self-efficacy is not concerned with the number of skills you have, but what you believe you can do with the skills you have. Banduras' cognitive theory suggests that, while successful performance enhances, repeated failures reduce perceived self-efficacy [23].

In this study, self-efficacy was assessed using a three-item questionnaire where each item was rated on a 7-grade Likert-type scale. The subjects completed the questionnaire before and after basic training as well as after the 2-day training course. Self-efficacy was calculated as the sum of all items [24].

Flow

Flow experience is reported to facilitate learning, encourage one to attempt a difficult task, promote the pace of creativity, increase the joy during an activity, and create meaning of involvement in an activity [25, 26].

Four categories of flow [27] were self-assessed using a 0–10 visual analog scale (enjoyment, four items; concentration, four items; control, three items; exploratory use, four items). A flow score was calculated as the sum of all items. Flow was assessed after the basic simulator set and after the 2-day simulator training.

Study design

The 28 OBGYN residents were first tested regarding visuospatial ability using MRT-A. They completed the self-efficacy evaluation before and after basic simulator training. The 19 participants taking the 2-day training course were additionally evaluated after the course. Flow was assessed following both basic and extensive simulator training (Fig. 1).

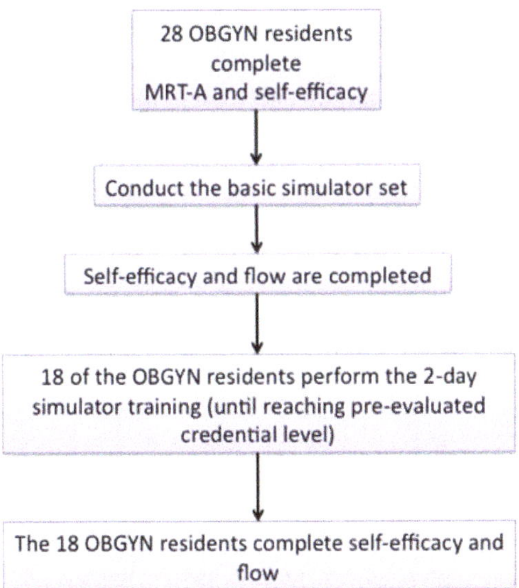

Fig. 1 Study design

Statistical analyses

Data analyses were carried out using JMP® version 9.0.0 (SAS Institute, Inc., Cary, NC, USA) for Mac OS X® version 10.5.7 (Apple, Inc., Cupertino, CA, USA). All the variables were tested for normality. Pearson's correlation was used to analyze the relationship between visuospatial ability, self-efficacy, and flow, respectively, and simulated laparoscopic performance. Student's t test was used to investigate differences in self-efficacy mean scores between the different sessions of simulator training. A level of $p<0.05$ was considered to be statistically significant.

Findings

The basic simulator set

The 28 subjects (23 females and five males; mean age of 34 years±5 SD) performed a basic set of tasks in the simulator. The first of two sets was performed to allow the subjects to familiarize themselves with the simulator.

We analyzed the performance of the second session of the task "lifting and grasping."

We first tested if visuospatial abilities and self-efficacy influenced the simulator performance. For this purpose, MRT-A scores were correlated with the parameter "total time" in the task "lifting and grasping." These two parameters were indeed inversely correlated with each other ($r=-0.40$, $p=.039$; Fig. 2). The visuospatial ability and self-efficacy were not intercorrelated.

No significant correlation was observed between self-efficacy, before or after the basic simulator set, and the simulator performance.

Next, we assessed whether the experience of flow correlated with the basic simulator performance. Flow correlated with four of the basic "lifting and grasping" simulator performance parameters analyzed (Table 1).

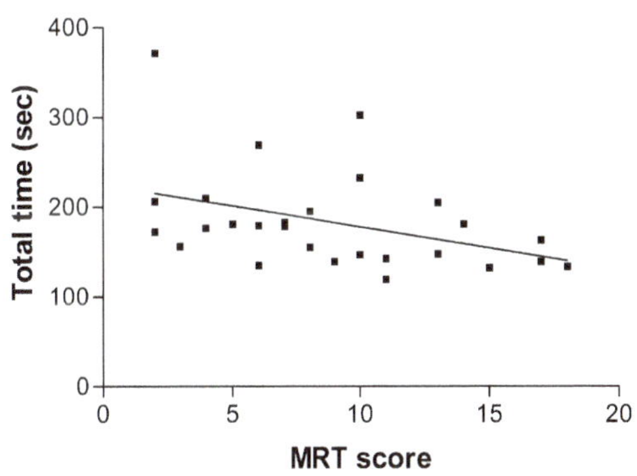

Fig. 2 Correlation between the visuospatial ability and the simulator performance in the basic set

Table 1 Correlation between basic simulator performance and flow

Simulator performance	Flow	
Lifting and grasping	*r*	*p* value
Right instrument angular path length (°)	−0.43	0.026
Left instrument angular path length (°)	−0.45	0.019
Right instrument path length (m)	−0.40	0.037
Left instrument path length (m)	−0.42	0.028

The 2-day simulator training

We next investigated whether visuospatial ability and self-efficacy had an impact on the simulator performance when subjects were trained. For this purpose, the 19 subjects (15 females and four males) who attended the 2-day course and who then all passed the pre-evaluated credential levels were further studied. Whereas the average number of sessions to reach the credential level in the task "lifting and grasping" was 31, the other tasks only required between four and 15 sessions, suggesting that "lifting and grasping "was the most demanding task. The average number of trials of all tasks, to reach credential level, was 69. When assessing simulator data from the 2-day course, we analyzed the number of trials until reaching the credential level in the task "lifting and grasping," as well as the sum of trials of all tasks until reaching credential level. The sum of trials of all tasks to reach credential level was calculated to generate an overall result from the 2-day training.

We also wanted to analyze the association between extensive simulator training and flow.

Performance in "lifting and grasping" and the overall result correlated with flow and self-efficacy, assessed after the course. Furthermore, the overall simulator results correlated with self-efficacy scores assessed before training (Table 2).

Table 2 Correlations between simulator performance, self-efficacy, and flow

	Self-efficacy before		Self-efficacy after		Flow	
Simulator performance after training	*r*	*p* value	*r*	*p* value	*r*	*p* value
Sessions of lifting and grasping until passed course	−0.40	0.089	−0.61	0.007	−0.48	0.042
Total sessions until passed course	−0.56	0.013	−0.74	0.001	−0.56	0.017

Self-efficacy was assessed before and after the 2-day simulator course. Flow was assessed after the 2-day simulator course

MRT-A, however, did not correlate with the simulator performance when subjects were trained.

A comparison of self-efficacy scores before basic training and after the 2-day simulator training suggested improvement in self-efficacy after intensive simulator training (Fig. 3).

Because of the gender imbalance, we also subanalyzed the female group. Most correlations became stronger, although when excluding the males, self-efficacy before the 2-day training and flow after did not significantly correlate to lifting and grasping. The correlations with the overall training result were still significant though.

Prior to the study, 14 of the residents had performed zero to one tubal occlusion, five of the residents had performed two to five, and ten of the subjects had performed six to ten laparoscopic tubal occlusion independently.

Discussion

In this study, we report correlations between visuospatial ability, flow, and self-efficacy, respectively, and the performance in image guided simulation, among residents in OBGYN. We also report an increase in self-efficacy after intense simulator training. To the best of our knowledge, these parameters have not previously been evaluated in OBGYN residents.

We chose to analyze the most difficult task in the simulator, "lifting and grasping" [21], in relation to self-efficacy, flow, and visuospatial ability. For this task, the average number of trials to reach the credential level was 31, whereas the typical gynecological procedures, "tubal occlusion" and "salpingectomy," were not as challenging, requiring only 4 and 8 trials, respectively. These procedures were, however, included when we analyzed the overall result, i.e., the sum of all tasks, to reach the credential level.

In this study, visuospatial ability correlated with the outcome of simulator performance only in the technically more demanding "lifting and grasping" in the basic simulator set.

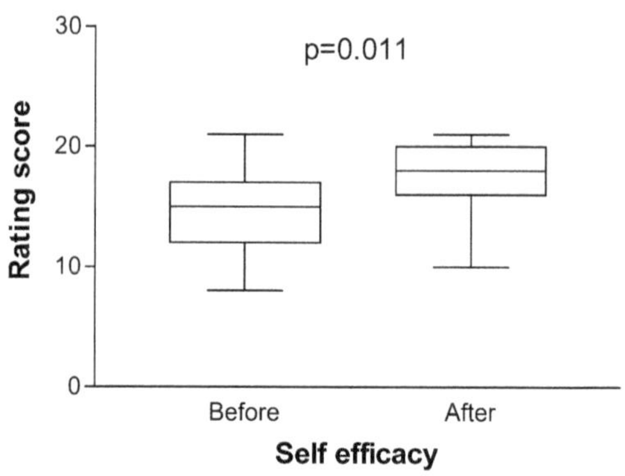

Fig. 3 Self-efficacy score before and after the 2-day training

This is in line with the study by Westman et al. [13] and Hedman et al. [14] who demonstrated that visuospatial abilities correlate positively with performance in the technically more demanding simulated colonoscopy and arthroscopy, respectively. Moreover, we previously reported that the visuospatial abilities of consultants in OBGYN correlated with the more demanding tasks during laparoscopic simulator training [12]. In the present study, visuospatial ability did not, however, correlate with simulator performance after training intensely during 2 days. These findings suggest that this type of training can compensate for a lesser visuospatial ability in novices. Testing the visuospatial ability can thus identify individuals who might benefit from such supplementary training and who need support in specific surgical tasks. It, however, remains to be established if visuospatial abilities also influence the actual surgical performance.

Others have reported that nontechnical factors play important roles in performing and learning the technical skills in surgery [8–10, 28]. Artino et al. reported that medical students who are bored and anxious achieve less theoretically. In their study, self-efficacy was positively correlated with enjoyment and negatively associated with boredom [29]. This is in line with Pain et al. [30] who reported that the performance of youth soccer players was negatively influenced by anxiety and boredom. Similarly, the findings of Maschuv et al. [16] suggest that surgical residents with low self-efficacy perform poorly during simulated laparoscopy.

In the present study, those who reported a high flow score, i.e., being able to concentrate and being engaged in and enjoying the task, performed better in the simulator, after the basic set as well as after extensive training, than those who reported low flow scores. This observation suggests that the simulator and the tasks are feasible and user friendly. One can speculate that the more the simulator task simulates an authentic operation, i.e., exhibit face validity, the greater the enjoyment, concentration, and performance will be. Simulators' accessibility and feasibility thus could be evaluated according to the flow experience. Future studies should therefore investigate the relationship between the face validity of simulator tasks and the flow experience.

Self-efficacy scores correlated positively with simulator performance suggesting that a high self-confidence level is important for the simulated surgical result. Moreover, self-efficacy increased after intense training, indicating a gain in confidence from the training. This is important because a higher confidence might lead to a better result in the next training session.

The majority of tasks for most OBGYN practitioners are outside of the operating room (OR). Because the tasks performed in the OR are discipline specific, procedures among surgical residents cannot always be generalized to OBGYN residents. We therefore think it is important to distinguish residents in OBGYN from the residents in surgery, when investigating performance in the simulator, as well as the nontechnical skills that might impact the surgical performance, and furthermore when designing a training program.

One limitation in this study was the gender imbalance. This reflects the situation in at least a Swedish gynecological setting. The gender aspect should be further explored in a future study.

The findings from this exploratory study should be replicated by also using other validated instruments for assessing self-efficacy and flow, as well as a control group design in order to analyze for cause–effect relationships.

Conclusions

When building a curriculum for residents in OBGYN, factors like enjoyment and concentration, as well as confidence, need to be considered. Flow and self-efficacy should be further investigated in relation to the actual performance in the operating theater.

Acknowledgments The authors wish to express their gratitude to Mr. Lars-Gunnar Andersson and Mr. Tomas Askerud, Department for Biomedical Engineering and CAMST, at Karolinska University Hospital, Stockholm, for excellent technical assistance. We thank Dr. Christian R. Larsen for letting us use his proficiency criteria setting in the simulator. We furthermore thank Sue and Steve Anderson for editing grammar and language in our manuscript. This study was supported by research grants from the Stockholm County Council (Pick Up and ALF).

Disclosure of interest None of the authors have any conflicts of interest to disclose.

References

1. Scott DJ (2006) Patient safety, competency, and the future of surgical simulation. Simul Healthc 1(3):164–170
2. Scott DJ, Dunnington GL (2008) The new ACS/APDS Skills Curriculum: moving the learning curve out of the operating room. J Gastrointest Surg 12(2):213–221
3. Stefanidis D, Arora S, Parrack DM, Hamad GG, Capella J, Grantcharov T, Urbach DR, Scott DJ, Jones DB (2012) Association for Surgical Education Simulation Committee. Research priorities in surgical simulation for the 21st century. Am J Surg 203 (1):49–53
4. Larsen CR, Soerensen JL, Grantcharov TP, Dalsgaard T, Schouenborg L, Ottosen C, Schroeder TV, Ottesen BS (2009) Effect of virtual reality training on laparoscopic surgery: randomised controlled trial. BMJ 338:b1802
5. Ahlberg G, Enochsson L, Gallagher AG, Hedman L, Hogman C, McClusky DA, Ramel S, Smith CD, Arvidsson D (2007) Proficiency-based virtual reality training significantly reduces the error rate for residents during their first 10 laparoscopic cholecystectomies. Am J Surg 193(6):797–804

6. Seymour NE, Gallagher AG, Roman SA, O'Brien MK, Bansal VK, Andersen DK, Satava RM (2002) Virtual reality training improves operating room performance: results of a randomized, double-blinded study. Ann Surg 236(4):458–463, discussion 463–4
7. Carthey J (2003) The role of structured observational research in health care. Qual Saf Health Care 12 (Suppl 2):ii13–ii16
8. Yule S, Flin R, Paterson-Brown S, Maran N, Rowley D (2006) Development of a rating system for surgeons' non-technical skills. Med Educ 40(11):1098–1104
9. Crossley J, Marriott J, Purdie H, Beard JD (2011) Prospective observational study to evaluate NOTSS (Non-Technical Skills for Surgeons) for assessing trainees' non-technical performance in the operating theatre. Br J Surg 98(7):1010–1020
10. Yule S, Flin R, Maran N, Rowley D, Youngson G, Paterson-Brown S (2008) Surgeons' non-technical skills in the operating room: reliability testing of the NOTSS behavior rating system. World J Surg 32(4):548–556
11. Just MA, Carpenter PA (1985) Cognitive coordinate systems: accounts of mental rotation and individual differences in spatial ability. Psychol Rev 92(2):137–172
12. Ahlborg L, Hedman L, Murkes D, Westman B, Kjellin A, Felländer-Tsai L, Enochsson L (2011) Visuospatial ability correlates with performance in simulated gynecological laparoscopy. Eur J Obstet Gynecol Reprod Biol 157(1):73–77
13. Westman B, Ritter EM, Kjellin A, Törkvist L, Wredmark T, Felländer-Tsai L, Enochsson L (2006) Visuospatial abilities correlate with performance of senior endoscopy specialist in simulated colonoscopy. J Gastrointest Surg 10(4):593–599
14. Hedman L, Ström P, Andersson P, Kjellin A, Wredmark T, Felländer-Tsai L (2006) High-level visual–spatial ability for novices correlates with performance in a visual-spatial complex surgical simulator task. Surg Endosc 20(8):1275–1280
15. Kneebone R (2005) Evaluating clinical simulations for learning procedural skills: a theory-based approach. Acad Med 80(6):549
16. Maschuw K, Schlosser K, Kupietz E, Slater EP, Weyers P, Hassan I (2011) Do soft skills predict surgical performance?: a single-center randomized controlled trial evaluating predictors of skill acquisition in virtual reality laparoscopy. World J Surg 35(3):480–486
17. Nakamura J, Csikszentmihalyi M (2002) The concept of flow. In: Snyder CR, Lopez SJ (eds) Handbook of positive psychology. Oxford University Press, Oxford, pp. 89–105
18. Creutzfeldt J, Hedman L, Medin C, Heinrichs WL, Felländer-Tsai L (2010) Exploring virtual worlds for scenario-based repeated team training of cardiopulmonary resuscitation in medical students. J Med Internet Res 12(3):e38
19. Peters M, Laeng B, Latham K, Jackson M, Zaiyouna R, Richardson C (1995) A redrawn Vandenberg and Kuse mental rotations test: different versions and factors that affect performance. Brain Cogn 28(1):39–58
20. Cosman PH, Hugh TJ, Shearer CJ, Merrett ND, Biankin AV, Cartmill JA (2007) Skills acquired on virtual reality laparoscopic simulators transfer into the operating room in a blinded, randomised, controlled trial. Stud Health Technol Inform 125:76–81
21. Larsen CR, Grantcharov T, Aggarwal R, Tully A, Sørensen JL, Dalsgaard T, Ottesen B (2006) Objective assessment of gynecologic laparoscopic skills using the LapSimGyn virtual reality simulator. Surg Endosc 20(9):1460–1466
22. van Dongen KW, Tournoij E, van der Zee DC, Schijven MP, Broeders IAMJ (2007) Construct validity of the LapSim: can the LapSim virtual reality simulator distinguish between novices and experts? Surg Endosc 21(8):1413–1417
23. Bandura A (1997) Self-efficacy: the exercise of control, 1st edn. Worth Publishers, New York
24. Pintrich PR, Smith DAF, Garcia T, Mckeachie WJ (1993) Reliability and predictive validity of the motivated strategies for learning questionnaire (Mslq). Educ Psychol Meas 53(3):801–813
25. Csıkszentmihályi M (1978) Beyond boredom and anxiety: experiencing flow in work and play. Jossey-Bass, San Francisco
26. Webster J, Trevino L (1993) Computers in human behavior: the dimensionality and correlates of flow in human-computer interactions. Comput Human Behav 9, 411–426
27. Ghani JA, Deshpande SP (1994) Task characteristics and the experience of optimal flow in human—computer interaction. J Psychol 128(4):381–391
28. Schaafsma BE, Hiemstra E, Dankelman J, Jansen FW (2009) Feedback in laparoscopic skills acquisition: an observational study during a basic skills training course. Gynecol Surg 6(4):339–343
29. Artino AR, La Rochelle JS, Durning SJ (2010) Second-year medical students' motivational beliefs, emotions, and achievement. Med Educ 44(12):1203–1212
30. Pain MA, Harwood C (2007) The performance environment of the England youth soccer teams. J Sports Sci 25(12):1307–1324

2

Intraperitoneal injection of cultured mesothelial cells decrease CO_2 pneumoperitoneum-enhanced adhesions in a laparoscopic mouse model

J. Verguts · A. Coosemans · R. Corona · M. Praet · K. Mailova · P. Koninckx

Abstract Mesothelial cells are involved in peritoneal repair, and they modulate adhesion formation. Intraperitoneal injection of cultured mesothelial cells can decrease adhesion formation. The importance of the amount of cells, of the culture methods or of the origin of the cells is still unknown. Female Balb/c mice were used in a CO_2 pneumoperitoneum-enhanced adhesion formation model. Mesothelial cells were obtained from Balb/c mice and cultured over a 3-week period. Following a pilot experiment (n=10) with injection of 400,000 mesothelial cells a dose–response study was performed with 400,000; 133,000; and 44,000 cells (n=40). Adhesion formation decreased after the injection of cultured mesothelial cells as evidenced in the first (proportion $p<0.046$, total adhesions: NS) and second experiment ($p<0.001$ for proportion and total adhesions). The reduction was moreover dose dependent with a half maximal effect with some 100,000 cells. Intraperitoneal injection of cultured mesothelial cells can decrease CO_2 pneumoperitoneum-enhanced adhesion formation in mice and the effect is dose dependent, the half maximum effect being obtained with some 100,000 cells, a number which is surprisingly similar to the number of cells harvested from one mouse.

J. Verguts · A. Coosemans · R. Corona · K. Mailova · P. Koninckx
Department of Obstetrics and Gynecology, UZ Leuven,
Campus Gasthuisberg,
Leuven, Belgium

M. Praet
Department of Pathology, UZ Gent,
Gent, Belgium

J. Verguts (✉)
Department of Obstetrics and Gynecology,
University Hospital Leuven,
Campus Gasthuisberg, Herestraat 49,
3000 Leuven, Belgium
e-mail: Jasper.Verguts@uz.kuleuven.ac.be

Keywords Laparoscopy · Adhesions · Mesothelial cells · Mouse model

Background

The pathophysiology of postoperative adhesions is not yet fully understood. Generally, peritoneal repair has been considered as a happening process at the traumatized areas consisting of an inflammatory reaction, exudation with fibrin deposition and appearance of macrophages, and mesothelial cells on the lesion within 24 h [1, 2]. Macrophages are believed to regulate healing through local secretion of cytokines and growth factors. They disappear within 8 days and are not incorporated into the repair [3]. When the fibrin matrix persists too long, constituting a scaffold for cellular ingrowth of fibroblasts, vessels and nerves, adhesion formation occurs.

Over the last decade, the entire peritoneal cavity has become recognized as a co-factor modulating adhesion formation at traumatized sites [4]. Identified as strongly adhesiogenic are pure CO_2 pneumoperitoneums, the addition of more than 4% oxygen to the CO_2 pneumoperitoneum, desiccation, and surgical trauma [5–8]. The mechanisms involved are believed to be mesothelial cell damage by hypoxia, by hyperoxia and reactive oxygen species, or directly by desiccation or trauma. These effects are moreover strongly attenuated at lower temperatures [9].

Prevention of adhesion formation in humans is based upon a model that considers interaction between traumatized areas. Since adhesions decreased when denuded areas were kept separated for more than 24–36 h, non-irritative and resorbable barriers were developed or traumatized areas were kept separated by flotation agents [10].

The recognition of the peritoneal cavity as a co-factor in adhesion formation has resulted in minimizing mesothelial trauma during surgery through cellular normoxia (a partial oxygen pressure of 28 mm of Hg achieved by adding 4% of oxygen to the CO_2 pneumoperitoneum), humidification, slight cooling, and minimal tissue handling [4]. Mesothelial cells obviously play an important role in peritoneal repair. Within hours, a peritoneal defect (i.e., caused by trauma during surgery) is covered with macrophages and mesothelial cells, previously described as tissue repair cells [11]. The healing process starts from multiple spots over the defect from where mesothelial cells proliferate. Hence, small and large defects heal in the same short time (7–10 days) [12]. It is an attractive concept that mesothelial cells at the edge of a lesion and mesothelial cells of the opposing mesothelial surface have an increased dividing capacity, a phenomenon being maximal within 2 days suggest locally secreted factors [13].

The origin of these mesothelial or repair cells remains unclear. Macrophages could transform to mesothelial cells when in contact with a defect, subserosal mesothelial cells could migrate into the wound, free-floating mesothelial cells could implant while these cells could originate from bone marrow precursors [14]. Indeed, subserosal mesothelial cells are pluripotent, since they can differentiate to mesenchymal and epithelial cells. After peritoneal injury, they differentiate and start expressing cytokeratin while losing expression of vimentin [15, 16]. The exudate after injury contains a high number of fibroblast and epithelioid-like cells. These cells have low proliferative activity for at least 48 h [17]. That free-floating mesothelial cells are important is attractive since they are present at all times, their number increases 12 times in 2 to 5 days after injury [2], these cells were demonstrated to implant at the peritoneal lesion, and since extensive lavage with removal of these free-floating cells slows down peritoneal healing [18]. That mesothelial cells might originate from bone marrow precursors in blood, probably is less important since total body radiation has no effect upon peritoneal wound healing [19].

Intraperitoneally, injected exogenous mesothelial cells can implant into the injured area and reduce adhesion formation in the human by injection of cultured mesothelial cells obtained from the omentum. This confirms the observations in a staphylococcal peritonitis rabbit model [20, 21]. In a rat abrasion model, the injection of cultured mesothelial cells or mesenchymal stem cells derived from skeletal muscles of newborn rats decreased adhesion formation [22, 23]. Recently, an artificial peritoneum with collagen gel, fibroblasts, and overlying mesothelial cells significantly reduced adhesions [24]. Mesothelial cells grown from adhesions moreover are different from fibroblasts derived from normal peritoneum [25].

The concept that cultured mesothelial cells can decrease adhesion formation in an abrasion model thus seems well established. The amount of cells required, however, the culture method and the origin of the cells are still unclear [22]. Since an abrasion model is a pure surgical lesion requiring laparotomy, we therefore wanted to evaluate whether cultured mesothelial cells also affected CO_2 pneumoperitoneum-enhanced adhesion formation.

Materials and methods

Collection and culture of mesothelial cells

Mesothelial cells were obtained from 9 to 16-week-old inbred female Balb/c mice. Following anesthesia with intradermal pentobarbital (Nembutal, Sanofi Sante Animale, Brussels, Belgium; 0.06 mg/g) the abdomen was shaved, the animal was secured to the table in supine position, and the skin disinfected with a 50% alcohol solution. A 14-gauge catheter (Insyte, Vialon, Becton Dickinson) was inserted into the abdomen at the umbilicus and fixed leak proof with a Prolene 5/0 purse suture.

The cells were collected via a two-step procedure per mouse. First, 10 ml of phosphate-buffered saline pH 7.3 (Dulbecco's phosphate-buffered saline, DPBS) was injected, of which at least 8 ml could be re-aspirated. This first set of "free-floating cells" was centrifuged at 200 g for 10 min and the pellet was then suspended in culture medium RPMI 1640 (Lonza, BioWhittaker) supplemented with 15% fetal calf serum (CSL UK Ltd., Andover, UK), 4 mML-glutamine (Gibco, Paisley, UK), 0.4 mg/ml of hydrocortisone (Sigma-Aldrich, Poole, UK), and antibiotics: penicillin, 120 mg/l, amphothericine (2.5 mg/l), and gentamicin (4 mg/l) as used by Foley-Comer et al. [3]. Secondly, 10 ml of DPBS with 0.25% trypsin and 1 mM EDTA 4Na at 37°C was injected through the same catheter and the mouse was softly shaken. After 10 min, the instilled fluid was re-aspirated. Next, the abdominal cavity was washed with 5 ml culture medium; to finish, the abdominal cavity was opened and gently rinsed eight times with 2 ml culture medium. All mesothelial cells obtained via this second procedure were collected together, centrifuged for 10 min at 200 g and re-suspended in culture medium. Each time two mice had undergone the procedure, cells of those mice were pooled, keeping cells of step 1 and 2 separately. Cells were then put in an incubator at 37°C with 5% CO_2. If cells were confluent, which was normally the case after 1 week, cells were split at a ratio of 1:2, after having them detached with trypsin–EDTA. After 3 weeks, cells were detached and counted for further use (pilot, 400,000 cells; dose–response, 400,000 cells; 133,000 cells; and 44,000 cells).

Immunohistochemistry

To ascertain the growing of mesothelial cells, cells from 3-week-old cultures were seeded on slides. After 2 days of culture, the slides were fixed and endogenous peroxidase activity was blocked by 0.5% H_2O_2 in methanol. Cells were evaluated for intercellular connections and for cytokeratin staining.

Mouse model

Laparoscopic surgery

Our laparoscopic mouse model has been described and validated extensively [5]. Briefly, a 2-mm endoscope with a 3.3-mm external sheath for insufflation (Karl Storz, Tuttlingen, Germany) was introduced into the abdominal cavity of 9–16-week-old inbred female Balb/c mice.

CO_2 pneumoperitoneum-enhanced adhesions were induced by performing two standardized 10×1.6-mm lesions in the antimesenteric border of both right and left uterine horns and on the pelvic sidewalls with bipolar coagulation (BICAPTM, bipolar hemostasis probe, BP-5200A, 5-Fr, 200 cm; IMMED Benelux, Linkebeek, Belgium) at 20 W (Autocon 200, Karl Storz, standard coagulation mode) after which the pneumoperitoneum with pure CO_2 was maintained for exactly 60 min without desiccation (using humidified gas) at 37°C in all mice. All mice in the first experiment were operated on by RC, in the second experiment some were operated by JV who was blind for the dose of mesothelial cells injected per mouse.

Adhesions were qualitatively and quantitatively scored blindly (the investigator was not informed of the group being evaluated) 1 week later by JV during laparotomy using a stereomicroscope (Wild Heerbrugg M7A, Gais, Switzerland). The quantitative scoring system assessed the percentage of the lesions covered by adhesions as follows: adhesion proportion (%)=(sum of the length of the individual attachments/length of the lesion)×100. The qualitative scoring system assessed: extent (0, no adhesions; 1, 1–25%; 2, 26–50%; 3, 51–75%; 4, 76–100% of the injured surface involved, respectively); type (0, no adhesions; 1, filmy; 2, dense; 3, capillaries present); tenacity (0, no adhesions; 1, easily fall apart; 2, require traction; 3, require sharp dissection). Total adhesion score was the sum of extent, type, and tenacity. All results represent the average of the adhesions formed at the four individual sites i.e., right and left visceral and parietal peritoneum.

Experimental design

All mice underwent four standard bipolar lesions and 1 h of CO_2 pneumoperitoneum as described above. After all laparoscopic ports had been closed, 1 ml of DPBS with or without mesothelial cells was injected intraperitoneally.

The first experiment was designed to prove that cultured mesothelial cells could prevent CO_2 pneumoperitoneum-enhanced adhesions. Mesothelial cells were collected in four mice, and cultured in eight flasks of 25 cm². Two weeks later, 2×10^6 cells were harvested. In order to investigate the effect in five mice, 400,000 cells per mouse were used. The control group, which only received DPBS, consisted of five mice. The second experiment was designed to obtain a dose–response curve of adding different amounts of cultured mouse mesothelial cells in adhesion reduction. Considering the effect of 400,000 cells from the first experiment and taking into account the number of cells available, we decided to inject per group of five mice 400,000 cells; 133,000; and 44,000 cells, i.e., a logarithmic decrease. The control group which only received DPBS consisted of five mice. The study was approved by the Institutional Review Animal Care Committee.

Statistics

Statistical analysis was performed with the SAS System (SAS Institute, Cary, NC) using the non-parametric Kruskal–Wallis test to compare individual groups. All data are presented as the mean±SE.

Findings

Culturing mesothelial cells

Culturing the harvested mesothelial cells did not provide any specific difficulty. Cultured cells were initially bipolar or multipolar in appearance, but at confluence they adopted a polygonal configuration as described by Yung et al. [26]. Viability of cells as estimated by trypan blue exclusion was over 95%. The cells had intercellular connections and were positive for cytokeratin staining confirming their mesothelial nature.

The cells from the first washing did not grow but remained viable as estimated by trypan blue exclusion after 3 weeks of culture. Their number, however, was too low for subsequent experiments.

Adhesion reduction

No mice died before the end of the experiment. In the first experiment, the injection of 400,000 cultured mesothelial cells caused a reduction of the proportion of adhesion formation from 19% to 7% ($p<0.046$), and a reduction of the total adhesion score from 3.1 (±1.74) to 1.7 (±1.68) (not significant (NS), $p<0.086$).

The second experiment confirmed that mesothelial cells can reduce CO_2 pneumoperitoneum-enhanced adhesion formation. With 44,000; 133,000; and 400,000 cells the proportion of adhesions dropped from 13.5% to 11.5% (NS), 8% ($p<0.055$), and 5% ($p<0.007$), respectively. The total adhesion score (Fig. 1) showed a similar decline being for the 44,000; 133,000; and 400,000 cells not significant, $p=0.0093$ and $p=0.0025$, respectively. When adhesions are plotted against the logarithm of the concentration of cells, the amount of cells required to decrease adhesion formation by half was estimated at 100,000 cells.

Discussion

Harvesting and growing mesothelial cells for 3 weeks is so time consuming that large scale experiments become difficult. These experiments confirm and extend the observations that cultured mesothelial cells obtained after trypsinization of the peritoneal cavity can reduce adhesion formation as described in rabbits and rats with mesothelial cells obtained from the omentum [20–22]. The effect, moreover, is not limited to pure surgical models such as the abrasion model [20, 21], but also in the CO_2 pneumoperitoneum-enhanced adhesion model. The effect is moreover dose dependent. Since we know that following a 60-min CO_2 pneumoperitoneum mesothelial cells retract thus exposing directly the basal membrane [27], we may speculate that injected mesothelial cells may fill the gaps between the retracted mesothelial cells thus attenuating the adhesion-enhancing effect of the CO_2 pneumoperitoneum by preventing the deleterious effect of the peritoneal cavity. Considering that 100,000 cells are needed for a half maximal effect, the hypothesis that the cells affect the entire peritoneal cavity seems attractive, as 100,000 cells exceed what is necessary to cover the injury which only measures 1 cm by 1.6 mm. These 100,000 cells indeed cover 10 cm^2 since a confluent culture flask of 25 cm^2 contains 250,000 cells. That 100,000 cells are similar to the number of cells recovered from the entire peritoneal cavity of one mouse further lends support to the hypothesis that these cells affect the entire peritoneal cavity. Whether this observation on CO_2 pneumoperitoneum-enhanced adhesions can be extended to hyperoxia, desiccation, or manipulation, enhanced adhesions are likely but remain to be established. Indeed, considering that the driving mechanisms of all these factors are micro-denuded areas all over the peritoneal cavity, the effect of cultured mesothelial cells is expected to be similar in all. A (surgical) trauma is essential to initiate adhesion formation, but these adhesions are enhanced by factors from the peritoneal cavity, the latter being quantitatively the most important. The importance of factors in the peritoneal cavity was unequivocally proven by the observation manipulation in the upper abdomen increased adhesions at the site of the surgical lesion [8]. This, moreover, was recently proven to be mediated by acute inflammation of the entire peritoneal cavity and also explains that de novo adhesions (outside the surgical lesion) were never observed.

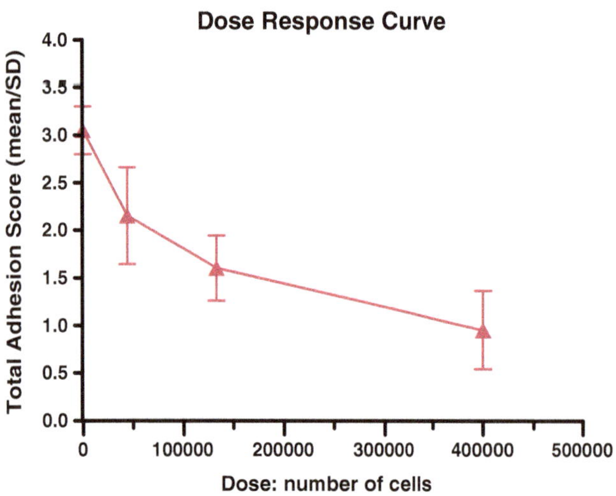

Fig. 1 Dose–response curve. *X*-axis, number of cells used per mouse

The mechanisms of adhesion reduction by cultured mesothelial cells can only be speculated upon. Whereas in pure surgical models, incorporation in the lesion as demonstrated in rats [3] seems logical, in the peritoneal cavity enhanced models incorporation in between retracted mesothelial cells of the entire peritoneal cavity cannot be excluded. Moreover, it is unclear whether the origin of the mesothelial cells and the culture conditions could be important or whether these cells actively secrete substances in the peritoneal fluid. We cannot even ascertain that the effect is specific for mesothelial cells since Alpay et al. demonstrated that also fibroblasts display different immunologic characteristics with an effect on adhesion formation [28].

It is unclear why the cells from the first washing did not grow although remaining viable. The same culture medium was used as for the detached mesothelial cells. The only difference between cells from the first washing and cells obtained after trypsinization is the fact that the former were kept for a much longer period in PBS, which indeed may damage mesothelial cells by making them lose their ability to divide (oral communication, S. Mutsaers).

The effect of mesothelial cells in reducing adhesion formation might seem less important in the pilot experiment (400,000 cells caused a 50% reduction in adhesions) than in the dose–response experiment where some 100,000 cells caused a 50% reduction in adhesions. This difference may be a consequence of the fact that cultured mesothelial cells probably stayed longer in PBS in the pilot study since our experience in handling cells was less at that moment. Also, variability in adhesion formation has to be taken into account. Indeed, although total adhesion scores were comparable in the two control groups of both experiments (3.1) the proportion of adhesions was lower in the second experiment (13.5%) than in the first experiment (19%). Although overall very reproducible, this variability in proportion of adhesions ranging from 45% to 15% between experiments had been observed previously [29, 30] This indeed prompted us to block randomize by day while standardizing all experimental conditions as temperature, pneumoperitoneum conditions and duration, anesthesia, and experience of the surgeon as much as possible.

The clinical implications of these experiments are far reaching, whereas the use of mesothelial cells for adhesion prevention becomes attractive. Extensive lavage during and after surgery might remove besides debris and fibrin also mesothelial cells and macrophages, and the latter might be detrimental. These animal experiments combined with clinical observation at least suggest that these effects should be evaluated in detail in specific experiments. Whereas collecting and culturing mesothelial cells for adhesion prevention in the same patient is not realistic today, this method could become useful if fibroblast would be useful or if some cell lines with similar effects could be developed. In case mesothelial cells could be preserved from the peritoneal lavage during surgery as is the case with peroperative cell salvage for blood, this could be a reliable method to prevent adhesions and the detrimental effects it may cause.

Conclusions

Cultured mesothelial cells can prevent adhesion formation in mice and the effect increases with the number of cells. In Balb/c mice, the number of cells needed to reduce adhesions by 50% seems to be around 100,000. Considering that 100,000 cells cover in culture 10 cm², this suggests that the effect is mediated by incorporation in the entire peritoneal cavity and not only at the lesion site

Acknowledgements We would like to thank Steven Mutsaers for his valued help in preparing the culture medium, Mercedes Binda in reviewing the manuscript, and the Research Foundation–Flanders (FWO) for their grant support (no. 1700409N).

Declaration of interest Drs. J. Verguts, A. Coosemans, R. Corona, M. Praet, K. Mailova, and P. Koninckx have no conflicts of interest or financial ties to disclose.

References

1. Mutsaers S, Whitaker D, Papadimitriou J (2002) Stimulation of mesothelial cell proliferation by exudate macrophages enhances serosal wound healing in a murine model. Am J Pathol 160(2):681–692
2. Fotev Z, Whitaker D, Papadimitriou JM (1987) Role of macrophages in mesothelial healing. J Pathol 151(3):209–219
3. Foley-Comer A, Herrick S, Al-Mishlab T, Prêle C, Laurent J, Mutsaers S (2002) Evidence for incorporation of free-floating mesothelial cells as a mechanism of serosal healing. J Cell Sci 115:1383–1389
4. Binda MM, Koninckx PR (2009) Prevention of adhesion formation in a laparoscopic mouse model should combine local treatment with peritoneal cavity conditioning. Hum Reprod 24(6):1473–1479
5. Molinas CR, Mynbaev O, Pauwels A, Novak P, Koninckx PR (2001) Peritoneal mesothelial hypoxia during pneumoperitoneum is a cofactor in adhesion formation in a laparoscopic mouse model. Fertil Steril 76(3):560–567
6. Elkelani OA, Binda MM, Molinas CR, Koninckx PR (2004) Effect of adding more than 3% oxygen to carbon dioxide pneumoperitoneum on adhesion formation in a laparoscopic mouse model. Fertil Steril 82(6):1616–1622
7. Binda MM, Molinas CR, Hansen P, Koninckx PR (2006) Effect of desiccation and temperature during laparoscopy on adhesion formation in mice. Fertil Steril 86(1):166–175
8. Schonman R, Corona R, Bastidas A, De Cicco C, Koninckx PR (2009) Effect of upper abdomen tissue manipulation on adhesion formation between injured areas in a laparoscopic mouse model. J Minim Invasive Gynecol 16(3):307–312
9. Peng Y, Zheng M, Ye Q, Chen X, Yu B, Liu B (2009) Heated and humidified CO_2 prevents hypothermia, peritoneal injury, and intra-abdominal adhesions during prolonged laparoscopic insufflations. J Surg Res 151(1):40–47
10. Ahmad G, Duffy JM, Farquhar C, Vail A, Vandekerckhove P, Watson A, Wiseman D (2008) Barrier agents for adhesion prevention after gynaecological surgery. Cochrane Database Syst Rev. (2):CD000475
11. di Zerega G, Campeau J (2001) Peritoneal repair and post-surgical adhesion formation. Hum Reprod Update 7:547–555
12. Hertzler AE (1919) In: Hertzler AE (ed) The peritoneum vol. 1. CV Mosby Company, St. Louis, pp 264–265
13. Yung S, Davies M (1998) Response of the human peritoneal mesothelial cell to injury: an in vitro model of peritoneal wound healing. Kidney Int 54(6):2160–2169
14. Mutsaers S, Prêle C, Lansley S, Herrick S (2007) The origin of regenerating mesothelium: a historical perspective. Int J Artif Organs 30(6):484–9410
15. Bolen J, Hammar S, McNutt M (1986) Reactive and neoplastic serosal tissue. A light-microscopic, ultrastructural, and immunocytochemical study. Am J Surg Pathol 10:34–47
16. Bolen J, Hammar S, McNutt M (1987) Serosal tissue: reactive tissue as a model for understanding mesotheliomas. Ultrastruct Pathol 11:251–262
17. Mutsaers S, Whitaker D, Papadimitriou J (2000) Mesothelial regeneration is not dependent on subserosal cells. J Pathol 190:86–92
18. Tolhurst Cleaver C, Hopkins A, Kee Kwong K, Raftery A (1974) The effect of postoperative peritoneal lavage on survival, peritoneal wound healing and adhesion formation following fecal peritonitis: an experimental study in the rat. Br J Surg 61:601–604
19. Whitaker D, Papadimitriou J (1985) Mesothelial healing: morphological and kinetic investigations. J Pathol 145:159–175
20. Di Paolo N, Vanni L, Sacchi G (1990) Autologous implant of peritoneal mesothelium in rabbits and man. Clin Nephrol 34:179–184
21. Di Paolo N, Sacchi G, Vanni L, Corazzi S, Terrana B, Rossi P, Gaggiotti E, Buoncristiani U (1991) Autologous peritoneal mesothelial cell implant in rabbits and peritoneal dialysis patients. Nephron 57:323–331
22. Betram P, Tietze L, Hoopmann M, Treutner KH, Mittermayer C, Schumpelick V (1999) Intraperitoneal transplantation of isologous mesothelial cells for prevention of adhesions. Eur J Surg 165:705–709

23. Lucas PA, Warejcka DJ, Zhang LM, Newman WH, Young HE (1996) Effect of rat mesenchymal stem cells on development of abdominal adhesions after surgery. J Surg Res 62:229–232
24. Kuga H, Morisaki T, Nakamura K, Onishi H, Matsuda T, Sueishi K, Tanaka M, Katano M (2004) Construction of a transplantable tissue-engineered artificial peritoneum. Eur Surg Res 36:323–330
25. Saed GM, Zhang W, Diamond MP (2001) Molecular characterization of fibroblasts isolated from human peritoneum and adhesions. Fertil Steril 75:763–8.22
26. Yung S, Li FK, Chan TM (2006) Peritoneal mesothelial cell culture and biology. Perit Dial Int 26:162–173
27. Volz J, Köster S, Spacek Z, Paweletz N (1999) Characteristic alterations of the peritoneum after carbon dioxide pneumoperitoneum. Surg Endosc 13(6):611–614
28. Alpay Z, Ozgönenel MS, Savaşan S, Buck S, Saed GM, Diamond MP (2006) Possible role of natural immune response against altered fibroblasts in the development of post-operative adhesions. Am J Reprod Immunol 55(6):420–427
29. Molinas CR, Binda MM, Campo R, Koninckx PR (2005) Adhesion formation and interanimal variability in a laparoscopic mouse model varies with strains. Fertil Steril 83 (6):1871–1874
30. Molinas CR, Binda MM, Carmeliet P, Koninckx PR (2004) Role of vascular endothelial growth factor receptor 1 in basal adhesion formation and in carbon dioxide pneumoperitoneum-enhanced adhesion formation after laparoscopic surgery in mice. Fertil Steril 82(Suppl 3):1149–1153

3

Laparoscopic tubal surgery for ectopic pregnancy: trainees' perspective in the UK

Rasiah Bharathan · Sarah Merritt · Hasib Ahmed

Abstract Ectopic pregnancies (EP) account for approximately 1% of all pregnancies. Surgical management of such patients should be accomplished through the laparoscopic route. Presently, available data from national studies suggest that only a minority of women benefit from such an approach. Regional studies and single institution reports suggest that trainee involvement in these procedures vary widely. Competency in laparoscopic surgery for EP is a mandatory requirement for independent practice in the UK. In a recent survey of UK trainees of all grades in obstetrics and gynaecology, 53.4% of trainees reported that they were trained or being trained in such procedures. This study examines the perspectives of the trainees. We performed a national questionnaire survey of intermediate- and advanced-level trainees in the UK During a 12-month period, 52% of trainees had performed at least one procedure independently; 80% of trainees performed most of the procedure on at least one occasion. The satisfaction with training was rated as 3 on a five-point Likert scale. Thirty percent of the trainees had access to a laparoscopy simulator. We found a high level of trainee engagement with laparoscopic tubal surgery. The intensity of experience is likely inadequate to satisfy the learning curve. A holistic approach s required to ensure surgical competence.

Keywords Training · Laparoscopy · Ectopic pregnancy

R. Bharathan (✉)
Nuffield Department of Obstetrics & Gynaecology,
John Radcliffe Hospital,
Headley Way,
Oxford OX3 9DU, UK
e-mail: r.bharathan@doctors.org.uk

S. Merritt
Department of Obstetrics & Gynaecology, St. Thomas' Hospital,
Westminster Bridge Road,
London SE1 7EH, UK

H. Ahmed
Department of Obstetrics & Gynaecology,
Medway Maritime Hospital,
Gillingham, Kent ME7 5NY, UK

Background

Ectopic pregnancies (EP) account for approximately 1% of all pregnancies, and 95% of these are located in the fallopian tube [1]. Optimal surgical management, based on the evidence of three randomised controlled trials, is achieved through the laparoscopic access [2–4]. In haemodynamically stable patients, current UK guidelines recommend laparoscopic surgery [5]. Presently, available data from two national studies suggest that only 27% and 35% of women were managed by laparoscopic surgery even though 90% of gynaecologists reported that if resources were available, laparoscopic approach could be adopted [6, 7]. In a recent regional study, 84% of patients were managed via laparoscopic surgery [8]. An earlier regional study revealed that 37% of trainees performed laparoscopic surgery for EP, but more recently, an urban single institution experience revealed that 53% of procedures were performed by trainees [9, 10]. With structured enthusiastic effort, over 90% of cases can be managed through laparoscopic route [11]. Competency in laparoscopic tubal surgery for EP is a mandatory requirement for the completion of training. Factors that have impeded rapid uptake and training include reduced exposure following the European Working Time Directive (EWTD), lack of appropriate trainers, theatre resources and implications of clinical governance. With ever wider provision of specialised early pregnancy assessment service and the subsequent conservative or medical management of patients with tubal pregnancy, the opportunities for training in the surgical management of such patients are further reduced. In a recent survey of UK trainees of all grades in obstetrics and gynaecology, 53.4% of trainees reported that they were trained or being trained to manage ectopic pregnancies laparoscopically; however, 47.3% said they had not performed surgery for ectopic pregnancy in the preceding 12 months [12]. In the same report, the proportion of trainees who said that supervision in theatre for all procedures was good or very good was 57%; this has remained stable since the first such survey in 1995. Since laparoscopic surgery for EP is a common procedure, a study of this from a trainee's perspective could be informative regarding the management of training.

Aims

Our questionnaire study aims to provide a measure of the surgical experience gained by the trainees and their perception of the quality of training across the specialty with regard to laparoscopic management of EP.

Materials and methods

With the approval of the Royal College of Obstetricians and Gynaecologists (RCOG) Honorary Secretary, a questionnaire was posted to specialist registrars or specialty trainees who had completed basic training for at least 2 years and were in the process of obtaining core (Specialty Trainee 3–5) or advanced level (Specialty Trainee 6–7) training within the UK in 2009. Each trainee was sent a cover letter, questionnaire (see Appendix) and a stamped addressed envelope for return. The postal communication was handled by the hospital clinical audit department. A reminder letter was not sent to non-responders; this preserves anonymity, and although a reminder may improve the response rate, it is unlikely to affect the overall findings. The questionnaire requested information from trainees regarding their grade, length of training, the extent and depth of their involvement in laparoscopic salpingectomy during the preceding 12 months, method of tubal salpingectomy, practice of salpingotomy, attendance at a laparoscopy course and availability of a laparoscopic simulator. In addition, our study illustrates the self-assessed competency level with regard to laparoscopic salpingectomy. In addition a five-point Likert scale, a widely used validated subjective assessment tool, was used to gauge the trainees' level of satisfaction with training and whether they anticipated attaining competency in laparoscopic tubal surgery prior to completion of training. On this scale, a score of 1 indicates a negative response and 5 indicates a positive response.

Findings

A total of 645 questionnaires were posted to registrar level trainees in obstetrics and gynaecology across the UK. Two hundred four responses were received (31.6%). Thirteen of the respondents had been appointed as consultants, and therefore, these responses were excluded from the analysis. Fourteen (7.3%) respondents were at specialist trainee (ST) level 3, 29 (15.2%) at ST4, 38 (19.9%) at ST5, 44 (23%) at ST6 and 56 (29.3%) were at ST7. A further ten (5.2%) were categorised as other as a grade was not specified, and their response is included in the analysis.

During the preceding 12 months, the median number of laparoscopic procedures for tubal ectopic pregnancies where a trainee was involved was four (interquartile range (IQR), 2–8). During the same period, the median number of procedures where the trainee performed the procedure at level 4 competency was three (IQR, 1–7). One hundred trainees had performed at least one laparoscopic tubal surgery at level 5 competence. Similarly, 54 trainees performed at least one procedure at level 4 competency, 26 trainees at level 3 and further ten trainees at level 2. One trainee did not respond to this question.

In terms of tubal preservation, 82 (43%) trainees reported that they performed salpingotomy when appropriate, whilst 98 (51%) did not perform such a procedure; 11

(6%) did not provide a response to that question. With regard to the method of excising the fallopian tube, 81 (42%) trainees reported that they preferred endoloop ligature and excision, 96 (50%) preferred diathermy excision, 6 (3%) used both of these techniques and the remaining 8 (4%) did not respond.

Ninety (47%) trainees had attended a level 2 RCOG-recognised or equivalent laparoscopy course within the preceding 2 years; the remaining 101 trainees had not attended such a course during this timeline. Fifty-seven (30%) trainees reported that they had access to a laparoscopic simulator at their place of work; the remaining134 (70%) trainees did not have such facility.

Figure 1 illustrates Likert scale responses to questions on whether the trainee anticipates reaching level 5 competence at completion of their training and secondly responses with regard to their level of satisfaction of training provided with regard to laparoscopic tubal surgery. Figure 1 demonstrates that 96 (50%) trainees felt it very likely that they would attain competence at level 5 prior to completion of training. However, the level of satisfaction with training is more uniformly distributed. The median Likert score for satisfaction with training was 2 (IQR, 1–3) for the junior group and 4 (IQR, 2–5) for the senior group in our study cohort. The median Likert score regarding their anticipation of attaining level 5 competency by completion of training was 4 (3–5) amongst the junior group and 5 (4–5) for the more senior group.

Free comments from the survey

In summary, comments suggested that university hospitals are more likely to provide a 'satisfactory' training. Additional factors which are perceived to influence the quality of laparoscopic training include rota arrangements which tend to favour the most senior trainees with respect to gynaecologic surgery, commitment from trainers and fluency of trainers in performing such procedures. Many trainees cited out of programme training in minimal access surgery as the most reliable solution.

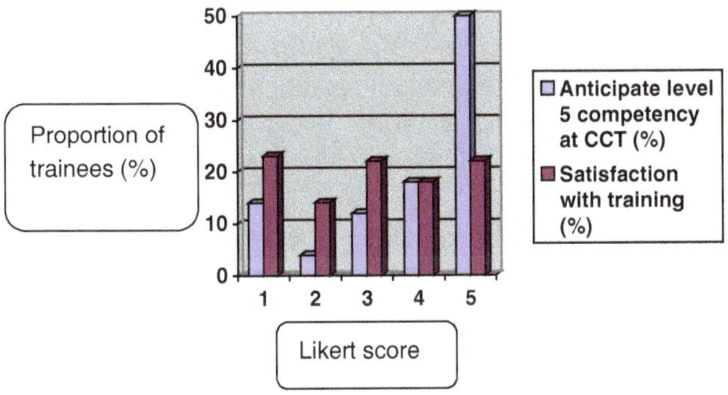

Fig. 1 Likert scale scores and their percentage distribution

Discussion

Clinical training, surgical education, workforce planning, patient safety and clinical governance are intertwined issues which concern all stakeholders. Composition, quality and delivery of training seem to preoccupy trainees as well as trainers. These issues are increasingly brought into focus as the duration and intensity of exposure of the trainees to clinical practice have declined. Legislation such as the EWTD and importantly the changing nature of gynaecological practice has had a major impact on training. In the UK presently, the emphasis on training is focused on improving the delivery of acute care such as intrapartum care and early pregnancy complications. Appropriate management of ectopic pregnancy is an important element of this care. This survey provides a 'snapshot' of trainees' perspective with regard to laparoscopic management of EP.

Overall response rate was 31.6%, and effective response rate was 29.6%. In this group, 42.4% of the respondents were within the junior registrar ranks, and 52.3% were senior registrars; the remaining 5.2% were non-career grade doctors who effectively function as registrars in the provision of service. During the preceding 12 months, 15 (7.9%) trainees said they had not been involved in a single procedure. The median number of procedures that a trainee was involved in was 4, and that where they performed at least most of the procedure was 3. During the same period, 147 (77%) trainees had performed most or all of at least one procedure under supervision. The RCOG survey had 1,001 respondents, which equated to about 66% of all trainees in the UK. Among this group of respondents, 30% were in 'basic' training and a further 10% represented a miscellaneous group of trainees who were lecturers, subspecialty trainees and research fellows; these subgroups were not targeted by our study as they would not have been suitable subjects. The target group of our study corresponds to the remaining 60% of that study. The RCOG trainees' survey reported that 47.3% of trainees had not performed any procedure during a 12-month period [12]. This discrepancy could be explained by the differing target groups of the surveys and potentially the phrasing of the question; in our survey, a graded response was possible with regard to the level of involvement, which was not the case with the RCOG survey. Further, amongst our group, 180 (94.2%) trainees had performed some component of at least one procedure. This lends weight to the finding that 90% of units felt that they could offer laparoscopic surgery for EP if adequate resources were available [7].

With regard to conservation of the tube, 51% of the respondents do not perform salpingotomy. A simulator-based assessment of salpingectomy revealed a learning curve in terms of time taken per procedure to reach a plateau to be up to 6 procedures for experts, 21 for intermediates and 27 for novices [13]. Although there are no similar data available for salpingotomy, but due to the need for a broader range of laparoscopic skills, it is our opinion that the likely learning curve for salpingotomy will be steeper. This will have implications for training and provision of such service by a generalist on an ad hoc basis. Conservation of the tube assumes clinical significance for psychological reasons or if the contralateral tube is diseased.

In this survey, 50% of the trainees preferred diathermy excision, whilst 42% preferred endoloop; the remainder used both techniques. A randomised controlled trial of salpingectomy by means of endoloop versus electrocautery demonstrated that with endoloop, operation takes shorter, a patient has less pain and lesser total analgesia requirement by day 7 [14]. Perhaps, trainees could be encouraged to utilise a technique which benefits the woman and optimises the use of operating theatre time. It is worth noting that Endoloop technique leads to a partial salpingectomy, whilst electrocautery offers the opportunity to perform total salpingectomy; tubal stump ectopic pregnancy could indeed be an extremely rare complication.

The RCOG-approved intermediate-level laparoscopy courses provide theoretical as well as practical teaching. There is some evidence that such courses can enable development and retention of skills [15, 16]. Longitudinal impact and potential need for reiteration have not been studied over a significant period, but at least annual verification would be necessary [17]. In our survey, only 47% of registrar level trainees had attended such a course within a 2-year period. Following instruction in laparoscopic surgery, consolidation in the form of practice would be required. It is well established in the literature that surgical complications decline with progression along the learning curve; this is indeed the case in laparoscopic surgery, where most problems tend to occur during the early learning phase [18, 19]. Both for logistical advantage and in the interest of patient safety, trainees should familiarise themselves with the instruments and make grounds on the learning curve prior to the clinical encounter of an acutely ill patient. In this respect, evidence from randomised clinical trials demonstrates that skills learnt with the aid of a simulator can be successfully transferred to the operating theatre [20–22]. In this study, 57 (30%) trainees reported having access to a simulator facility. This confirms the similar finding in a regional study regarding access to a simulator [23]. The same study revealed that although 81% of the respondents felt simulator training was essential in improving laparoscopic skills, trainees did not make adequate use of facilities where they existed [23].

So, how can we improve the training, performance and satisfaction of the trainees? The concept of surgical competence frames components in surgical practice which can optimise the performance (Fig. 2), namely psychomotor skills, communication skills, knowledge base and evaluation and continuing development. This could be a useful framework both for the trainer and the trainee since it provides a scaffolding for surgical education. A better understanding of the environment, needs of the health care system and the methods of training and assessment will help the trainees to manage their own expectation and progress.

Psychomotor skills can be learnt through courses and refined through simulation practice and later in the operating theatre. One option that might increase usage of simulators is if they are made available at a regional level with nominated supervisors for dedicated sessions. RCOG is currently examining the role of simulators in formal training. A regional study from the UK revealed that all hospitals had the necessary laparoscopic equipment; so, simulator training could be a meaningful adjunct in augmenting training across the board [24]. The potential value of a simulator in such training is

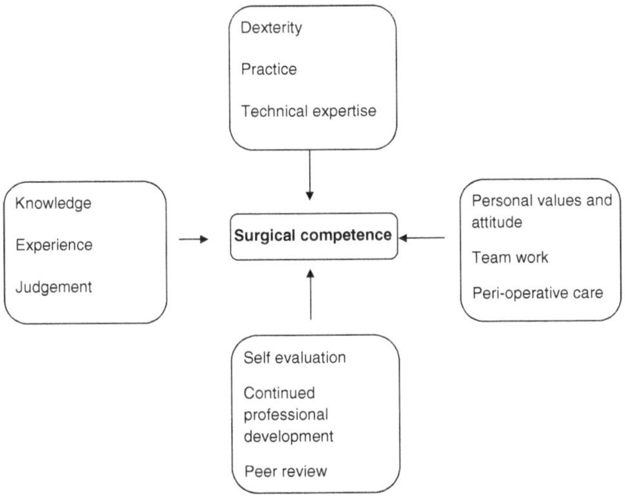

Fig. 2 Components of surgical competence

further emphasised by the anecdotal evidence that increasing medical or conservative management of patients with ectopic pregnancy reduces the opportunity for surgical training in theatre.

Knowledge base should be expanded by courses, local educational activities and web-based resources, to name a few. In this study, only 47% of the trainees had attended a suitable course within a defined time period.

In the UK, trainees are required to undergo regular objective assessment—OSATS. Implementation of this tool creates an interaction between the trainee and the supervisor, where various aspects of trainees' performance are assessed. This tool has proven its value in improving the trainees' understanding and improvement in performance [25]. The secondary effect of this tool in increasing the direct supervision and systematic discussion of trainees' performance is a key feature facilitating 'formative assessment'.

In Table 1, we have summarised the published data regarding trainee involvement in the laparoscopic management of tubal pregnancy in the UK over the last decade. It would appear from these articles that a high proportion of tubal pregnancies can be managed through the laparoscopic route. From this limited information, it is not clear how the trainee involvement is changing in the wider context. Of course, practitioners' willingness to submit their data and publication bias must be borne in mind when interpreting the wider trend.

Conclusion

Our national survey of trainees demonstrates that there is a high level of trainee engagement in laparoscopic surgery for ectopic pregnancy. Despite the variable satisfaction with the training aspects, majority anticipate attainment of competency by the end of the training period. With increasing standardisation of training, use of objective assessment tools and increasing consultant presence, we anticipate all trainees will become versed in laparoscopic surgery for ectopic pregnancy. This would be more likely to be achieved if simulators are formally integrated within the gynaecological surgery training syllabus. This will be realised once a steady state of all the necessary resources has been established.

Declaration of interest The authors report no conflicts of interest. The authors alone are responsible for the content and writing of the paper.

Table 1 Summary of UK literature regarding surgical access and trainee involvement in tubal pregnancy surgery

Authors	Year	No. of cases	Laparoscopy (%)	Trainee surgeon (%)
Olagundoye et al. [26]	2000	106	66	68
Mohamed et al. [27]	2002	209	84	50
Davidson and Nicholson [28]	2002	50	62	90
Odejinmi et al. [29]	2003	62	90	16
Subair et al. [10]	2004	40	64	53
Karri and Harris [30]	2005	114	89	33
Odejinme et al. [8]	2010	179	84	51

References

1. Hoover KW, Tao G, Kent CK (2010) Trends in the diagnosis and treatment of ectopic pregnancy in the United States. Obstet Gynecol 115:495–502
2. Lundorff P, Thorburn J, Hahlin M, Kallfelt B, Lindblom B (1991) Laparoscopic surgery in ectopic pregnancy: a randomized trial versus laparoscopy. Acta Obstet Gynecol Scand 70:343–348
3. Murphy AA, Nager CW, Wujek JJ, Kettel LM, Torp VA, Chin HG (1992) Operative laparoscopy versus laparotomy for the management of ectopic pregnancy. Fertil Steril 57:1180–1185
4. Vermesh M, Silva P, Rosen G, Stein AL, Fossum GT, Sauer MV (1989) Management of unruptured ectopic gestation by linear salpingostomy: a prospective, randomized clinical trial of laparoscopy versus laparotomy. Obstet Gynecol 73:400–404
5. The Royal College of Obstetricians and Gynaecologists (2004) Guideline number 21: the management of tubal pregnancy. RCOG Press, London
6. Saidi SA, Butler-Manuel S, Poweel M (1998) Laparoscopic treatment of ectopic pregnancy in the UK: a nationwide survey of consultant gynaecologists. Proceedings of the 28th British Congress in Obstetrics and Gynaecology. Br J Obstet Gynaecol 105(Supplement 17):48
7. Toozs-Hobson P, Bidmead J, Khalid A, Cardozo L, Hill S (2000) Current trends in management of ectopic pregnancy in the United Kingdom. J Obstet Gynaecol 20:74–77
8. Odejinmi F, Rizzuto I, Ballard KD (2010) Potential barriers to the laparoscopic management of ectopic pregnancies: a regional U.K study. Acta Obstet Gynecol Scand 89(10):1350–1353
9. Bancroft K, Whittaker MD, Clayton RD, Garry R (1999) The availability of training in the laparoscopic management of ectopic pregnancy. Gynaecol Endos 8:85–87
10. Subair O, Omojole F, Mistry N, Morgan H (2004) Trainees and the management of ectopic pregnancy. J Obstet Gynaecol 24:811–812
11. Odejinme FO, Rizzuto MI, MacRae RE, Thakur V (2008) Changing trends in the laparoscopic management of ectopic pregnancy in a London district general hospital: 7-year experience. J Obstet Gynaecol 28:614–617
12. The Royal College of Obstetricians and Gynaecologists (2009) Trainee survey report. RCOG Press, London
13. Aggarwal R, Tully A, Grantcharov T, Larsen CR, Miskry T, Farthing A, Darzi A (2006) Virtual reality simulation training can improve technical skills during laparoscopic salpingectomy for ectopic pregnancy. BJOG 113:1382–1387
14. Lim YH, Ng SP, Ng PH, Tan AE, Jamil MA (2007) Laparoscopic salpingectomy in tubal pregnancy: prospective randomized trial using endoloop versus electrocautery. Obstet Gynaecol Res 33:855–862
15. Torkington J, Smith SG, Rees B, Darzi A (2001) The role of the basic surgical skills course in the acquisition and retention of laparoscopic skill. Surg Endosc 15:1071–1075
16. Pareek G, Hedican SP, Bishoff JT, Shichman SJ, Wolf JS Jr, Nakada SY (2008) Skills-based laparoscopy training demonstrates long-term transfer of clinical laparoscopic practice: additional follow-up. Urology 72:265–267
17. Maagaard M, Sorensen JL, Oestergaard J, Dalsgaard T, Grantcharov TP, Ottesen BS, Larsen CR (2011) Retention of laparoscopic procedural skills acquired on a virtual-reality surgical trainer. Surg Endosc 25:722–727
18. Crist DW, Gadacz TR (1993) Complications of laparoscopic surgery. Surg Clin North Am 73:265–289
19. Gadacz TR (2000) Update on laparoscopic cholecystectomy, including a clinical pathway. Surg Clin North Am 80:1127–1149
20. Seymour NE, Gallagher AG, Roman SA, O'Brien MK, Bansal VK, Andersen DK, Satava RM (2002) Virtual reality training improves operating room performance: results of a randomized, double-blinded study. Ann Surg 236:458–463
21. Grantcharov TP, Kristiansen VB, Bendix J, Bardram L, Rosenberg J, Funch-Jensen P (2004) Randomized clinical trial of virtual reality simulation for laparoscopic skills training. Br J Surg 91:146–150
22. Larsen CR, Soerensen JL, Grantcharov TP, Dalsgaard T, Schouenborg L, Ottosen C, Schroeder TV, Ottesen BS (2009) Effect of virtual reality training on laparoscopic surgery: randomised controlled trial. BMJ 338:b1802–b1808
23. Majmudar T, Slack M (2009) Laparoscopy training for obstetrics and gynaecology trainees? A pilot study in the Eastern Deanery, UK. Gynaecol Surg 6:45–50
24. Qureshi NS, Wiener JJ, Weerakkody ANA (2006) Laparoscopic management of tubal ectopic pregnancy: availability of training. Obstet Gynaecol 8:251–255
25. Lentz GM, Mandel LS, Goff BA (2005) A six-year study of surgical teaching and skills evaluation for obstetric/gynecologic residents in porcine and inanimate surgical models. Am J Obstet Gynecol 193:2056–2061
26. Olagundoye V, Adeghe J, Guirguis M, Cox C, Murphy D (2000) Laparoscopic surgical management of ectopic pregnancy: a district general hospital experience. J Obstet Gynaecol 20:620–623
27. Mohamed H, Maiti S, Phillips G (2002) Laparoscopic management of ectopic pregnancy: a 5-year experience. J Obstet Gynaecol 22:411–414
28. Davidson E, Nicholson SC (2002) Management of ectopic pregnancy in a Scottish teaching hospital: implications for training. J Obstet Gynaecol 22:197–200
29. Odejinmi F, Madhuvrata P, Naftalin A, Boulton J, Chenoy R, Raveendran M (2003) Enthusiasm and teamwork—the basis for increase in laparoscopic surgery for ectopic pregnancy: an Inner London district hospital experience. J Obstet Gynaecol 23:645–647
30. Karri K, Harris CP (2005) Successful laparoscopic management of ectopic pregnancy in a district hospital. J Obstet Gynaecol 25:769–771

4

Efficacy of polyethylene glycol adhesion barrier after gynecological laparoscopic surgery

R. P. G. ten Broek · N. Kok-Krant · H. R. Verhoeve · H. van Goor · E. A. Bakkum

Abstract Postoperative adhesions are the most frequent complication of peritoneal surgery, causing small bowel obstruction, female infertility and chronic pain. This pilot study assessed the efficacy of a sprayable polyethylene glycol (PEG) barrier in the prevention of de novo adhesions. 16 patients undergoing laparoscopic gynecological surgery were randomly assigned by shuffled sealed envelopes to receive either the adhesion barrier or no adhesion prevention. Incidence and severity of adhesions were scored at eight sites in the pelvis and reassessed by second look laparoscopy. Adhesion prevention was considered successful if no de novo adhesion were found at second look laparoscopy. One patient was excluded before randomization. Nine patients were randomized to treatment and six patients to control group. De novo adhesions were found in 0/9 patients who received the PEG barrier compared to 4/6 without adhesion prevention (0% vs. 67%, P=0.01). Reduction in adhesion score was significantly greater in patients receiving PEG barrier (−2.6 vs. −0.06, P=0.03). Meta-analysis of three randomized trials demonstrated that PEG barrier reduces the incidence of adhesions (odds ratio [OR]= 0.27; 95% CI 0.11–0.67). From this study, PEG barrier seems effective in reducing postoperative formation of de novo adhesions.

R. P. G. ten Broek · H. van Goor
Department of Surgery,
Radboud University Nijmegen Medical Centre,
Nijmegen, The Netherlands

N. Kok-Krant · H. R. Verhoeve · E. A. Bakkum (✉)
Department of Gynaecology and Obstetrics,
Onze Lieve Vrouwe Gasthuis,
P.O. Box 95500, 1090 HM Amsterdam, The Netherlands
e-mail: E.A.Bakkum@olvg.nl

Keywords Tissue adhesions · Laparoscopy · Polyethylene glycol · Hydrogels · Randomized controlled trial

Background

Adhesions develop after gynecological surgery in the pelvic cavity in almost all cases and cause significant morbidity [1]. In a large population-based study of gynecological pelvic surgery, the readmission rate directly or probably related to adhesions was 13.9%, and the introduction of less invasive techniques, such as laparoscopy, did not seem to reduce this adhesion related morbidity [2]. The incidence of adhesive small bowel obstruction (ASBO) after oncologic gynecological surgery is about 11% [3]. Adhesions are the leading cause of secondary female infertility worldwide [4, 5], and an important cause of chronic pelvic pain [6, 7]. In addition, adhesiolysis during reoperation is time-consuming and exposes the patient to the risk of unintended injury such as enterotomy [1, 8].

Adhesion barriers or anti-adhesive agents are needed because refinements in surgical techniques do not seem to be sufficient in reducing adhesion-related morbidity. Several products have come to the market ranging from membranes for selective coverage of injured peritoneal areas to liquids for broad nonspecific coverage. An important drawback of the available membranous adhesions barriers is the difficulty of handling them during laparoscopic procedures. Alternatives to membranes for laparoscopic use are sprays that are easily applied intraperitoneally through trocars at sites that need to be covered. Recently, a sprayable polyethylene glycol (PEG) anti-adhesion barrier was developed for anti-adhesive purposes (SprayGel; Confluent Surgical Inc., Waltham, MA). The PEG adhesion barrier consists of two liquid precursor solutions that quickly react to form a hydrogel after being sprayed and mixed in the abdomen. One of the precursors contains a small concentration of methylene blue allowing visualization of the area covered and the thickness of the hydrogel layer during laparoscopy. The hydrogel is biodegradable and physically separates the injured peritoneal sites in order to promote adhesion free peritoneal regeneration.

The PEG anti-adhesion spray proved to be effective in rodent and porcine models with 75% reduction of the incidence of adhesions in a rat cecal abrasion model and 60% reduction in a porcine uterine horn model [9, 10]. Four human randomized controlled trials (RCTs) have been performed: two in patients undergoing laparoscopic or open myomectomy and two in patients undergoing loop ileostomy closure [11–14]. No RCT has included patients undergoing laparoscopic surgery alone, and all RCTs included a specific group of patients rather than investigating the various common types of laparoscopic benign gynecological surgery. The use of PEG spray was correlated with a reduction in extend and tenacity of adhesions in these RCTs. However, reductions in adhesion incidence — in contrast to reduction in adhesion extend or tenacity — is particularly important for predicting the value of an anti-adhesive product reducing ASBO and unintended organ injury during adhesiolysis. We undertook a small prospective randomized controlled study to evaluate the PEG spray on adhesion formation in women undergoing common laparoscopic gynecological procedures. In addition, we performed a meta-analysis of reported studies, including the present one, focusing on the efficacy of PEG spray in reducing the incidence of adhesions.

Materials and methods

The study was a randomized single-blinded (patient) study. Patients who were scheduled for laparoscopic treatment of benign gynecologic disease involving ovaries, pelvic sidewalls, fallopian tubes or uterus were assessed for eligibility between September 2002 and March 2004. Inclusion criteria were as follows: age ≥18 years; the patient might benefit from and agrees to return for second look laparoscopy (SLL); and the patient agrees to use contraception until SLL was conducted.

Pregnant and lactating patients were excluded, as well as patients with known or suspected malignancy. Peroperative exclusion criteria were endometriosis classified as stage IV, using the Revised American Society for Reproductive Medicine Classification of Endometriosis scoring system and if complete adhesiolysis was not possible [15].

At the end of index laparoscopic surgery and before removal of all instruments, patients were randomly assigned — via shuffled sealed envelopes — to treatment with PEG or no treatment groups. The PEG barrier was sprayed at all sites of surgical injury with the potential for adhesion formation. SLL was planned to evaluate adhesion formation. The surgeon performing SLL was blinded for the treatment group.

The study protocol was approved by the local Medical Ethical Committee and designed according to the ethical considerations described in the revised version of the Declaration of Helsinki (October 2008, Seoul). All patients gave written informed consent. The study was investigator-driven. PEG was kindly donated by Confluent, Surgical Inc (Waltham, MA, USA). The trial was registered at clinical trials.gov with identifier: NCT01187680.

Adhesion scoring

The incidence of patients with and without any adhesion was assessed in both initial and second look laparoscopies. All surgical procedures were performed by the same surgeons (EB and HV). Adhesions at SLL were classified as de novo adhesions or reformed adhesions. De novo adhesions are adhesions that are newly formed following the first laparoscopy at sites without any former adhesions. Reformed adhesions are adhesions that formed at the sites of adhesiolysis during the first laparoscopy [16].

Adhesions were graded using the Local Adhesion Barrier Scoring System (LABS) score, based on the modified version of the American Fertility Society score system [17]. The LABS is an integrated score system comprising the adhesion's morphology and extend of the site covered with adhesions (Table 1). The LABS score differs from the modified version of the American Fertility Society score system; adhesions are scored at a lower number of sites that are more specific to gynecologic surgery. Adhesions were systematically evaluated for incidence and LABS score at eight sites: both left and right tubes, ovaries and pelvic sidewall and the anterior and posterior uterus. For each patient, the total LABS score was calculated as the mean of LABS scores at these eight separate locations.

Table 1 Local Adhesion Barrier Scoring (LABS) system

LABS adhesion score		
Tenacity	Extend	Score
None	None (0% covered)	0
Mild	Localized (<33% covered))	1
Mild	Moderate (33–67% covered)	2
Mild	Extensive (>67% covered)	4
Severe	Localized (<33% covered))	4
Severe	Moderate (33–67% covered)	8
Severe	Extensive (>67% covered)	16

Safety aspects

All patients were treated in day care. Postoperatively, patients were controlled for temperature, pain, hemodynamic changes and signs of bleeding in the recovery area.

Outcomes

The primary outcome for this pilot study was the number of patients with de novo adhesions. Secondary outcomes were change in the number of sites covered with adhesions and change in LABS adhesion score.

The number of patients with any adhesions is the most preferable outcome of adhesion prevention studies. However, as the sample size of this pilot study would be inadequate to provide in sufficient power on this outcome, we addressed this outcome in meta-analysis of systematically searched studies on PEG adhesion barrier.

Power analysis

Based on animal studies, the incidence of de novo adhesions was estimated at 30% in the PEG group and 90% in the control group [10]. Fourteen patients in each arm of the study were needed to detect such difference with 80% power and 5% two-tailed significance threshold at 1:1 randomization. Accounting for loss to follow-up, a minimum of 30 patients were to be randomized.

Statistical analysis

All statistical tests performed were two-tailed with significance was determined at the 5% level. Unpaired *t*-test was used for the testing of continuous data and Fisher's exact test for dichotomous data. All statistical analyses were performed using SPSS 16.0.2 (SPSS inc., Chicago, ILL).

Meta-analysis

A comprehensive search of Pubmed and Embase search was performed on July 1, 2011 to identify papers published in peer-reviewed journals from RCTs in surgical or gynaecological patients for the intervention with PEG and outcome adhesions. In Pubmed, randomized trials were identified via the Cochrane Highly Sensitive Search Strategy for identifying randomized trials (sensitivity- and precision-maximizing version) [18]. We selected randomized trials in Embase using the top performing search strategy (minimizing difference between sensitivity and specificity version) described by Wong et al. [19]. Relevant RCTs were searched for data on the number of patients with any adhesions. The incidence of adhesions was expressed in odds ratio (OR) for meta-analysis. A fixed-effects model was applied for meta-analysis. In the presence of significant heterogeneity, the random-effects model was applied. Heterogeneity was tested with Cochrane Q-test and I^2 test. An I^2 value ≥50% or P value <0.05 was considered significant. Meta- analysis was carried out using Review Manager 5.0 (The Cochrane Collaboration, Copenhagen, Denmark).

End of study

The study was prematurely ended due to financial and organizational reasons. During the conduct of the study, the clinical trial insurance unexpectedly required a separate fee for both laparoscopic procedures in each patient.

Results

A total of 16 eligible patients gave informed consent. Fifteen underwent successful laparoscopic gynecological or fertility surgery and were randomized. One patient had severe pelvic adhesions that could not be lysed completely and was excluded before randomization. There were no significant differences between the PEG and control group at index laparoscopy in age, type of surgical procedure, history of prior surgery, Chlamydia serology and smoking status at baseline (Table 2). Adhesiolysis was performed in 14 patients.

At index laparoscopy, there was a non-significant trend towards more sites covered with adhesions (5.1±2.3 vs. 3± 2.2; P=0.10) and higher LABS score (3.7±2.8 vs. 2.4±3.0; P=0.40) in the PEG group (Table 3). Time of surgery was comparable between the PEG and control group at index laparoscopy. Time period between initial and second look laparoscopies was similar for both groups: 27.9±11.5 days in the PEG group and 28.0±17.6 in the control group (P>0.99).

All 15 randomized patients underwent SLL. De novo adhesions were found in 0/9 patients in the PEG group (0%) compared to 4/6 (67%) of patients in the control group (P=0.01). Patients in the PEG group had a decrease in LABS score compared to an increase in the control group (−2.6±2.1 vs. 0.1±1.7; P=0.03). This decrease was most prominent at the ovaries and fallopian tubes sites. The change in the number of sites covered with adhesions was −2.4±2.0 for patients treated with PEG spray compared to 0.8±2.3 for control patients (P=0.01). There were no significant differences in the absolute incidence, sites covered with adhesions and LABS scores between the PEG group and controls at SLL (Table 4). There were no post- operative complications in both groups.

Although no significant differences were found in the incidence of adhesions at any of the specific sites at SLL,

Table 2 Baseline characteristics

	PEG	Control	*P* value
Number of randomized patients	9	6	
Age	30.1±5.7[a]	34.5±4.3[a]	0.12
Type of surgical procedures performed			
Adhesiolysis	8 (89%)	5 (83%)	>0.99
Salpingotomy/salpingectomy	4 (44%)	2 (33%)	>0.99
Cystectomy	2 (22%)	3 (50%)	0.33
Laparotomy	0/9 (0%)	0/6 (0%)	>0.99
Laparoscopy	5/9 (56%)	5/6 (83%)	0.58
Positive Chlamydia serology	4/9 (44%)	1/6(17%)	0.58
Smoker	1/9 (11%)	0/6 (0%)	>0.99
Completed SLL	9 (100%)	6 (100%)	>0.99

[a]Mean±SD

the effect of PEG appeared maximal at the ovaries. The incidence of adhesions around the ovaries was reduced between index laparoscopy and SLL in the PEG treated group by 33% and 44% for the right and left ovaries, respectively. On the contrary, a 17% and 33% increase in incidence of adhesions around the right and left ovaries, respectively, was seen in control patients.

Meta-analysis of adhesion incidence

A total of 85 papers from peer-reviewed journals were identified using the search strategy. Five papers were identified studying the efficacy of PEG on adhesion formation after peritoneal surgery in an RCT [11–14, 20]. The number of patients with any adhesions could be assessed from three papers investigating patients undergoing myomectomy [11, 13, 20]. One paper was excluded because it described an interim analysis and results from the completed study were described in another paper [11, 20]. Thus, two RCTs and the present study remained for meta-analysis. In all here studies a trend towards a lower overall incidence of adhesions was demonstrated in PEG treated patients. Pooled data, using a fixed effects model, showed a significant reduction of the incidence of adhesions with an OR of 0.27 (95% CI 0.11–0.67; *P*=0.005, Fig. 1).

Discussion and conclusion

From this study, PEG anti-adhesion barrier seems effective in the prevention of de novo adhesions in common gynecological laparoscopic procedures, but especially in fertility enhancing procedures. Furthermore, there was a significant difference in change of LABS score favoring patients treated with PEG adhesion barrier. Meta-analysis also showed a significant reduction in the total incidence of adhesions.

The PEG anti-adhesion barrier has a set of unique characteristics compared to other existing barriers. The

Table 3 Adhesions at initial laparoscopy

	PEG	Control	*P* value
Patients with any adhesion	8/9 (89%)	5/6 (83%)	>0.99
Adhesion sites	5.1±2.3[a]	3±2.2[a]	0.10
LABS score (mean)	3.7±2.8[a]	2.4±3.0[a]	0.44
• Left ovary	5.1±4.9	2.0±3.3	0.17
• Right ovary	5.8±6.0	4.0±6.2	0.59
• Left fallopian tube	6.4±5.8	2.0±3.3	0.08
• Right fallopian tube	6.2±5.7	3.5+6.3	0.42
• Left pelvic side wall	3.3±3.2	1.3±3.3	0.27
• Right pelvic side wall	1.6±2.8	4.3±6.5	0.36
• Anterior uterus	0.2±0.7	0.0±0.0	0.35
• Posterior uterus	1.2±1.7	2.7±2.1	0.19
Time of surgery (min)	151.9±29.5[a]	146.7±47.8[a]	0.82
Time to SLL (days)	27.9±11.5[a]	28.0±17.6[a]	>0.99

SLL second look laparscopy
[a]Mean±SD

Table 4 Adhesions at second look laparoscopy

Outcome	PEG	Control	*P* value
Patients with any adhesion	7/9 (78%)	6/6 (100%)	0.49
Patients with de novo adhesions	0/9 (0%)	4/6 (67%)	0.01
Adhesions (number of sites)	2.7±2.4[a]	3.8±1.7[a]	0.29
Δ Adhesions (number of sites)[a]	−2.4±2.0[a]	0.8±2.3[a]	0.01
LABS score (Mean)	1.2±1.3[a]	2.4±2.4[a]	0.29
• Left ovary	0.7±0.9	2.2±3.0	0.28
• Right ovary	2.9±5.2	5.5±6.4	0.43
• Left fallopian tube	2.2±3.3	1.7±1.4	0.66
• Right fallopian tube	2.3±2.8	2.8±6.5	0.86
• Left pelvic side wall	1.0±2.6	0.7±1.0	0.74
• Right pelvic side wall	0.0±0.0	4.0±6.7	0.20
• Anterior uterus	0.0±0.0	0.0±0.0	1.00
• Posterior uterus	0.3±0.5	2.5±3.1	0.15
Δ LABS score[b] (mean)	−2.6±2.1[a]	0.1±1.7[a]	0.03
• Left ovary	−4.4±5.1	0.2±2.2	0.03
• Right ovary	−2.9±4.8	1.5±5.3	0.13
• Left fallopian tube	−4.2±5.0	−0.3±4.0	0.12
• Right fallopian tube	−3.9±4.0	−0.7±1.2	0.05
• Left pelvic side wall	−2.3±2.8	−0.7±3.7	0.38
• Right pelvic side wall	−1.6±2.8	−0.3±0.8	0.24
• Anterior uterus	−0.2±0.7	0.0±0.0	0.35
• Posterior uterus	−0.9±1.5	−0.2±2.7	0.57

[a]Mean±SD

[b]Δ = difference between index laparoscopy and second look laparoscopy

formula of two liquid PEG precursors that rapidly polymerize into a solid hydrogel, allows the surgeon to laparoscopically apply a barrier with the characteristics of a site specific barrier and the ease of application of a liquid [12]. Most site specific barriers are solid membranes that are difficult to apply laparoscopically. Site specific adhesion barriers seem most efficacious against adhesion (re)formation as they remain on the exact place of application during mesothelial healing. In the study of Ferland et al. both uterine horns and opposing peritoneum in a porcine model were abraded. One side was randomly assigned to coverage with a 1- to 2-mm-thick layer of PEG adhesion barrier. The barrier remained in place, and at SLL a significantly lower incidence of adhesion was found at the treated sides, demonstrating that the PEG adhesion barrier acts as a site-specific adhesion barrier [10]. The methylene blue dye makes it easy to assess if an area is sufficiently covered with the PEG anti-adhesion barrier. PEG molecules polymerize without the need of an external energy source or excess heat production and the hydrogel remains intact for 5–6 days, which is long enough for peritoneal layers to heal [21]. When degrading, the hydrogel falls apart in water-soluble PEG molecules that are easily resorbed and cleared in the urine [22].

Although a small number of patients could be included in this trial, our findings support those of earlier studies demonstrating that PEG spray is a highly efficacious site specific barrier for laparoscopic use. The incidence of adhesions could be assessed from two previous RCTs in patients undergoing myomectomy [11, 13]. In the present study and the two RCTs, a trend towards a lower overall

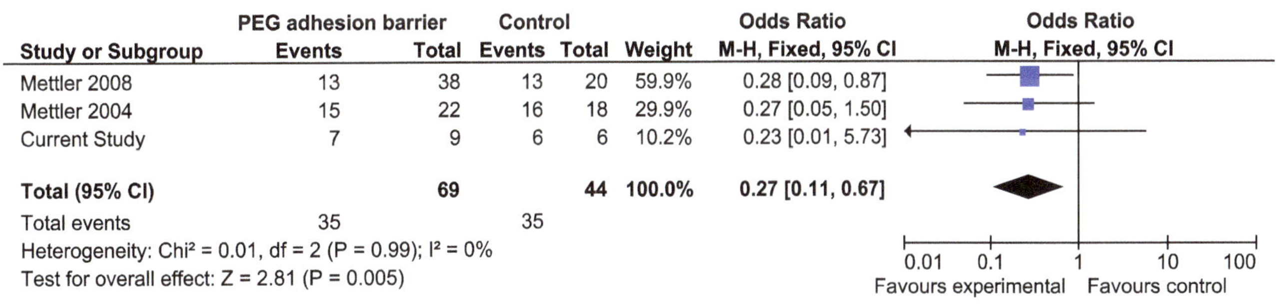

Fig. 1 Results from meta-analysis on the efficacy of PEG adhesion barrier reducing the total incidence of adhesions

incidence of adhesions was demonstrated in PEG treated patients. Pooled data showed a significant reduction of the incidence of adhesions in our meta-analysis. Complete adhesion prevention is of particular importance as it is the only means of providing a definitive protection against all adhesion related complications, such as infertility, ASBO and inadvertent enterotomies.

A limitation of this study is the analysis of adhesion prevention and not the clinical complications of adhesions, such as infertility or ASBO. Infertility as an endpoint is difficult to assess because failure to attain pregnancy is a multi-factorial endpoint. To assess the efficacy of adhesion barriers on fertility, a randomised trial is required in subfertile patients due to tubal pathology, which compares use of a barrier to no treatment after adhesiolysis and compares time to natural conception. Oxidized regenerating cellulose (Interceed®, Ethicon, Sommerville, NJ) is the only adhesion barrier that was proven to increase pregnancy rate in an RCT [23]. However, oxidized regenerating cellulose has limitations because it is difficult to handle laparoscopically and can cause adverse adhesiogenic effects in the presence of blood [24, 25]. Studies evaluating the efficacy of adhesion barriers in reducing the number of ASBO and enterotomies are rare. The incidence of these complications is relative low, thus a large number of patients is needed to demonstrate a significant effect. Modified sodium hyaluronic acid (HA) and carboxymethyl-cellulose (Seprafilm®; Genzyme Corporation, Cambridge, MA) reduced the number of ASBO requiring reoperation or found at autopsy by 45% in a study of 1,701 patients who underwent benign colorectal surgery [26]. This barrier has limitations because it cannot easily be applied at laparoscopy.

Change in adhesion score can be difficult to interpret as an outcome measure for adhesion prevention because the adhesion score at baseline influences the maximal effect. However, in our study, not only the size but also the direction of the effect differed between the groups. There was a marked decrease in LABS adhesion score in PEG treated group, while patients in the control group had a slight increase in adhesion score.

To study the efficacy of adhesion barriers by means of a second look procedure is becoming increasingly difficult. First, it is deemed more and more unethical to perform an invasive second procedure just for scientific purposes. Second, the benefit of SLL as part of fertility surgery is questionable. Today, women have more access to alternative treatment modalities to become pregnant such as in vitro fertilization [27]. Future adhesion prevention studies expectedly have to rely on non-invasive techniques to evaluate adhesion formation. For long, this has been considered impossible but recent studies show promising results of cine-MRI as a non-invasive diagnostic tool for the detection of adhesions [28]. More experience is needed to delineate the value of cine-MRI as an alternative to SLL in adhesion prevention studies.

Sprayable barriers that can be introduced via a laparoscopic trocar and handled with ease in the abdominal-pelvic cavity are of surplus value in the therapeutic arsenal of adhesion preventive agents. Clinical trials have demonstrated that laparoscopy only reduces the extend of adhesions but does not decrease the incidence of adhesions [29, 30]. Maximal efforts to prevent adhesion formation in fertility surgery should therefore comprise laparoscopy as well as an adhesion barrier. Although a large number of agents show adhesion reduction in animal models, only a few demonstrated such effects in RCT in humans [31–33]. PEG is one of a few barriers that has been evaluated in both gynecological and gastrointestinal patients and was found to be effective in both our study and previous RCTs [11, 13, 14, 20]. However, more research is needed to investigate the effect on adhesion related complications, such as ASBO and infertility.

Conflict of interest The study was investigator-initiated. Confluent Surgical Inc. (Waltham, MA) kindly provided the PEG adhesion barrier and paid the trial insurance fees of patients participating in this study. There were no further financial ties to Confluent Surgical Inc.

References

1. van Goor H (2007) Consequences and complications of peritoneal adhesions. Colorectal Dis 9(Suppl 2):25–34
2. Lower AM, Hawthorn RJ, Clark D et al (2004) Adhesion-related readmissions following gynaecological laparoscopy or laparotomy in Scotland: an epidemiological study of 24 046 patients. Hum Reprod 19:1877–1885
3. Montz FJ, Holschneider CH, Solh S et al (1994) Small bowel obstruction following radical hysterectomy: risk factors, incidence, and operative findings. Gynecol Oncol 53:114–120
4. Kaminski P, Gajewska M, Wielgos M et al (2006) The usefulness of laparoscopy and hysteroscopy in the diagnostics and treatment of infertility. Neuro Endocrinol Lett 27:813–817
5. Cates W, Farley TM, Rowe PJ (1985) Worldwide patterns of infertility: is Africa different? Lancet 2:596–598
6. Swank DJ, van Erp WF, Repelaer Van Driel OJ et al (2003) A prospective analysis of predictive factors on the results of laparoscopic adhesiolysis in patients with chronic abdominal pain. Surg Laparosc Endosc Percutan Tech 13:88–94
7. Mettler L, Alhujeily M (2007) Role of laparoscopy in identifying the clinical significance and cause of adhesions and chronic pelvic pain: a retrospective review at the Kiel School of Gynecological Endoscopy. JSLS 11:303–308
8. Van Der Krabben AA, Dijkstra FR, Nieuwenhuijzen M et al (2000) Morbidity and mortality of inadvertent enterotomy during adhesiotomy. Br J Surg 87:467–471
9. Dunn R, Lyman MD, Edelman PG et al (2001) Evaluation of the SprayGel adhesion barrier in the rat cecum abrasion and rabbit uterine horn adhesion models. Fertil Steril 75:411–416

10. Ferland R, Mulani D, Campbell PK (2001) Evaluation of a sprayable polyethylene glycol adhesion barrier in a porcine efficacy model. Hum Reprod 16:2718–2723
11. Mettler L, Audebert A, Lehmann-Willenbrock E et al (2004) A randomized, prospective, controlled, multicenter clinical trial of a sprayable, site-specific adhesion barrier system in patients undergoing myomectomy. Fertil Steril 82:398–404
12. Johns DA, Ferland R, Dunn R (2003) Initial feasibility study of a sprayable hydrogel adhesion barrier system in patients undergoing laparoscopic ovarian surgery. J Am Assoc Gynecol Laparosc 10:334–338
13. Mettler L, Hucke J, Bojahr B et al (2008) A safety and efficacy study of a resorbable hydrogel for reduction of post-operative adhesions following myomectomy. Hum Reprod 23:1093–1100
14. Tjandra JJ, Chan MK (2008) A sprayable hydrogel adhesion barrier facilitates closure of defunctioning loop ileostomy: a randomized trial. Dis Colon Rectum 51:956–960
15. Revised American Society for Reproductive Medicine (1997) Classification of endometriosis: 1996. Fertil Steril 67:817–821
16. Diamond MP, Wexner SD, diZereg GS et al (2010) Adhesion prevention and reduction: current status and future recommendations of a multinational interdisciplinary consensus conference. Surg Innov 17:183–188
17. American Fertility Society (1988) The American Fertility Society classifications of adnexal adhesions, distal tubal occlusion, tubal occlusion secondary to tubal ligation, tubal pregnancies, Mullerian anomalies and intrauterine adhesions. Fertil Steril 49:944–955
18. Higgins J, Green S (2009) Cochrane handbook for systematic reviews of interventions. The Cochrane Collaboration
19. Wong SS, Wilczynski NL, Haynes RB (2006) Comparison of top-performing search strategies for detecting clinically sound treatment studies and systematic reviews in MEDLINE and EMBASE. J Med Libr Assoc 94:451–455
20. Mettler L, Audebert A, Lehmann-Willenbrock E et al (2003) Prospective clinical trial of SprayGel as a barrier to adhesion formation: an interim analysis. J Am Assoc Gynecol Laparosc 10:339–344
21. Reijnen MM, Bleichrodt RP, van Goor H (2003) Pathophysiology of intra-abdominal adhesion and abscess formation, and the effect of hyaluronan. Br J Surg 90:533–541
22. Yamaoka T, Tabata Y, Ikada Y (1994) Distribution and tissue uptake of poly(ethylene glycol) with different molecular weights after intravenous administration to mice. J Pharm Sci 83:601–606
23. Sawada T, Nishizawa H, Nishio E et al (2000) Postoperative adhesion prevention with an oxidized regenerated cellulose adhesion barrier in infertile women. J Reprod Med 45:387–389
24. Wiseman DM, Gottlick-Iarkowski L, Kamp L (1999) Effect of different barriers of oxidized regenerated cellulose (ORC) on cecal and sidewall adhesions in the presence and absence of bleeding. J Invest Surg 12:141–146
25. Wiseman DM, Gottlick LE, Diamond MP (1992) Effect of thrombin-induced hemostasis on the efficacy of an absorbable adhesion barrier. J Reprod Med 37:766–770
26. Fazio VW, Cohen Z, Fleshman JW et al (2006) Reduction in adhesive small-bowel obstruction by Seprafilm adhesion barrier after intestinal resection. Dis Colon Rectum 49:1–11
27. Duffy JM, Johnson N, Ahmad G et al (2009) Postoperative procedures for improving fertility following pelvic reproductive surgery. Cochrane Database Syst Rev CD001897
28. Lienemann A, Sprenger D, Steitz HO et al (2000) Detection and mapping of intraabdominal adhesions by using functional cine MR imaging: preliminary results. Radiology 217:421–425
29. Lundorff P, Hahlin M, Kallfelt B et al (1991) Adhesion formation after laparoscopic surgery in tubal pregnancy: a randomized trial versus laparotomy. Fertil Steril 55:911–915
30. Audebert AJ, Gomel V (2000) Role of microlaparoscopy in the diagnosis of peritoneal and visceral adhesions and in the prevention of bowel injury associated with blind trocar insertion. Fertil Steril 73:631–635
31. Metwally M, Watson A, Lilford R et al (2006) Fluid and pharmacological agents for adhesion prevention after gynaecological surgery. Cochrane Database Syst Rev CD001298
32. Kumar S, Wong PF, Leaper DJ (2009) Intra-peritoneal prophylactic agents for preventing adhesions and adhesive intestinal obstruction after non-gynaecological abdominal surgery. Cochrane Database Syst Rev CD005080
33. Ahmad G, Duffy JM, Farquhar C et al (2008) Barrier agents for adhesion prevention after gynaecological surgery. Cochrane Database Syst Rev CD000475

5

Entry techniques in gynecologic laparoscopy

Johannes Ott · Agnes Jaeger-Lansky · Gunda Poschalko · Regina Promberger · Eleen Rothschedl · René Wenzl

Abstract Laparoscopy is one of the most common surgical procedures in gynecologic medicine. Major complications associated with gynecologic laparoscopy are relatively rare, with up to 50% related to laparoscopic entry. Several entry techniques have been developed, all of which aim to provide a safe and easy entry to the abdominal cavity. In this article, we aim to review the available evidence on laparoscopic entry techniques in gynecologic surgery. We found no evidence that the Hasson (open) technique is superior to the Veress needle entry, the preferred method of most gynecologists all over the world. When entering the abdomen using the Veress needle, an intraperitoneal pressure <10 mmHg is a reliable predictor of correct intraperitoneal placement. Entry at Palmer's point (left upper quadrant laparoscopy) is recommended for patients with suspected or known periumbilical adhesions, or a history or presence of umbilical hernia, or after three failed insufflation attempts at the umbilicus. Recently published trials suggest that direct trocar entry, especially when using optical trocar systems, might be superior to both the Hasson open technique and the Veress needle entry to avoid extraperitoneal insufflation and failed entry. Moreover, blood loss can be reduced and the mean entry time shortened. Laparoscopic entry techniques are still a controversial topic in gynecologic surgery. Many studies are underpowered in order to assess the risk for rare but life-threatening complications. In conclusion, there is no solid evidence proving the superiority of any method of laparoscopic entry.

J. Ott · A. Jaeger-Lansky · G. Poschalko · E. Rothschedl · R. Wenzl (✉)
Department of Gynecology and Obstetrics,
Medical University of Vienna,
Waehringer Guertel 18-20,
1090 Vienna, Austria
e-mail: rene.wenzl@meduniwien.ac.at

R. Promberger
Department of Surgery, Medical University of Vienna,
Vienna, Austria

Keywords Laparoscopy · Entry techniques · Gynecology · Complications · Veress needle · Hasson technique · Direct trocar entry

Background

Laparoscopy is one of the most common surgical procedures in gynecologic medicine and has become the method of choice over the last few decades for treating benign diseases that require surgery [1, 2]. Major complications from gynecologic laparoscopy are relatively rare, occurring in three to six per 1,000 cases. However, complications related to access represent one third to one half of these adverse events [1, 3]. These complications include serious and potentially life-threatening adverse events in about 0.4 of 1,000 laparoscopic procedures, such as perforation of the bowel, major abdominal vessels, and vessels of the anterior abdominal wall. These factors make the access phase the most critical step of a laparoscopic procedure. Less serious complications include postoperative infection, extraperitoneal insufflations, and subcutaneous emphysema [4].

In a large survey of 506 patients with entry access injuries, gynecologic procedures accounted for 63% of claims outside the USA and for at least 47% of all cases. The structures injured most frequently during primary entry access were the small bowel, the iliac artery, and the colon, together accounting for more than 50% of injuries [5]. These data present a more severe spectrum of injuries than those described in procedure-based studies and underline the severity and possible lethality of entry access injuries.

Several entry techniques exist [6–8]. However, there is no clear consensus on the optimal method of entry to the peritoneal cavity [8, 9]. Even a recent Cochrane database systematic review showed no evidence of benefit with regard to the safety of one technique over another [9]. We aimed to review the available evidence on laparoscopic entry techniques.

Methods

A computerized search of the medical literature was conducted with the MedLine database. Articles published up until February 2011 were searched for the keywords laparoscopy, laparoscopic entry, Veress needle, Hasson technique, open trocar entry, complications, and adverse events. The selected articles' bibliographies were also manually examined for any articles not captured by the computerized search. Case reports, abstracts, and letters were excluded. Randomized, quasi-randomized, and non-randomized, or cohort, studies on human patients were included if they compared access methods and provided relevant information on safety and efficacy outcome that had to be defined a priori.

Findings

Challenges during laparoscopic entry

Adhesions at the umbilical area are a major concern with regard to the safety of laparoscopic entry. Rates of up to 21% and 28% have been reported for women with previous laparoscopy and previous laparotomy, respectively [10, 11]. Patients with prior midline incisions, in particular, are at high risk (up to 42%) [12]. Entry techniques other than the classic CO_2 insufflation using a subumbilical Veress needle might be useful in these patients.

In very thin patients, especially in those with an android pelvis or a prominent sacral promontory, the great vessels have been reported to lie about 1 to 2 cm underneath the umbilicus [13, 14]. In obese patients, the umbilicus is shifted caudally toward the aortic bifurcation [15]. These patients are believed to be at an increased risk for major vessel injury during the course of a closed laparoscopic entry [16].

The Veress needle

Basic data on various entry techniques are provided in Table 1. The Veress needle technique is the preferred method of most gynecologists all over the world [17, 18]. The Veress needle is used to establish a pneumoperitoneum by blind insertion into the abdomen, which is then followed by trocar insertion. The classic insertion site in gynecologic laparoscopy is in the umbilical area in the midsagittal plane, used by 98% of gynecologists [9].

Alternative Veress needle insertion sites

Alternative sites for Veress needle insertion have been reported: Insertion in the left upper quadrant (LUQ, Palmer's point) has been mentioned to be useful in obese and very thin patients, as well as in those with a history of previous open abdominal surgery. In the presence of a large uterine or pelvic mass, it may be also advantageous [19]. The Veress needle is inserted 3 cm below the left subcostal border in the midclavicular line [20]. The method should not be applied in patients with previous splenic or gastric surgery, portal hypertension, hepatosplenomegaly, and gastropancreatic masses [21]. Laparoscopic entry using Palmer's point has been reported to be safe and effective, with a low failure rate of about 1.5%. Complications, mainly puncture of the left lobe of the liver, have been found in about 1% of cases [19, 22, 23].

Insertion of the Veress needle directly through the ninth or tenth intercostal space, at the anterior axillary line along the superior surface of the lower rib, has also been reported to be safe. A retrospective analysis of more than 900 cases of

Table 1 Overview of different entry techniques

Entry technique	First published in	Rates of major visceral injury (%)	Rates of major vascular injury (%)
Veress needle entry (classic)	*Gastroenterologia*, 1961 [89]	0.04–0.08	0.02–0.07
Optical Veress needle (minilaparoscopy)	*Endosc Surg Allied Technol*, 1995 [45]	1.1	Uncertain
Pressure sensor-equipped Veress needle	*J Am Assoc Gynecol Laparosc*, 1994 [47]	Uncertain	Uncertain
Hasson technique (open entry)	*Am J Obstet Gynecol*, 1971 [64]	0.05–0.1	0–0.005
Direct trocar entry	*Obstet Gynecol*, 1983 [90]	0	0

pneumoperitonization through the ninth intercostal space revealed only two major complications directly related to the laparoscopic entry [24]. The same indications apply to this method as to the entry at the Palmer's point [11].

Last but not the least, one might insufflate CO_2 through the posterior vaginal fornix ("trans cul-de-sac insufflation") or transvaginally through the fundus of the uterus. Both methods are indicated in extremely obese women [25–32]. For the transuterine route, there was a lower ratio between punctures and establishment of a pneumoperitoneum, when prospectively compared to the classical intraumbilical approach in obese women with a BMI >25 kg/m^2 [30].

Additional considerations with the Veress needle entry

The following tests that attempt to determine the correct intra-abdominal placement of the Veress needle have been described: the double click sound of the Veress needle; the Palmer's test (aspiration test); the hanging drop of saline test [33]; the "hiss" sound test [34]; the syringe test [35–38]; and the pressure profile test, of which the first five pressures registered by the gas insufflator are recorded at 5-s intervals and pressures less than 10 mmHg are assumed to indicate correct intraperitoneal placement [17, 39]. A prospective analysis demonstrated that the double click, aspiration, and hanging drop tests provided very little useful information about the placement of the Veress needle [40]. These findings are supported by the fact that, despite the implementing of these tools in the clinical routine, serious complications occur. Especially in women with previous open abdominal surgery, the pressure profile test is more specific and sensitive than the Palmer's test [39]. However, performing the Palmer's test is still recommended because of its value in warning the surgeon if any blood or feces is aspirated.

Many gynecologists elevate the anterior lower abdominal wall at the time of the Veress needle insertion either by hand or with the use of towel clips [11]. However, only with the use of towel clips a sufficient elevation of about 7 cm above the level of the viscera can be achieved [41]. Moreover, by lifting the abdominal wall by hand, one might also elevate the omentum in rare cases, causing omental perforations [42]. However, in a recent Cochrane database analysis, the authors concluded that lifting the abdominal wall resulted in an increased rate of entry failure (odds ratio 5.17) without an increase in the complication rate [9].

The literature reports successful Veress needle entry into the abdominal cavity on the first attempt in about 85% of cases. This is of particular importance since higher numbers of attempts are associated with increased complication rates including extraperitoneal insufflation, omental injuries, bowel injuries, and failed laparoscopy [41, 43].

The optical Veress needle

Entry using the optical Veress needle is also called "minilaparoscopy." A modified Veress needle of 2.1 mm diameter and a 10.5-cm-long cannula are used, allowing insertion of a thin, zero-degree, semirigid, fiberoptic minilaparoscope. During insertion of the Veress cannula with the telescope, one observes a cascade of color sequences on the monitor that represent the different abdominal wall layers. No randomized trials have been published as yet. Therefore, the relative risks of this procedure remain unclear [44]. However, in a prospective study of 184 cases, two bowel perforations occurred (Table 1) [45].

As another modification of the classical Veress needle, a pressure sensor-equipped Veress needle has been described [46]. However, no further studies evaluating the risk profile of this method have been published to date. It would be reasonable to conclude that these Veress needle modifications have not proven themselves in practice.

Insertion of the camera trocar after establishment of the pneumoperitoneum

Pneumoperitonization using the Veress needle is followed by trocar insertion. The force applied to the anterior abdominal wall during this procedure might put the viscera at risk for damage.

An adequate pneumoperitoneum is considered useful to prevent visceral damage during trocar insertion. Traditionally, the pneumoperitoneum has been defined as sufficient after insufflation of 1 to 4 L of CO_2 or the establishment of an intraperitoneal pressure of 10 to 15 mmHg [43]. It has been demonstrated that the use of the "pressure technique," using a median pressure of 14 mmHg, leads to a reduction in the complication rate of 50% when compared to the "volume technique" [43].

Based on these considerations, one might consider the pressure-controlled "high-pressure entry" (HIP entry) technique of benefit in order to decrease the complication rate. Three prospective studies on the safety of HIP entry using median intra-abdominal pressure values of 25–30 mmHg included nearly 9,000 female subjects. Only four bowel injuries (0.04%) and one major vessel injury (0.01%) were reported. Although the method leads to a significant decline in pulmonary compliance of about 20%, the maximum respiratory effects at 25 to 30 mmHg did not differ from the effect of the Trendelenburg position with intra-abdominal pressures of 15 mmHg [2, 44, 47, 48].

In order to minimize the risk for entry-associated complications following Veress needle insufflation, disposable shielded trocars and optical access trocars have been developed. Disposable shielded trocars are designed with a shield that partially retracts, exposing the sharp tip as it encounters resistance through the abdominal wall. After the shield enters the abdominal cavity, it springs forward and covers the sharp tip of the trocar [44]. The rationale for this method is to avoid intra-abdominal injuries. However, evidence proves that major complications, including death from trocar entry, cannot be avoided by using disposable shielded trocars [49, 50]. There is a lack of evidence in the literature about the safety of these instruments when used after establishment of the pneumoperitoneum.

There are two available disposable visual entry systems: the Endopath Optiview optical trocar (Ethicon Endo-Surgery, Inc., Cincinnati, OH) and the Visiport optical trocar (Tyco-United States Surgical, Norwalk, CT). Both are inserted through a 5-mm incision in the anterior rectus fascia after having withdrawn the Veress needle and dissected off the fatty tissue. However, with regard to trocar entry after pneumoperitonization by the Veress needle, most reports did not show superiority of visual entry trocars over other trocars, based on entry-associated complications, since these trocars cannot avoid vascular or visceral injury [44, 51–53]. Only in one retrospective study, the rate of major complications during insertion of the primary trocar in the blind insertion group was five of 1,000 (0.5%), whereas there were no major complications in the optical-guided insertion group (0.0%) [54].

Another visual entry system is the EndoTIP visual cannula (ENDOTIP; Karl Storz, Tuttlingen, Germany). The cannula has no cutting or sharp end. Thus, tissue layers are not transsected [55]. However, there are no randomized trials that compare this entry method to any other method.

Radially expanding access system

The radially expanding access system (Step; InnerDyne, Sunnyvale, CA) consists of a 1.9-mm Veress surrounded by an expanding polymeric sleeve. The abdomen can be insufflated prior to removal of the Veress needle and subsequent dilatation of the sleeve by inserting a blunt obturator with a twisting motion [56–58]. The advantages of this system arise from the elimination of sharp trocars [44, 56]. In a number of case series and randomized trials, there were no major vessel injuries and no procedure-related deaths [56]. Randomized controlled trials have demonstrated less postoperative pain and more patient satisfaction with the radially expanding device than with the conventional trocar entry techniques [59–62].

Hasson technique (open laparoscopic entry)

Hasson first described his technique of open access to the peritoneal cavity in 1971 (Table 1) [63]. He suggested that the method might result in less adverse events, such as gas embolism, preperitoneal insufflation, visceral and major vascular injury, and that it thus might be superior to the blinded entry. Thus, it has been recommended for patients with previous abdominal surgery, especially for those with longitudinal abdominal wall incisions.

In their large 2002 meta-analysis on laparoscopic entry techniques, Molloy et al. reported a rate of 0.1% bowel injuries and 0.005% major vascular injuries for the Hasson technique out of a total of 21,547 procedures, with the vast majority of reviewed studies providing only level III evidence [64]. However, several case reports of vascular injuries with the open technique have been published [5, 65, 66].

The Veress needle vs. the Hasson open technique

Many studies have been conducted comparing the safety of the Hasson technique vs. entry using the Veress needle. Hasson himself conducted a review that included 17 publications of open laparoscopy (20,691 patients), comparing them to studies of closed laparoscopy (669,662 patients). This detailed analysis revealed an interesting result: General surgeons had experienced higher complication rates than gynecologists with the closed technique, whereas gynecologists had reported similar complication rates with both techniques [67].

Several other reviews of studies comparing open and closed entry techniques have been published.

Bonjer et al. reviewed 12 trials on laparoscopy in general surgery (6 about the closed and 6 about the open technique, including 489,335 and 12,444 patients, respectively). The rates of visceral and vascular injury were, respectively, 0.08% and 0.07% after closed laparoscopy, and 0.05% and 0% after open laparoscopy (p=0.002). Mortality rates did not differ significantly [68]. Similar findings in general surgery were reported by Sigman et al. [69] and Zaraca et al. [70].

However, other studies did not report any significant differences, in terms of major complication rates, between the Veress needle entry and the Hasson technique. The Swiss Association for Laparoscopic and Thoracoscopic Surgery prospectively collected data on 14,243 low-risk patients undergoing standard laparoscopy between 1995 and 1997. Only eight visceral injuries (0.06%) after primary port insertion were found (six after blind insertion vs. two after a Hasson entry; not significant) [71]. However, in a meta-analysis of a mixed study population including gynecologic and general surgical trials, the risk of bowel injury was higher with open access compared to needle/trocar access (relative risk=2.17). However, the authors noted that selection bias may have influenced the results: open procedures may be more likely chosen for patients with previous abdominal surgery. On the other side, in nonobese patients, a 57% reduced risk of minor complications was seen with open access (relative risk=0.43).

Considering serious adverse events secondary to gas insufflation, open laparoscopy seems superior to the closed entry. The rate of carbon dioxide embolism was 0.001% in a review of 489,335 closed laparoscopies [69]. Several case reports have reported coronary, cerebral, or other gas embolism with fatal or near fatal outcomes [67, 72]. Such complications have not been reported at open laparoscopy.

The evidence does not provide a definitive answer to the question of whether the open technique is superior or inferior to the Veress needle entry. One might also consider other Veress needle insertion sites, such as the Palmer's point, more appropriate than the Hasson entry in high-risk patients with obesity or previous abdominal surgery.

Laparoendoscopic single-site surgery/single-incision laparoscopic surgery

Laparoendoscopic single-site surgery (LESS) is a novel and rapidly advancing minimally invasive technique, developed to result in improved cosmesis for patients and even decreased postoperative analgesia requirements when compared to conventional laparoscopy [73]. The access point for these surgeries is typically the umbilicus [73]. There are various multiaccess single-port systems provided by various manufacturers. The open Hasson entry is used to install these subumbilical access systems. Comparisons between the single-incision approach and conventional multipuncture procedures have demonstrated similar complication rates. However, the sample sizes were too small to draw valid conclusions about the safety profile of LESS in gynecologic studies.

Direct trocar entry

This technique was developed to reduce or avoid various complications related to the Veress needle use, such as a failed pneumoperitoneum, preperitoneal insufflation, intestinal insufflation, or the more serious CO_2 embolism [44]. Moreover, it is faster than any other method of laparoscopic entry [74, 75]. Recently, a large prospective study that included 17,350 patients undergoing gynecologic laparoscopy in China using the "Yan's open technique" was published. Laparoscopic entry was performed by making an umbilical incision with a scalpel followed by direct entry of a 10-mm trocar into the abdominal cavity through direct trocar puncture or insertion of the cannula sheath via the opened umbilicus. As a control group, 4,570 patients were enrolled, who were undergoing the traditional Veress needle entry. The use of the Veress needle was associated with a significantly higher complication rate (0.09% vs. 0.01%) [76].

Several randomized controlled trials, comparing direct trocar access to the Veress needle, have been published, most of them demonstrating lower minor complication rates and/or a shorter entry time. The largest trial (n=1,000) was published by Zakherah, which showed a significantly lower minor complication rate for the direct trocar access (0.4% vs. 14%, p<0.0001) [77]. Agresta et al. compared direct trocar insertion to the Veress needle access in nearly 600 patients. Obesity, major abdominal distension, and two or more previous abdominal operations were the exclusion criteria. There were no minor complications in the direct access group, in contrast to a rate of 5.9% in the Veress needle group (p<0.01) [7]. Similar results concerning the rate of minor complications were reported by Nezhat et al., who excluded past abdominal surgery but took into account BMI, and by Byron et al. [74, 78]. A study by Altun et al. showed higher rates for both major and minor complications in the Veress needle group, which, however, were not significant due to the small sample size [79].

Direct access can also be performed using optical access trocars to achieve visual guidance during direct entry. Only a few randomized trials prospectively evaluated the risk profile of direct optical access and compared it to other entry techniques.

Two trials compared the direct optical access to the Veress needle technique [80, 81]. The first study was performed in postmenopausal women. Estrogen loss at menopause is known to have a profound influence on skin, with postmenopausal atrophy and loss of tone and elasticity. The study demonstrated significantly lower entry time (65.7±11.9 vs. 192.8±5.6 s) and lower overall blood loss in the direct optical access group (9.6±8.1 19.2±7.3 ml) [80]. Similar results were found, in premenopausal women, by the same group of investigators. Direct optical access led to a shorter entry time [81]. When comparing the direct optical access to the Hasson technique, there was lower blood loss (9.6±8.1 vs. 19.2±7.3 ml) and a shorter mean entry time (61.8±10.4 vs. 163.1±9.2 s) [82]. Based on these results, the direct optical access can be considered a feasible and safe alternative for first laparoscopic entry in both pre- and postmenopausal women.

One recent prospective study evaluated direct primary visual entry using the EndoTIP visual cannula (ENDOTIP; Karl Storz) in 165 urologic patients [83]. Access to the peritoneum with the EndoTIP was successful in all consecutive transperitoneal cases. No complications were registered. The method seems feasible and safe in a gynecologic patient collective. Direct optical access has also been mentioned as a possible future entry technique at Palmer's point when adhesions are suspected [84].

Study weaknesses

Several study weaknesses have to be considered when drawing conclusions from the reported results. First and foremost, surgeons might be experienced in either one of the techniques—this issue has not been properly assessed in most of the studies. Thus, learning curves must be taken into account when surgeons are recommended to start using a technique that has been considered superior in studies. The existence of learning curves for laparoscopic entry techniques has already been proven, and the incidence of related complications is higher among inexperienced surgeons. Surgeons might experience fewer adverse events if they use the technique with which they are most familiar [85–87]. This might also be considered when recommending alternative Veress needle entry sites in obese patients or women with previous abdominal surgery. The use of alternative Veress insertion sites by gynecologists is limited as is the literature on this issue.

Furthermore, only very few studies have evaluated the safety profile of alternative entry techniques including the optical Veress needle and the radially expanding access system. Thus, the incidences of rare but possibly life-threatening complications can hardly be assessed for these procedures. The same is true for direct trocar access. However, more prospective randomized studies will hopefully be published in the near future providing a reliable overview on the technique's safety profile. Whether LESS procedures might be widely accepted will depend on other outcome parameters than just an improved cosmesis: reduced pain, perioperative morbidity, and convalescence could justify both the increased technical demands and the increased costs [85].

Literature on cosmetic considerations is also scarce. To the best of our knowledge, only one study has directly addressed this issue. This trial dealt with the general population's view on the aesthetic importance of the umbilicus with regard to single-incision techniques [88]. From that point of view, one might consider direct trocar entry using 5-mm trocars superior to the Hasson technique. Keeping in mind that most of the entry techniques are similar in terms of major complication rates, future research might also want to focus on the cosmetic aspects of these techniques.

Conclusions

All in all, there is no solid evidence proving the superiority of any method of laparoscopic entry. In general, the guidelines set forth by the Society of Obstetricians and Gynecoogists of Canada in 2007 [44] remain valid. Among other recommendations, we chose to underline the following: in gynecologic procedures, there is no evidence that the Hasson technique is superior to the Veress needle entry. When entering the abdomen using the Veress needle, an intraperitoneal pressure <10 mmHg is a reliable predictor of correct intraperitoneal placement. Entry at the Palmer's point (LUQ laparoscopy) is recommended in patients with suspected or known periumbilical adhesions or a history or presence of umbilical hernia, or after three failed insufflation attempts at the umbilicus.

However, recently published trials suggest that direct trocar entry, especially when using optical trocar systems, might be superior to both the Hasson open technique and the Veress needle entry in terms of avoiding extraperitoneal insufflation and failed entry. Moreover, blood loss can be reduced and the mean entry time shortened.

Much work has been done in order to make laparoscopy a safe procedure. However, further investigation is needed in order to shed some new light into the "hot topics" of laparoscopic entry. Will there be hard evidence for a certain technique on how to deal with obese patients or suspected anterior wall adhesions? Will any new strategies be developed in order to avoid major complications, such as major vessel or bowel injury? Hopefully, researchers will be able to clarify these and other concerns in the future. Notably, cosmetic results have not been considered in the literature as yet and might also be a focus of interest in the near future for the older Veress needle and the Hasson entry techniques.

Declaration of interest The authors report no conflicts of interest. The authors alone are responsible for the content and writing of the paper.

References

1. Makai G, Isaacson K (2009) Complications of gynecologic laparoscopy. Clin Obstet Gynecol 52:401–411
2. Garry R (1999) Towards evidence based laparoscopic entry techniques: clinical problems and dilemmas. Gynaecol Endosc 8:315–326
3. Jansen FW, Kolkman W, Bakkum EA, de Kroon CD, Trimbos-Kemper TC, Trimbos JB (2004) Complications of laparoscopy: an inquiry about closed- versus open-entry technique. Am J Obstet Gynecol 190:634–638
4. Varma R, Gupta JK (2008) Laparoscopic entry techniques: clinical guideline, national survey, and medicolegal ramifications. Surg Endosc 22:2686–2697
5. Chandler JG, Corson SL, Way LW (2001) Three spectra of laparoscopic entry access injury. J Am Coll Surg 192:478–491
6. Tinelli A, Malvasi A, Schneider AJ, Keckstein J, Hudelist G, Barbic M, Casciaro S, Giorda G, Tinelli R, Perrone A, Tinelli FG (2006) First abdominal access in gynaecological laparoscopy: which method to utilize? Minerva Ginecol 58:429–440
7. Agresta F, De Simone P, Ciardo LF, Bedin N (2004) Direct trocar insertion vs Veress needle in nonobese patients undergoing laparoscopic procedures: a randomized prospective single-center study. Surg Endosc 18:1778–1781
8. Merlin TL, Hiller JE, Maddern GJ, Jamieson GG, Brown AR, Kolbe A (2003) Systematic review of the safety and effectiveness of methods used to establish pneumoperitoneum in laparoscopic surgery. Br J Surg 90:668–679

9. Ahmad G, Duffy JM, Phillips K, Watson A (2008) Laparoscopic entry techniques. Cochrane Database Syst Rev 16(2):CD006583
10. Sepilian V, Ku L, Wong H, Liu CY, Phelps JY (2007) Prevalence of infraumbilical adhesions in women with previous laparoscopy. JSLS 11:41–44
11. Vilos AG, Vilos GA, Abu-Rafea B, Hollett-Caines J, Al-Omran M (2006) Effect of body habitus and parity on the initial Veres intraperitoneal CO_2 insufflation pressure during laparoscopic access in women. J Minim Invasive Gynecol 13:108–113
12. Audebert AJ, Gomel V (2000) Role of microlaparoscopy in the diagnosis of peritoneal and visceral adhesions and in the prevention of bowel injury associated with blind trocar insertion. Fertil Steril 73:63163–63165
13. Hurd WW, Bude RO, DeLancey JO, Pearl ML (1992) The relationship of the umbilicus to the aortic bifurcation: implications for laparoscopic technique. Obstet Gynecol 80:48–51
14. Nezhat F, Brill AI, Nezhat CH, Nezhat A, Seidman DS, Nezhat C (1998) Laparoscopic appraisal of the anatomic relationship of the umbilicus to the aortic bifurcation. J Am Assoc Gynecol Laparosc 5:135–140
15. Hurd WW, Bude RD, De Lancey JOL, Gavin JM, Aisen AM (1991) Abdominal wall characterization with magnetic resonance imaging and computed tomography: the effect of obesity in the laparoscopic approach. J Reprod Med 26:473–476
16. McIlwaine K, Cameron M, Readman E, Manwaring J, Maher P (2011) The effect of patient body mass index on surgical difficulty in gynaecological laparoscopy. Gynaecol Surg 8:145–149
17. Azevedo JL, Azevedo OC, Miyahira SA, Miguel GP, Becker OM Jr, Hypólito OH, Machado AC, Cardia W, Yamaguchi GA, Godinho L, Freire D, Almeida CE, Moreira CH, Freire DF (2009) Injuries caused by Veress needle insertion for creation of pneumoperitoneum: a systematic literature review. Surg Endosc 23:1428–1432
18. Perissat J, Vitale GC (1991) Laparoscopic cholecystectomy: gateway to the future. Am J Surg 161:408
19. Granata M, Tsimpanakos I, Moeity F, Magos A (2010) Are we underutilizing Palmer's point entry in gynecologic laparoscopy? Fertil Steril 94:2716–2719
20. Palmer R (1974) Safety in laparoscopy. J Reprod Med 13:1–5
21. Tulikangas PK, Nicklas A, Falcone T, Price LL (2000) Anatomy of the left upper quadrant for cannula insertion. J Am Assoc Gynecol Laparosc 7:211–214
22. Tulikangas PK, Robinson DS, Falcone T (2003) Left upper quadrant cannula insertion. Fertil Steril 79:411–412
23. McDanald DM, Levine RL, Pasic R (2005) Left upper quadrant entry during gynecologic laparoscopy. Surg Laparosc Endosc Percutan Tech 15:325–327
24. Agarwala N, Liu CY (2005) Safe entry technique during laparoscopy: left upper quadrant entry using the ninth intercostal space: a review of 918 procedures. J Minim Invasive Gynecol 12:55–61
25. Sanders RR, Filshie GM (1994) Transfundal induction of pneumoperitoneum prior to laparoscopy. J Obstet Gynaecol Br Cmwlth 107:316–317
26. Morgan HR (1979) Laparoscopy: induction of pneumoperitoneum via transfundal puncture. Obstet Gynecol 54:260–261
27. Wolfe WM, Pasic R (1990) Transuterine insertion of Veress needle in laparoscopy. Obstet Gynecol 75:456–557
28. Trivedi AN, MacLean NE (1994) Transuterine insertion of Veress needle for gynecological laparoscopy at Southland Hospital. NZ Med J 107:316–317
29. Pasic R, Levine RL, Wolfe WM Jr (1999) Laparoscopy in morbidly obese patients. J Am Assoc Gynecol 6:307–312
30. Santala M, Jarvela I, Kauppila A (1999) Transfundal insertion of a Veress needle in laparoscopy of obese subjects: a practical alternative. Hum Reprod 14:2277–2278
31. Neely MR, McWilliams R, Makhlouf HA (1975) Laparoscopy: routine pneumoperitoneum via the posterior fornix. Obstet Gynecol 45:459–460
32. van Lith DA, van Schie KJ, Beekhuizen W, du Plessis M (1980) Cul-de-sac insufflation: an easy alternative route for safely inducing pneumoperitoneum. Int J Gynaecol Obstet 17:375–378
33. Fear RE (1968) Laparoscopy: a valuable aid in gynecologic diagnosis. Obstet Gynecol 31:297–309
34. Lacey CG (1976) Laparoscopy: a clinical sign for intraperitoneal needle placement. Obstet Gynecol 47:625–627
35. Rosen DM, Lam AM, Chapman M, Carlton M, Cario GM (1998) Methods of creating pneumoperitoneum: a review of techniques and complications. Obstet Gynecol Surv 53:167–174
36. Brill AJ, Cohen BM (2003) Fundamentals of peritoneal access. J Am Assoc Gynecol Laparosc 10:287–297
37. Marret H, Harchaoui Y, Chapron C, Lansac J, Pierre F (1998) Trocar injuries during laparoscopic gynaecological surgery. Report from the French Society of Gynecological Laparoscopy. Gynaecol Endosc 7:235–241
38. Semm K, Semm I (1999) Safe insertion of trocars and Veress needle using standard equipment and the 11 security steps. Gynaecol Endosc 8:339–347
39. Yoong W, Saxena S, Mittal M, Stavoulis A, Ogbodo E, Damodaram M (2010) The pressure profile test is more sensitive and specific than Palmer's test in predicting correct placement of the Veress needle. Eur J Obstet Gynecol Reprod Biol 152:210–213
40. Teoh B, Sen R, Abbott J (2005) An evaluation of four tests used to ascertain Veress needle placement at closed laparoscopy. J Minim Invasive Gynecol 12:153–158
41. Roy GM, Bazzurini L, Solima E, Luciano AA (2001) Safe technique for laparoscopic entry into the abdominal cavity. J Am Assoc Gynecol Laparosc 8:519–528
42. Hill DJ, Maher PJ (1996) Direct cannula entry for laparoscopy. J Am Assoc Gynecol Laparosc 4:77–79
43. Richardson RF, Sutton CJG (1999) Complications of first entry: a prospective laparoscopic audit. Gynaecol Endosc 8:327–334
44. Vilos GA, Ternamian A, Dempster J, Laberge PY, The Society of Obstetricians and Gynaecologists of Canada (2007) Laparoscopic entry: a review of techniques, technologies, and complications. J Obstet Gynaecol Can 29:433–465
45. Schaller G, Kuenkel M, Manegold BC (1995) The optical Veress needle—initial puncture with a minioptic. Endosc Surg Allied Technol 3:55–57
46. Janicki TI (1994) The new sensor-equipped Veress needle. J Am Assoc Gynecol Laparosc 1:154–156
47. Phillips G, Garry R, Kumar C, Reich H (1999) How much gas is required for initial insufflation at laparoscopy? Gynaecol Endosc 8:369–374
48. Abu-Rafea B, Vilos GA, Vilos AG, Ahmad R, Hollett-Caines J (2005) High pressure laparoscopic entry does not adversely affect cardiopulmonary function in healthy women. J Minin Invasive Gynecol 12:475–479
49. Champault G, Cazacu F, Taffinder N (1996) Serious trocar accidents in laparoscopic surgery: a French survey of 103,852 operations. Surg Laparosc Endosc 6:367–370
50. Saville LE, Woods MS (1995) Laparoscopy and major retroperitoneal vascular injuries (MRVI). Surg Endosc 9:1096–1100
51. McKernan J, Finley C (2002) Experience with optical trocar in performing laparoscopic procedures. Surg Laparosc Endosc 12:96–99
52. Angelini L, Lirici M, Papaspyropoulos V, Sossi F (1997) Combination of subcutaneous abdominal wall retraction and optical trocar to minimize pneumoperitoneum-related effects and needle and trocar injuries in laparoscopic surgery. Surg Endosc 11:1006–1009

53. Visiport Optical Trocar information booklet (Internet). Norwalk CY: AutoSuture. http://www.autosuture.com/AutoSuture/pagebuilder.aspx?contentID=39263&topicID=31737&breadcrumbs=0:63659,30780:0,65365:0#. Accessed 4 April 2007
54. Jirecek S, Dräger M, Leitich H, Nagele F, Wenzl R (2002) Direct visual or blind insertion of the primary trocar. Surg Endosc 16:626–629
55. Ternamian AM (2001) How to impove laparoscopic access safety: ENDOTIP. Min Invasive Ther Allied Technol 10:31–39
56. Turner DJ (1999) Making the case for the radially expanding access system. Gynaecol Endosc 8:391–395
57. Bhoyrul S, Mori T, Way LW (1995) A safer cannula design for laparoscopic surgery: results of a comparative study. Surg Endosc 9:227–229
58. Turner DJ (1996) A new radially expanding access system for laparoscopic procedures versus conventional cannulas. J Am Assoc Gynecol Laparosc 3:609–615
59. Yim SF, Yuen PM (2001) Randomized double-masked comparison of radially expanding access device and conventional cutting tip trocar in laparoscopy. Obstet Gynecol 97:435–438
60. Lam TY, Lee SW, So HS, Kwok SP (2000) Radially expanding trocars: a less painful alternative for laparoscopic surgery. J Laparoendosc Adv Surg Tech A 19:269–273
61. Bhoyrul S, Payne J, Steffes B, Swanstrom L, Way LW (2000) A randomized prospective study of radially expanding trocars in laparoscopic surgery. J Gastrointest Surg 4:392–397
62. Feste JR, Bojahr B, Turner DJ (2000) Randomized trial comparing a radially expandable needle system with cutting trocars. J Soc Laparosc Endosc Surg 4:11–15
63. Hasson HM (1971) A modified instrument and method for laparoscopy. Am J Obstet Gynecol 110:886–887
64. Molloy D, Kalloo PD, Cooper M, Nguyen TV (2002) Laparoscopic entry: a literature review and analysis of techniques and complications of primary port entry. Aust N Z J Obstet Gynaecol 42:246–254
65. Vilos GA (2000) Litigation of laparoscopic major vessel injuries in Canada. J Am Assoc Gynecol Laparosc 7:503–509
66. Hanney RM, Carmalt HL, Merrett N, Tait N (1999) Use of the Hasson cannula producing major vascular injury at laparoscopy. Surg Endosc 13:1238–1240
67. Hasson HM (1999) Open laparoscopy as a method of access in laparoscopic surgery. Gynaecol Endosc 8:353–362
68. Bonjer HJ, Hazebroek EJ, Kazemier G, Giuffrida MC, Meijer WS, Lange JF (1997) Open versus closed establishment of pneumoperitoneum in laparoscopic surgery. Br J Surg 84:599–602
69. Sigman HH, Fried GM, Garzon J, Hinchey EJ, Wexler MJ, Meakins JL (1993) Risks of blind versus open approach to celiotomy for laparoscopic surgery. Surg Laparosc Endosc 3:296–299
70. Zaraca F, Catarci M, Gosselti F, Mulieri G, Carboni M (1999) Routine use of open laparoscopy: 1,006 consecutive cases. J Laparoendosc Adv Surg Tech A 9:75–80
71. Schafer M, Lauper M, Krahenbuhl L (2001) Trocar and Veress needle injuries during laparoscopy. Surg Endosc 15:275–280
72. Neudecker J, Sauerland S, Nengebauer F, Bergamaschi R, Bonjer HJ, Cuschieri A (2002) The European Association for Surgery Clinical Practice Guideline on the pneumoperitoneum for laparoscopic surgery. Surg Endosc 16:1121–1143
73. Fader AN, Cohen S, Escobar PF, Gunderson C (2010) Laparoendoscopic single-site surgery in gynecology. Curr Opin Obstet Gynecol 22:331–338
74. Byron JW, Markenson G, Miyazawa K (1993) A randomized comparison of Veress needle and direct trocar insertion for laparoscopy. Surg Gynecol Obstet 177:259–262
75. Borgatta L, Gruss L, Barad D, Kaali SG (1990) Direct trocar insertion vs Veress needle use for laparoscopic sterilization. J Reprod Med 35:891–894
76. Liu HF, Chen X, Liu Y (2009) A multi-center study of a modified open trocar first-puncture approach in 17 350 patients for laparoscopic entry. Chin Med J (Engl) 122:2733–2736
77. Zakherah MS (2010) Direct trocar versus Veress needle entry for laparoscopy: a randomized clinical trial. Gynecol Obstet Invest 69:260–263
78. Nezhat FR, Silfen SL, Evans D, Nezhat C (1991) Comparison of direct insertion of disposable and standard reusable laparoscopic trocars and previous pneumoperitoneum with Veress needle. Obstet Gynecol 78:148–150
79. Altun H, Banli O, Kavlakoglu B, Kücükkayikci B, Kelesoglu C, Erez N (2007) Comparison between direct trocar and Veress needle insertion in laparoscopic cholecystectomy. J Laparoendosc Adv Surg Tech A 17:709–712
80. Tinelli A, Malvasi A, Guido M, Istre O, Keckstein J, Mettler L (2009) Initial laparoscopic access in postmenopausal women: a preliminary prospective study. Menopause 16:966–970
81. Tinelli A, Malvasi A, Istre O, Keckstein J, Stark M, Mettler L (2010) Abdominal access in gynaecological laparoscopy: a comparison between direct optical and blind closed access by Verres needle. Eur J Obstet Gynecol Reprod Biol 148:191–194
82. Tinelli A, Malvasi A, Hudelist G, Istre O, Keckstein J (2009) Abdominal access in gynaecologic laparoscopy: a comparison between direct optical and open access. J Laparoendosc Adv Surg Tech A 19:529–533
83. Hickey L, Rendon RA (2006) Safe and novel technique for peritoneal access in urologic laparoscopy without prior insufflation. J Endourol 20:622–626
84. Aust TR, Kayani SI, Rowlands DJ (2010) Direct optical entry through Palmer's point: a new technique for those at risk of entry-related trauma at laparoscopy. Gynaecol Surg 7:315–317
85. Fader AN, Rojas-Espaillat L, Ibeanu O, Grumbine FC, Escobar PF (2010) Laparoendoscopic single-site surgery (LESS) in gynecology: a multi-institutional evaluation. Am J Obstet Gynecol 203:501.e1–501.e6
86. Lalchandi S, Phillips K (2005) Laparoscopic entry technique—a survey of practices of consultant gynaecologists. Gynaecol Surg 2:245–249
87. Burke C, Nathan E, Karthigasu K, Garry R, Hart R (2009) Laparoscopic entry—the experience of a range of gynaecological surgeons. Gynaecol Surg 6:125–133
88. Iranmanesh P, Morel P, Inan I, Hagen M (2011) Choosing the cosmetically superior laparoscopic access to the abdomen: the importance of the umbilicus. Surg Endosc 25(8):2578–2585
89. Veress J (1961) A needle for the safe use of pheumoperitoneum. Gastroenterologia 96:150–152
90. Copeland C, Wing R, Hulka JF (1983) Direct trocar insertion at laparoscopy: an evaluation. Obstet Gynecol 62:655–659

6

Mini-laparotomy in advanced ovarian cancer

S. Sircar · G. J. Robson · J. A. Davis · J. K. Kennedy · F. Alexander-Sefre

Abstract Optimal cytoreduction (OCR) remains the gold standard treatment of ovarian cancer. Current radiological imaging has limited sensitivity and specificity in prediction of achieving OCR prior to surgery. This prospective pilot study included 50 patients with advanced ovarian carcinoma. Prior to the main laparotomy, a mini-laparotomy—just large enough to allow a hand in—was performed. A decision was then made as to whether achieving OCR is "possible", "not possible" or lastly "unsure". Formal laparotomy then followed. At the end of the formal laparotomy, cytoreduction was regarded as either "optimal" or "suboptimal" based on residual disease. Out of 45 cases where results were deemed suitable for analysis, 27 were regarded as "OCR possible", out of which OCR was achieved in 24 cases following full laparotomy. Ten were commented upon as "unsure" and only in three cases OCR was feasible. Eight were classed as "OCR not possible" and in none of these OCR was obtained. The only noted complication associated with mini-laparotomy was bleeding in just three cases (6%). The sensitivity, specificity, PPV and NPV of mini-laparotomy were 100%, 73%, 89% and 100%, respectively. However, when "unsure", only in 30% OCR was achieved. We concluded that mini-laparotomy is a safe, simple and effective technique for predicting feasibility of OCR. This simple technique could obviate the need for full laparotomy in patients who may benefit from neo-adjuvant chemotherapy.

S. Sircar · G. J. Robson · J. A. Davis · J. K. Kennedy · F. Alexander-Sefre
Department of Gynaecological Oncology,
Glasgow Royal Infirmary,
Glasgow G4 0SF Scotland, UK

F. Alexander-Sefre (✉)
Ward 56B, Glasgow Royal Infirmary,
Castle Street,
Glasgow G4 0SF Scotland, UK
e-mail: f.alexander.sefre@ggc.scot.nhs.uk

Keywords Mini-laparotomy · Optimal · Resectability · Advanced ovarian malignancy · Ovarian cancer

Background

Ovarian cancer is the most common gynaecological malignancy in the United Kingdom with nearly 7,000 reported cases per year [1]. The mainstay of treatment remains cytoreductive surgery followed by adjuvant chemotherapy. Most patients present with omental and peritoneal metastasis, hence making complete surgical resection a challenge [2]. Overall survival greatly depends on the possibility of resecting most of the diseased areas with little residual disease (optimal cytoreduction [OCR]). In early stages (I and II), when the disease is confined to the pelvis, the overall survival exceeds 70% whilst in advanced stages (III and IV) the 5-year survival is less than 40% [3]. In Scotland alone, there are over 600 reported cases per annum, of which over 400 succumb to the disease, hence an overall reported survival of 30% [4].

Achievement of OCR is the single most important factor for survival in patients with ovarian cancer [5]. Currently the preoperative selection of patients for primary surgery is mainly based on detailed imaging [6, 7]. The commonest imaging modality is computer tomography (CT) in most centres. CT accuracy varies greatly in assessment of resectability and prediction of OCR in advanced stage ovarian cancer [8]. Other preoperative assessment methods such as laparoscopy have not as yet been established in most centres.

This pilot study aims to evaluate the role of mini-laparotomy as an alternative or complementary (to CT imaging) means of determining tumour resectability and the chances of achieving OCR in advanced stage ovarian cancer.

Methods

A total of 50 consecutive patients with stage III/IV ovarian cancer were included in this prospective study. The study was conducted in the department of gynaecological oncology at Glasgow Royal Infirmary, over a period of 18 months. They had all undergone CT imaging and clinical examination by the three gynaecological oncologists who performed the operations (FAS, JD and JK). Their CT images were reviewed in our regular multidisciplinary team meetings (MDT), involving our lead radiologist and all the above operating surgeons. Following this review, only selected patients in whom OCR was deemed possible on CT imaging were then admitted for surgery. All subjects had also been previously examined and were regarded as fit and potentially suitable for up-front surgical intervention. These were therefore regarded as the inclusion criteria. Patients with advanced metastatic stage (stage IV), unfit or in cases OCR was deemed unfeasible, were excluded from the study.

Data gathering and documentation were pro-forma based, recording the operative findings from both mini-laparotomy and formal laparotomy. The details of mini-laparotomy included the site, length of mini-laparotomy incision, time taken to enter the peritoneal cavity, time taken to finish the procedure and any operative or post operative complication.

Prior to operation, an examination under anaesthesia was performed in all of the cases. A mini-laparotomy incision was made through a midline incision. The incision was sited below, over or above the umbilicus, depending on where the surgeon deemed it most appropriate for full intra-abdominal assessment. The length of the incision was kept to the minimum, allowing only the insertion of one hand after some negotiation. This length usually corresponded to the surgeon's glove size or width of the palm at metacarpophalangeal joint (Fig. 1). To keep the incision length to the minimum, the surgeon placed his hand over the preferred site of incision and marked either side of his knuckles with a marker pen. The length between the two marked points was measured prior to incision and starting time noted.

The palpation findings were charted as main tumour mass, other pelvic and abdominal organs, peritoneal and omental disease. This was followed by visual inspection, usually using a Morris retractor to allow lifting of the anterior abdominal wall. The time taken to enter abdomen, and to complete both palpation and inspection was recorded.

The criteria for OCR were regarded as residual tumour less than 2 cm in volume. This criteria still remains an acceptable standard in most UK centres. Following inspection and palpation through the mini-laparotomy, the surgeon's impression of achieving OCR was recorded as "possible" (meaning that it may be possible to reduce the volume of disease to less than 2 cm), "not possible" or "unsure". The impression was mainly based on palpation findings, as the visual inspection in most cases was limited.

Formal laparotomy was then carried out by the same operator, extending the mini-laparotomy incision, both caudally and cranially. On completion of the surgery, the operating surgeon documented whether "optimal" or "suboptimal" cytoreduction had been achieved.

Findings and analysis

Data was collected for a total of 50 consecutive patients with suspected stage III/IV ovarian cancer, over a span of 18 months. Data from five cases was regarded as either

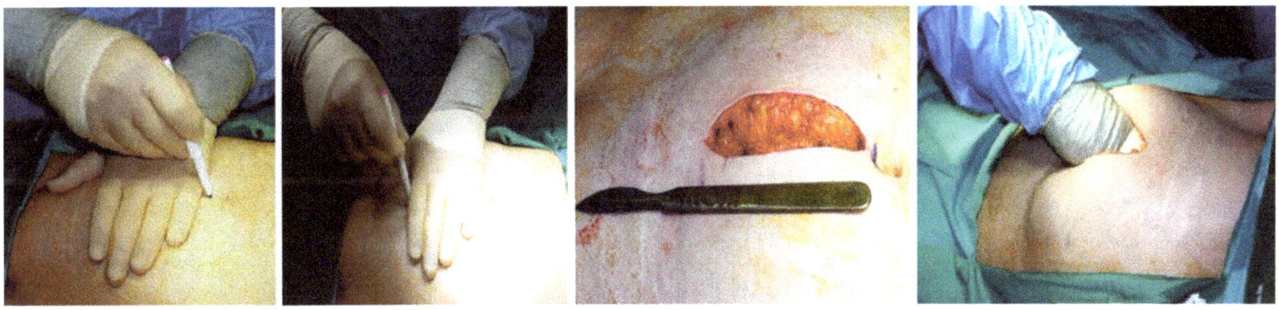

a b c d

Fig. 1 The steps involved in minilaparotomy: demarcation of a suitable midline site and length corresponding to the width of the palm at meta-carpo-phalygeal joint (**a** and **b**), formation of minilaparotomy was limited to the site marked (**c**), systemic intraabdominal palpation, examination and assessment of resectability (**d**)

inadequate or retrospective and hence excluded. Hence results from 45 cases were analysed. The median age of the patients was 64 years (mean 62.5 years, range 34–80, SD 11.71). The median BMI was 29.1 kg/m^2 (mean 29.9 kg/m^2, range 18.7–67.5, SD 7.55). The median abdominal girth was 95 cm (mean 95.87 cm, range 42–148, SD 16.79). Fifteen patients (33%) had previously undergone abdominal surgery for various gynaecological and non gynaecological reasons. Based on clinical and radiological imaging, stage III disease was suspected in thirty eight (84.44%) and stage IV in seven cases (5.56%). The majority of these patients (n=40, 89%) underwent upfront surgery prior to adjuvant chemotherapy. Only five patients had received neo-adjuvant chemotherapy (11%) prior to their delayed primary surgery.

The median length of the mini-laparotomy incision was 9 cm (mean 8.59 cm, range 5–12, SD 1.16). The median time to enter the peritoneal cavity, starting from knife to skin, was 4 min (mean 5.10 min, range 1–15, SD 3.04) while the median time taken to complete the palpation and visual exploration was 6.5 min (mean 7.52 min, range 2–30, SD 4.83).The total median time for making the incision and completion of examinations was 10 min (with mean of 12.62 min, range 5–45, SD 7.23).

Satisfactory palpation of pelvis and upper abdomen, through the mini-laparotomy incision, was proven to be possible in all cases (100%) but visual inspection was limited, particularly for upper abdominal organs.

Following formation of mini-laparotomy, 27 out of the 45 cases were deemed optimally cyto-reducible or "OCR possible". From this "possible" group, OCR was achieved in 24 cases. In eight cases, OCR was regarded as "not possible" and in none of these cases was OCR achieved. In the remaining ten patients, the surgeon was "unsure" and in only three of these cases was OCR achieved (Table 1).

The specificity of mini-laparotomy to predict OCR was noted to be 73% and sensitivity was 100%. Positive predictive value (PPV) of mini-laparotomy in assessment of OCR was calculated to be 89% and negative predicative value (NPV) of 100%.

In three cases, OCR was not possible despite initial assessment through mini-laparotomy. In one patient, part of ovarian capsule could not be fully resected away from pelvic side wall. In the second case, failure to achieve OCR was due to tumour plaques in Pouch of Douglas (POD) and over rectum. The third patient had previous total abdominal hysterectomy and residual tumour plaques could not be fully resected from vaginal vault and bladder base.

Out of ten cases commented as "unsure" at mini-laparotomy, in only three cases (30%) was OCR achieved at laparotomy. Each of these three cases required radical surgery, including bowel resection in two patients.

In eight cases OCR was regarded as not possible after mini-laparotomy examinations and in none of these was OCR achieved after full laparotomy. In four of these patients (50%) the main reason was fixed central pelvic mass densely adherent to the adjacent pelvic and abdominal structures. In the other four patients (50%), extensive upper abdominal disease involving diaphragmatic surfaces, spleen, stomach and porta hepatis were the main reasons precluding OCR. In addition to the above eight cases, there were ten patients that OCR was not achieved (3 falsely predicted as "OCR possible" and in seven cases the operator was "unsure"). This was due to following reasons: fixed and densely adherent pelvic mass, extensive supracolic omental mass, significant peritoneal disease and involvement of upper abdominal organs.

There were no complications associated with mini-laparotomy. However, excess bleeding according to the surgeon's judgment was reported in three cases (6%). The bleeding in all three cases was noted to be from central tumour mass that was adherent to the peritoneum over the site of mini-laparotomy incision.

Discussion

OCR remains the gold standard treatment for all stages of ovarian cancer. In advanced ovarian malignancy, achievement of OCR has been shown to have a direct impact on patient's disease-free interval and overall survival [9–11]. The definition of OCR has greatly changed over the years: from residual disease of less than 2 cm to resection or ablation of all macroscopic disease in recent years [12]. However, in most UK centres, a residual disease of less than 2 cm remains an acceptable goal. Currently the mainstay of preoperative assessment of such patients with regards to resectability and likelihood of achieving OCR are based on clinical examinations, tumour marker levels and CT findings [8–11, 13–16]. It is also common practice in UK to administer neo-adjuvant chemotherapy prior to

Table 1 Comparison of outcome of mini-laparotomy and laparotomy

	OCR achieved after full laparotomy	OCR not achieved after full laparotomy	Total
OCR predicted possible on mini-laparotomy	24 (true positive)	3 (false positive)	27
OCR predicted not possible on mini-laparotomy	0 (false negative)	8 (true negative)	8
Unsure following mini-laparotomy	3	7	10

delayed primary surgery in patients that OCR may not appear feasible on initial assessment.

Current preoperative assessments have limited predictability in selection of patients suitable for OCR. The sensitivity of CT in identifying patients that OCR can be achieved is around 60–70%, with varying reported specificity between 70% and 100% [17, 18]. The main drawbacks of CT imaging is the inability to reliably assess the extent of disease in the supra colic compartment, porta hepatis, miliary disease over bowel mesentery and peritoneum, especially in absence of ascites [8–11, 19].

In order to overcome the limitations associated with CT, a few centres routinely perform laparoscopic staging in all their ovarian cancer patients prior to formal laparotomy. This modality of assessment, in experienced hands, has been shown to have PPV of 87% and NPV of 100% [20–22]. However, laparoscopic assessment requires an experienced surgical team and laparoscopic resources. In addition, it is associated with increased theatre time and possible increased morbidity. Furthermore, there are reported technical difficulties with the laparoscopic procedure, particularly when intra abdominal adhesions are present in advanced stage disease [23–26]. More importantly, there is a lack of tactile sensation which is of great importance in assessment of resectability and achievement of OCR [27–29]. We believe such shortcomings can be avoided by using a simple mini-laparotomy as described in this paper. Furthermore, time required to perform mini-laparotomy would be much less than laparoscopic method due to its simplicity and greater familiarity with the technique. There is no need for a learning curve in mini-laparotomy unlike laparoscopic techniques and is clearly more cost effective.

In our group of patients, all 45 patients were regarded as suitable candidates for OCR following MDT review. However, OCR was achieved in only 27 out of the 45 patients (60%). This finding is consistent with reported suboptimal CT accuracy in predicting OCR in the literature [30]. In contrast, following intra-abdominal palpation through mini-laparotomy, the accuracy for predicting OCR was much higher at 89% (24 of 27cases). More importantly, OCR was not achieved in any of the eight patients where it was predicted that OCR would not be possible at mini-laparotomy, reflecting an NPV of 100%. This has great clinical importance in avoiding unnecessary major laparotomy. In addition, considering small size and lack of morbidity associated with mini-laparotomy, it should result in much quicker recovery and hence shorten delay in receiving neo-adjuvant chemotherapy.

We acknowledge the principle shortcoming of the study to be the small sample size, hence potential for type II statistical error. However, despite this limitation, we believe the findings to be of clinical importance.

In mini-laparotomy, one could encounter a degree of visual and tactile restriction as compared with abdominal and pelvic assessment following full laparotomy. This may explain the reason why in nearly 20% of cases the operating surgeon was unsure of ability to obtain OCR. However, it is of interest to note that in this group of patients OCR was only achieved in 30%. One therefore could conclude that mini-laparotomy may also help surgeon in making a balanced decision, as to proceed or not in the "unsure" group of patients.

In order to overcome the visual limitation of mini-laparotomy, one may consider a combination of the techniques of laparoscopy and mini-laparotomy, better known as hand-assisted laparoscopy. However such technique will be inevitably associated with increased theatre time and operative complexity. In future, it is anticipated that integrated FDG-PET/CT may have a role in assessment of disease spread and decision with regards to best therapeutic strategy in ovarian cancer. FDG-PET/CT has been shown to have a higher sensitivity (91%) than PET, CT or MRI in assessment of disease spread [31, 32]. Hence, it may further assist in early identification of patients who are not suitable for up front surgery.

Conclusions

Despite our small sample size, this study has shown mini-laparotomy to be a safe, simple and effective technique in assessment of tumour resectability and chances of obtaining OCR. More importantly it is very accurate in identifying patients unsuitable for primary cytoreduction. By avoiding an unnecessary full laparotomy, patients' recovery will be expedited and chemotherapy could be initiated earlier.

Conflicts of interest The authors report no conflicts of interest. The authors alone are responsible for the content and writing of the paper.

References

1. Information Services Division, NHS National Services Scotland: Cancer in Scotland. Sept 2008, page 4
2. Junor EJ, Hole DJ, McNulty L, Mason M, Young J (1999) Specialist gynaecologists and survival outcome in ovarian cancer: a Scottish national study of 1866 patients. Br J Obstet Gynaecol 106:1130–1136
3. Kristensen GB, Trope C (1997) Epithelial ovarian carcinoma. Lancet 349:113–117
4. Information Services Division, NHS National Services Scotland: Cancer in Scotland. Sept 2008, p 13
5. Hunter RW, Alexander NDE, Soutter WP (1992) Meta-analysis of surgery in advanced ovarian carcinoma: is maximum cytoreductive surgery an independent determinant of prognosis? Am J Obstet Gynecol 166:504–511

6. Hoskins WJ, Bundy BN, Thigpen JT et al (1992) The influence of cytoreductive surgery on recurrence-free interval and survival in small-volume stage III epithelial ovarian cancer: a Gynecologic Oncology Group study. Gynecol Oncol 47:159–166
7. Allen DG, Heintz AP, Touw FW (1995) A meta-analysis of residual disease and survival in stage III and IV carcinoma of the ovary. Eur J Gynaecol Oncol 16(5):349–356
8. Hacker NF, Berek JS, Lagasse LD, Nieberg RK, Elashoff RM (1983) Primary cytoreductive surgery for epithelial ovarian cancer. Obstet Gynecol 61:413–420
9. Hogberg T (1995) Primary surgery in ovarian cancer: current opinions. Ann Med 27:95–100
10. Voest EE, van Houwelingen JC, Neijt JP (1989) A meta-analysis of prognostic factors in advanced ovarian cancer with median survival and overall survival (measured with the log [relative risk]) as main objectives. Eur J Cancer Clin Oncol 25:711–720
11. Chen SS, Bochner R (1985) Assessment of morbidity and mortality in primary cytoreductive surgery for advanced ovarian carcinoma. Gynecol Oncol 20:190–195
12. Winter WE, Maxwell GL, Tian C et al (2007) Prognostic factors for stage III epithelial ovarian cancer: a Gynecologic Oncology Group Study. J Clin Oncol 25:3621–3627
13. Bristow RE, Duska LR, Lambrou NC, Fishman EK, O'Neill MJ, Trimble EL, Montz FJ (2000) A model for predicting surgical outcome in patients with advanced ovarian carcinoma using computed tomography. Cancer 89:1532–1540
14. Nelson B, Rosenfeld AT, Schwartz PE (1993) Preoperative abdominopelvic computed tomographic prediction of optimal cytoreduction in epithelial ovarian carcinoma. J Clin Oncol 11:166–172
15. Forstner R, Hricak H, Occhipinti KA, Powell CB, Frankel SD, Stern JL (1995) Ovarian cancer: staging with CT and MR imaging. Radiology 197:619–626
16. Sanders RC, McNeil BJ, Finberg HJ et al (1983) A prospective study of computed tomography and ultrasound in the detection and staging of pelvic masses. Radiology 146:439–442
17. Kurtz AB, Tsimikas JV, Tempany CM et al (1999) Diagnosis and staging of ovarian cancer: comparative values of Doppler and conventional US, CT, and MR imaging correlated with surgery and histopathologic analysis—report of the Radiology Diagnostic Oncology Group. Radiology 212:19–27
18. Bristow RE (2006) Predicting unresectable ovarian cancer: taking aim at a moving target. Editorial. Gyn Oncol 100(3):449–450
19. Kubik-Huch RA, Dörffler W, von Schulthess GK, Marincek B, Köchli OR, Seifert B, Haller U, Steinert HC (2000) Value of (18 F)-FDG positron emission tomography, computed tomography, and magnetic resonance imaging in diagnosing primary and recurrent ovarian carcinoma. Eur Radiol 10:761–767
20. Funt SA, Hricak H, Abu-Rustum N, Mazumdar M, Felderman H, Chi DS (2004) Role of CT in the management of recurrent ovarian cancer. AJR Am J Roentgenol 182:393–398
21. Axtell AE, Lee MH, Bristow RE et al (2007) Multi-institutional reciprocal validation study of computed tomography predictors of suboptimal primary cytoreduction in patients with advanced ovarian cancer. J Clin Oncol 25:384–389
22. Dowdy S, Mullany S, Brandt K, Huppert B, Cliby W (2004) The utility of computed tomography scans in predicting suboptimal cytoreductive surgery in women with advanced ovarian carcinoma. Cancer 101:346–352
23. Meyer JI, Kennedy AW, Friedman R (1995) Ovarian carcinoma: value of CT in predicting success of debulking surgery. Am J Roentgenol 165:875–878
24. Deffieux X, Castaigne D, Pomel C (2006) Role of laparoscopy to evaluate candidates for complete cytoreduction in advanced stages of epithelial ovarian cancer. Int J Gynecol Cancer 16:35–40
25. Angioli R, Palaia I, Zullo MA, Muzii L, Manci N, Calcagno M, Panici PB (2006) Diagnostic open laparoscopy in the management of advanced ovarian cancer. Gynecol Oncol 100:455–461
26. Fagotti A, Fanfani F, Ludovisi M, Lo Voi R, Bifulco G, Testa AC, Scambia G (2005) Role of laparoscopy to assess the chance of optimal cytoreductive surgery in advanced ovarian cancer patients: a pilot study. Gynecol Oncol 96:729–735
27. Fagotti A, Ferrandina G, Longo R, Mancuso S, Scambia G (2002) Minilaparotomy in early endometrial cancer: an alternative to standard and laparoscopic treatment. Gynecol Oncol 86:177–183
28. Nicoletto MO, Tumolo S, Talamini R et al (1997) Surgical second look in ovarian cancer: a randomized study in patients with laparoscopic complete remission—a Northeastern Oncology Cooperative Group–Ovarian Cancer Cooperative Group Study. J Clin Oncol 15:994–999
29. Abu-Rustum NR, Barakat RR, Siegel PL, Venkatraman E, Curtin JP, Hoskins WJ (1996) Second-look operation for epithelial ovarian cancer: laparoscopy or laparotomy? Obstet Gynecol 88:549–553
30. Clough KB, Ladonne JM, Nos C, Renolleau C, Validire P, Durand JC (1999) Second look for ovarian cancer: laparoscopy or laparotomy? Prospective comparative study. Gynecol Oncol 72:411–417
31. Risum S, Høgdall C, Loft A, Berthelsen AK, Høgdall E, Nedergaard L, Lundavall L, Engelholm SA (2008) Prediction of suboptimal primary cytoreduction in primary ovarian cancer with combined positron emission tomography/computed tomography—a prospective study. Gyn Oncol 108:265–270
32. Kitajima K, Murakami K, Sakamoto S, Kaji Y, Sugimura K (2011) Present and future of FDG-PET/CT in ovarian cancer. Ann Nucl Med 25:155–164

7

The influence of a 'take home' box trainer on laparoscopic performance for gynaecological surgeons

Kushal Chummun · John P. Burke · Ray O'Sullivan · Walter Prendiville

Abstract Laparoscopic surgery requires a unique set of technical skills. There is emphasis on increasing patient safety, and therefore, a growing need to improve laparoscopic training. The aim of this study is to determine if the use of a 'take-home' box trainer would improve gynaecological surgeon performance. Thirteen obstetricians and gynaecologists (consultants and registrars) were enrolled to receive 6 months formal laparoscopic training using a 'take-home' box trainer. Laparoscopic skills were objectively assessed using a virtual reality haptic-enhanced simulator prior to commencement and at the completion of the course utilising three defined exercises (locating and coordinating, tissue manipulation and object positioning) where task duration, path length, economy of movement, hand dominance and overall score were assessed. Data is presented as mean± SEM and differences between groups evaluated with ANOVA. All 13 gynaecologists completed the programme. For tissue manipulation, laparoscopic training using the box trainer reduced the task duration (214.8±16.5 s vs. 147.7± 12.6 s, P=0.04) and increased economy of movement (22± 7.1% vs. 78.9±2.3%, P<0.001) and overall score (11.7± 3.1% vs. 33.7±1.8%, P<0.001). For object positioning, laparoscopic training with the box trainer reduced task duration (280.1±40.3 s vs. 106.6±5.1 s, P<0.001) and path length (825.3±48.3 cm vs. 463.4±16.8 cm, P<0.001) and increased overall score (4.15±1.7% vs. 15.2±2%, P< 0.001). The box trainer did not significantly affect laparoscopic locating and coordinating or change hand dominance. Formal training and continuous practice using the box trainer model improves surgical skills required for laparoscopic surgery. The box trainer could be a more accessible and preferred tool for those training to become laparoscopic surgeons.

Keywords Laparoscopic training · Box trainers · Virtual reality · Simulation

Background

An increasing number of surgical procedures are being performed via a laparoscopic approach, which requires a unique set of technical skills. Laparoscopy can be problematic for surgical training as the learning curve is steep and significant experience is required before competency is achieved [1–4]. Reasons include altered depth perception by a two-dimensional video imaging system, new cues must be learned before spatial relationships can be reliably established, long instruments diminish tactile feedback, range of motion is limited by trocars, fulcrum effect of the body wall and video eye–hand coordination must be developed to correctly position instruments in the operative field.

The different methods of laparoscopic surgical training include traditional mentorship training in the operating theatre, live animal training, human and animal cadaver training, training using a box trainer and virtual reality training (training using computer simulation) [5].

Traditional training is not without costs and risk to the patient. The operating time has been shown to increase significantly for junior surgeons compared to senior surgeons [6–9]. Cadavers provide training outside the operating

K. Chummun · R. O'Sullivan · W. Prendiville (✉)
National Clinical Skills Centre,
Coombe Women and Infants, University Hospital,
Dublin, Ireland
e-mail: fidelma.kavanagh@gmail.com

J. P. Burke
Department of Surgery, Beaumont Hospital,
Dublin, Ireland

theatre, but have cost implications, are of limited availability, and have noncompliant tissue that may be difficult to use [10]. Live animal models are useful but problem includes difference in anatomy from humans, cost, structural facilities, ethical issues and European legislation [11, 12]. Virtual reality training shortens the time to skill acquisition in different surgical procedures and offers an ethical way of assessing the competency of a surgeon in performing a procedure without a risk to the patient [5, 13–17]. However, significant cost implications are a deterrent for many institutions.

'Take home' box trainers are alternative tools used for laparoscopic training. They are economical and can be easily acquired not only by institutions but also by trainees in laparoscopic surgery. This allows the trainee to not only practise while in hospital or on a course but also at home. The aim of the current study was to evaluate the use of a 'take home' box trainer as a learning tool in laparoscopic surgical skills for gynaecological surgeons.

Methods

Thirteen gynaecologists (10 registrars and 3 consultants) were enrolled at the National Clinical Skills Centre (NCSC) for a 6-month laparoscopic training course using a 'take home' box trainer. A maximum of 16 places are available for each course at the NCSC as it allows a one to one training and monitoring. Our participants were neither laparoscopic novices nor experts and would on average perform about one to two laparoscopic procedures per week at their respective place of work.

The box trainer, evolved from a need to provide a novel take home system. Initially the 'box' consisted of storage boxes and cheaply available webcams. This system has been refined into the LaProTrain® (Fig. 1) laparoscopic simulator (Endosim Ltd, Belfast, Northern Ireland). The box trainer is light, non cumbersome and portable which encourages a long-term use even after completion of the course.

At the beginning of the course, each delegate's laparoscopic skills were assessed using a virtual reality ProMIS® enhanced laparoscopic simulator (Haptica Ltd, Dublin, Ireland).

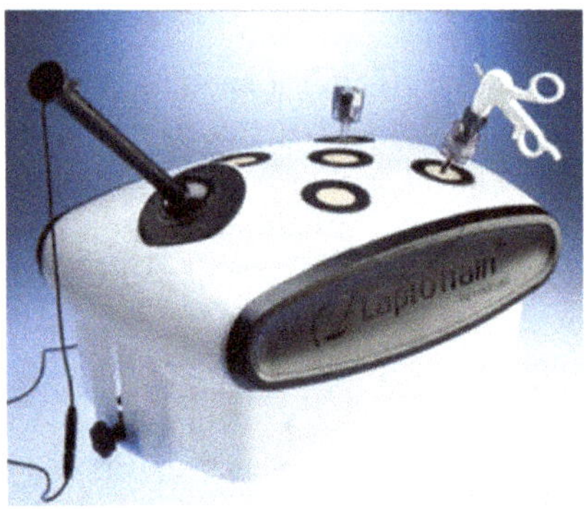

Fig. 1 The LaProTrain® box trainer

The assessment involved three precise, computer-controlled exercises (locating and coordinating, tissue manipulation and object positioning). Task duration, path length, economy of movement, change in hand dominance and the overall score were recorded.

In locating and coordinating exercise, the user must touch and/or track a series of fixed and dynamic objects in a virtual environment, while trying to avoid colliding with tissue. Audio cues and on-screen directions provide guidance. Tissue manipulation involved the user to stretch simulated tissue from one marked point to another, learning to judge tissue strength and appropriate force. Lastly, the object positioning exercise involved the user to pick up a number of objects, transfer them from one hand to another and place them in a specified target area.

The participants then attended the NCSC course once a month for 6-month period where new techniques and exercises were taught using their own individual box trainer. After each of the six training sessions, the delegates took their box trainer home where they were encouraged to practise the exercises for at least 1 h each day and also apply the newly learnt technique during laparoscopy. At the start of each course, prior to learning new techniques, the exercises taught previously were reviewed to identify weakness points in each participant and therefore allow targeting practice at home.

Examples of exercises (Fig. 2) on the box trainer included:

- Basic tasks such as
  - touching different points on a piece of paper using graspers with the camera fixed and again with the camera tracking the grasper,
  - passing beans from one grasper to another and placing beans on designated spot and
  - assembling and disassembling puzzles.
- Complex drills such as
  - using grasper and scissors to cut a circle marked on a surgical glove;
  - performing a simulated ovarian cystectomy—this involved removing a liquid washing tablet placed inside a partially glue stuck deflated balloon without bursting the tablet;
  - suturing exercises which included

    extracoporal suturing,
    endoloop placement,
    intra-corporeal knot suturing.
  - Specimen retrieval exercises involve using an endo-bag to retrieve different objects (e.g. liquid washing tablet) from the box trainer.

At the end of the sixth month, the participants were reassessed using the same three exercises on the ProMIS®

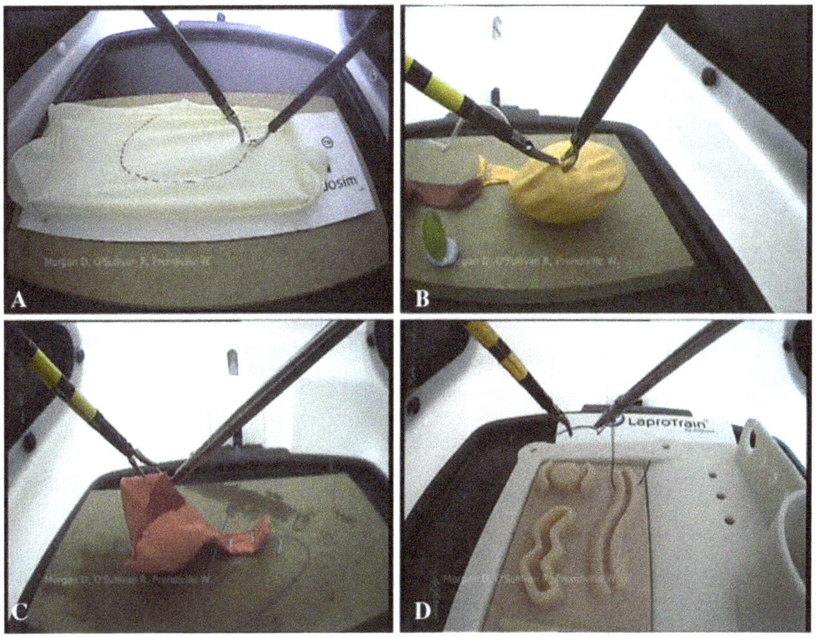

Fig. 2 **a** Cutting exercise. **b** Ovarian cystectomy simulation. **c–d** Suturing exercises

enhanced laparoscopic simulator. The task duration, path length, economy of movement, change in hand dominance and overall score were again recorded and the data compared to that at the start of the course. Data is presented as mean±SEM and differences between groups evaluated with ANOVA using SPSS V.12 (Chicago, IL, USA).

Findings

All 13 gynaecologists completed the programme and 100% data was available on all participants. Results are presented under the subcategories of locating and coordinating, tissue manipulation and object positioning.

Locating and coordinating

In this subcategory, there was no significant difference between the assessment before and after training in all the measured parameters:

- task time (410.9±29.7 s vs. 398.5±30.6 s, P=0.772) (Fig. 3a),
- path length (925.7±86.5 cm vs. 963.2±71.9 cm, P=0.742) (Fig. 3b),
- percentage change in hand dominance (8.4±1.6% vs. 6.8±2.1%, P=0.633) (Fig. 3c),
- overall score (9.9±2.3 vs 6.3±3.2, P=0.492) (Fig. 3d).

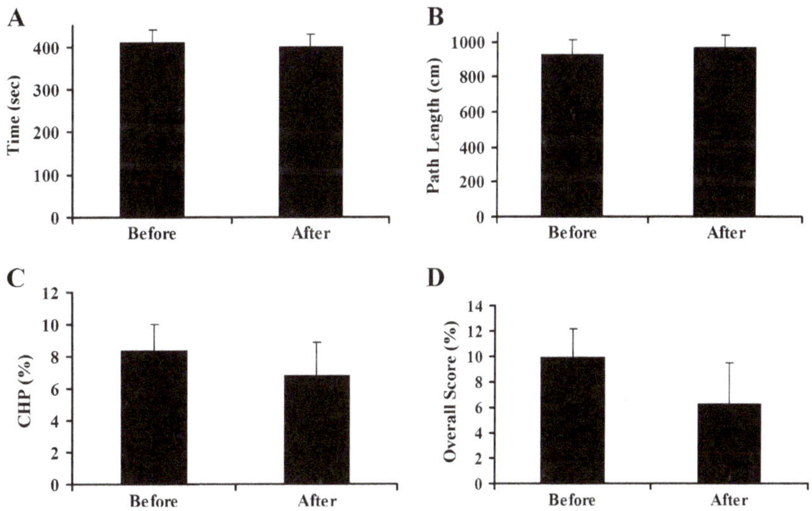

Fig. 3 Change in locating and coordinating skills following box trainer use. *CHP* change in hand preference. No significant difference between groups, ANOVA

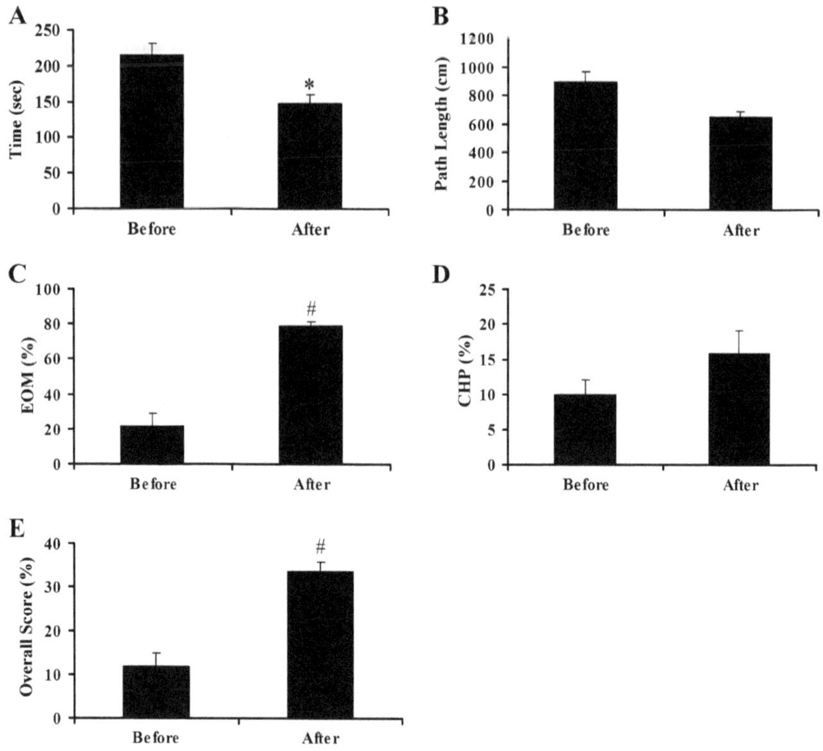

Fig. 4 Change in tissue manipulation skills following box trainer use. *CHP* change in hand preference, *EOM* economy of movement. *P<0.05, #P<0.001, ANOVA

Tissue manipulation

In this subcategory, significant improvement was noted in terms of:

- total task time (214.8±16.5 s vs. 147.7±12.6 s, P=0.04) (Fig. 4a),
- economy of movement (22±7.1% vs. 78.9±2.3%, P< 0.001) (Fig. 4c) and
- overall score (11.7±3.1% vs. 33.7±1.8%, P<0.001) (Fig. 4e).

There was however no difference between the assessment before and after training in terms of path length (892.8±68.3 cm vs. 652.9±40.5 cm, P=0.079) (Fig. 4b) or percentage change in hand dominance (10.1±2.1% vs. 15.8±3.3%, P=0.169) (Fig. 4d).

Object positioning

In this subcategory, there was a significant improvement between the assessment before and after training in terms of:

- task time (280.1±40.3 s vs. 106.6±5.1 s, P=0.028) (Fig. 5a),
- path length (825.3±48.3 cm vs. 463.4±16.8 cm, P< 0.001) (Fig. 5b) and

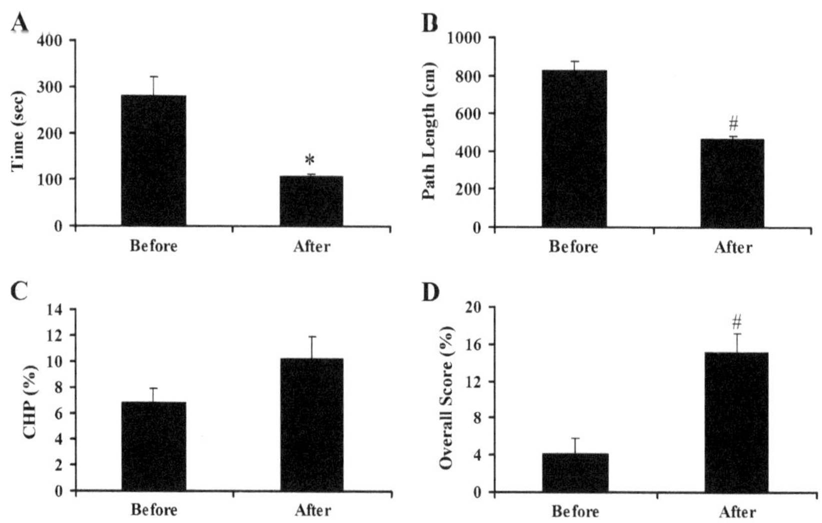

Fig. 5 Change in object positioning skills following box trainer use. *CHP* change in hand preference, *EOM* economy of movement. *P<0.05, #P<0.001, ANOVA

- overall score (4.2±1.7% vs. 15.2±2.0%, $P<0.001$) (Fig. 5d).

There was however no difference between the assessment before and after training in terms of percentage change in hand dominance (6.8±1.1% vs. 10.2±1.7%, $P=0.127$) (Fig. 5c).

Discussion

Globally, increasing number of gynaecological surgeries is being performed laparoscopically. Because of the European Working Time Directive, there is decreasing time to train surgeons. It is now more important than ever to improve the surgical skills in the least time with maximum efficiency [18].

Virtual reality has been proven to improve surgical skills [14, 16, 19]. However, virtual reality training is expensive and is not readily available to most trainees. In that respect, training using a 'take home' box trainer becomes more attractive. Our study has clearly supported the fact that skills acquired using a 'take home' box trainer would improve laparoscopic skills as measured by performance on a virtual reality laparoscopic simulator.

In this study, significant improvement was demonstrated in tissue manipulation and object positioning exercises. This was expressed by a reduction in total task time and an increase in overall score for both exercises as well as an improvement in economy of movement in tissue manipulation exercise and a decrease in path length in object positioning.

In the tissue manipulation exercise, there was no change in path length. This may be explained by the fact that, in this exercise, simulated tissue is stretched from one fixed point to another as directed by the computer. Hence, the overall path length would remain the same. However, a better measurement of skill in this exercise was economy of movement, which analysed how effective the tissues were moved from one point to another with the least tissue manipulation and instrument handling.

In the object positioning exercise, besides reduction in task time and overall score, there was also a reduction in path length. A reduction in path length may suggest that there was a more fluent and successful first time transfer of objects between one hand and the other and less accidental drop of the objects. This is further supported by the fact that task time was also reduced. These demonstrate an overall improvement on laparoscopic dexterity.

In regards to locating and coordinating exercise, there was no statistically significant difference in task time, path length, hand dominance or overall score. This can be explained by the fact that the participants were not laparoscopic 'novices' and because this exercise is basic, such that the performance at the start of the course was good with small room for improvement in this particular group. As regards to percentage change in hand dominance, the lack of improvement in all three exercises may indicate that a 6-month training period may not be sufficient enough time to cause significant change in the non-dominant hand. It may also show a need to develop exercises on the box trainer to increase dexterity in the non-dominant hand.

Studies have reported that an improvement on performance on a virtual reality laparoscopic simulator as indicated by improved score on different exercises translates into improved operative performance [20, 21]. Our study has shown that practice on a 'take home' box trainer also improved performance on the laparoscopic simulator and should logically be reflected in improved laparoscopic skill in vivo. Moreover, assessing performance on the virtual laparoscopic simulator at regular intervals after practising on a box trainer may be a more reliable way of assessing improvement in surgical skills as improved score on the simulator after repeating the exercises on the simulator itself may be due to increased familiarity with the exercises rather than improved surgical skills.

Those two hypotheses can be explored by having a group of registrars train on the virtual reality simulator and another on the box trainer. Their progress can then be assessed during laparoscopic surgery by independent viewers (consultants and nurses) blinded as to which group they belong. This will directly measure if training on box trainers improves laparoscopic skill in vivo and whether the degree of improvement on the virtual simulator is comparable to the improvement noted during laparoscopic surgery.

In retrospect, our study was limited by the fact that we did not have a control group. However, we did not identify any other factors such as increase in number of laparoscopic procedures performed per week by each participant, during the 6-month period that would have contributed to an improved score on the virtual reality machine other than the course itself and training on the box trainer.

Conclusion

In conclusion, we have shown that a 'take home' box trainer improves laparoscopic performance on many exercises as scored by the virtual reality simulator and could therefore be a more accessible, realistic and cost-effective tool for those training to become laparoscopic surgeons.

Acknowledgements We would like to thank all the participants of the course and study.

Declaration of interest Walter Prendiville and Ray O'Sullivan are directors of Endosim Ltd and possess patents related to Laprotrain. Kushal Chummun and John Burke have no conflicts of interest or financial ties to disclose.

References

1. Jones DB, Brewer JD, Soper NJ (1996) The influence of three-dimensional video systems on laparoscopic task performance. Surg Laparosc Endosc 6:191–197
2. Wolfe BM, Szabo Z, Moran ME, Chan P, Hunter JG (1993) Training for minimally invasive surgery: need for surgical skills. Surg Endosc 7:93–95
3. Melvin WS, Johnson JA, Ellison EC (1996) Laparoscopic skills enhancement. Am J Surg 172:377–379
4. Dent TL (1992) Training, credentialing, and evaluation in laparoscopic surgery. Surg Clin North Am 72:1003–1010
5. Munz Y, Kumar BD, Moorthy K, Bann S, Darzi A (2004) Laparoscopic virtual reality and box trainers: is one superior to the other? Surg Endosc 18(3):485–494
6. Farnworth LR, Lemay DE, Wooldridge T, Mabrey JD, Blaschak MJ, DeCoster TA, Wascher DC, Schenck RC Jr (2001) A comparison of operative times in arthroscopic ACL reconstruction between orthopaedic faculty and residents: the financial impact of orthopaedic surgical training in the operating room. Iowa Orthopedic Journal 21:31–35
7. Babineau TJ, Becker J, Gibbons G, Sentovich S, Hess D, Robertson S, Stone M (2004) The "cost" of operative training for surgical residents. Archives of Surgical Research 139(4):366–370
8. Wilkiemeyer M, Pappas TN, Giobbie-Hurder A, Itani KM, Jonasson O, Neumayer LA (2005) Does resident postgraduate year influence the outcomes of inguinal hernia repair? Ann Surg 241(6):879–884
9. Kauvar DS, Braswell A, Brown BD, Harnisch M (2006) Influence of resident and attending surgeon seniority on operative performance in laparoscopic cholecystectomy. J Surg Res 132(2):159–163
10. Anastakis DJ, Regehr G, Reznick RK, Cusimano M, Murnaghan J, Brown M, Hutchison C (1999) Assessment of technical skills transfer from the bench training model to the human model. Am J Surg 177:167–170
11. Hunter JG, Sackier JM, Berci G (1994) Training in laparoscopic cholecystectomy: quantifying the learning curve. Surg Endosc 8:28–31
12. Rowan AN (1993) Is justification of animal research necessary? JAMA 269:1114
13. Hyltander A, Liljegren E, Rhodin PH, Lonroth H (2002) The transfer of basic skills learned in laparoscopic simulator to the operating room. Surg Endosc 16(9):13248
14. Seymour NE, Gallagher AG, Roman SA, O'Brien MK, Bansal VK, Andersen DK, Satava RM (2002) Virtual reality training improves operating room performance: results of a randomized, double-blinded study. Ann Surg 236(4):458–464
15. Watterson JD, Beiko DT, Kuan JK, Denstedt JD (2002) Randomized prospective blinded study validating acquistion of ureteroscopy skills using computer based virtual reality endourological simulator. J Urol 168(5):1928–1932
16. Grantcharov TP, Kristiansen VB, Bendix J, Bardram L, Rosenberg J, Funch-Jensen P (2004) Randomized clinical trial of virtual reality simulation for laparoscopic skills training. Br J Surg 91 (2):146–150
17. Moorthy K, Munz Y, Jiwanji M, Bann S, Chang A, Darzi A (2004) Validity and reliability of a virtual reality upper gastrointestinal simulator and cross validation using structured assessment of individual performance with video playback. Surg Endosc 18 (2):328–333
18. Chikwe J, de Souza AC, Pepper JR (2004) No time to train the surgeons. BMJ 328(7437):418–419
19. Aggarwal R, Tully A, Grantcharov T, Larsen CR, Miskry T, Farthing A, Darzi A (2006) Virtual reality simulation training can improve technical skills during laparoscopic salpingectomy for ectopic pregnancy. BJOG 113(12):1382–1387
20. Scott DJ, Bergen PC, Rege RV, Laycock R, Tesfay ST, Valentine RJ, Euhus DM, Jeyarajah DR, Thompson WM, Jones DB (2000) Laparoscopic training on bench models: better and more cost effective than operating room experience? J Am Coll Surg 191 (3):272–283
21. Kirby TO, Numnum TM, Kilgore LC, Straughn JM (2008) A prospective evaluation of a simulator- based laparoscopic training program for gynecology residents. J Am Coll Surg 206(2):343–348

8

Laparoscopy in the public health system in Ecuador: an evaluation of the status quo and the education in minimally invasive surgery

Harald Krentel · Mercedes Almagro Ruiz

Abstract The following study describes the use of laparoscopic surgery in the public hospitals of the Ecuadorian ministry of public health in Quito, Ecuador in the year 2008. The aim of the present study was the description of the recent situation of laparoscopic surgery in the public sector of the Ecuadorian capital, the level of training and education of laparoscopists, and the determination of missing factors in the educational programs in minimally invasive surgery in Ecuador. We analyzed the use of laparoscopic approach in correlation to the specialty and the diagnosis. The results revealed that in many diagnoses, the standard surgical approach still is the laparotomy. The discrepancy between general surgery, gynecology, and urology in the use of minimally invasive surgery in the public health system shows the different educational levels and the need of training programs at university level and in the hospitals especially in gynecology.

Keywords Gynecologic endoscopy · Training and education

H. Krentel
CEGPA, Centro de Endoscopía Ginecológica Peruano Aleman, Lima, Peru

H. Krentel (✉)
Städtisches Krankenhaus Eisenhüttenstadt, Gynecology and Obstetrics, Friedrich-Engels-Str. 39, 15890 Eisenhüttenstadt, Germany
e-mail: krentel@cegpa.org

M. A. Ruiz
Hospital Eugenio Espejo, Quito, Ecuador

Background

Minimally invasive surgery has become the most important surgical approach in the last two decades in the surgical treatment of benign and malign intraabdominal diseases in general surgery, gynecology, and urology. Especially in gynecology in various centers of laparoscopy and hysteroscopy, more than 90% of the interventions are realized by endoscopic approaches. However there is a big discrepancy between the use of laparoscopy in different countries, especially in correlation with the status of general development. The success of laparoscopy in developed regions like North America and Europe is correlated with the demand of this minimally invasive procedure by the patients due to the well-known benefits—faster recuperation, less pain, and small incisions with a good cosmetic result. However only a well-informed patient can demand a new procedure and laparoscopic interventions can only be realized by trained surgeons. The present evaluation analyzes the educational level of Ecuadorian laparoscopists in the public sector, the use of laparoscopy in comparison with laparotomy, and the training situation in Ecuador.

Methods and aim

In a first step, we evaluated the daily practice and the personal experience of the surgeons with laparoscopy using a questionnaire. One hundred seven general surgeons, gynecologists, and urologists from the following hospitals were included to the study: Eugenio Espejo, Baca Ortiz, Isidro Ayora, Pablo Arturio Suarez, and Enrique Garces. In the second step, the database of the five public hospitals in Quito, Ecuador were analyzed comparing laparoscopy versus laparotomy in general surgery, gynecology, and urology.

Finally we analyzed the postgraduate courses of all Ecuadorian universities with medical faculties. The aim of the study was to answer the following questions:

- What is the recent training level of laparoscopists working in the public hospitals in Quito, Ecuador?
- Do the surgeons participate in training workshops?
- Does an Ecuadorian certification system in laparoscopy exists?
- What is the status quo in laparoscopy in the public hospitals in Quito, Ecuador?
- What is the status quo in gynecologic laparoscopy in the public hospitals in Quito, Ecuador?
- Is there a quality standard in laparoscopy in Ecuador?
- How many Ecuadorian universities offer postgraduate programs in laparoscopy?
- Do the surgeons wish to continue their individual training?

Results

Evaluation of surgeons working in the public hospital of Quito, Ecuador

Fifty-eight out of 107 (54%) physicians (surgeons, gynecologists, urologists) working at the public hospitals in the Ecuadorian capital responded to the questionnaire. Almost 90% of the interviewed surgeons already realize laparoscopies in their daily practice. However 44% of the laparoscopists perform a laparoscopic surgery only one to three times a month, while 40% answered to realize a laparoscopy one to three times a week and 16% only occasionally laparoscope their patients. All interviewed surgeons participated in one or more workshops of laparoscopic surgery in Ecuador or another country. The duration of the training in 69% of the cases was less than a month. Only 14% of the physicians commented to have participated a training program for more than 7 months. Half of the surgeons received a certification of participation (53%), while 38% did not receive any certification after the training program. Only 9% of the realized laparoscopic educational programs were linked to an university including a respective certification. Before operating on humans, 76% of all interviewed surgeons exercised laparoscopy with animal models. However all physicians would like to continue their education in laparoscopy.

Evaluation of postgraduate courses at Ecuadorian universities

We analyzed the type of postgraduate courses the universities in Ecuador offer. The database of information in this case was the CONESUP (Consejo Nacional de Educación Superior). This analyzation reveals that there is no postgraduate program at any of the eight Ecuadorian universities in laparoscopic surgery (Table 1).

Comparison of laparoscopy versus laparotomy in all realized surgeries in 2008

We analyzed all realized surgeries in the five public hospitals in Quito in the year 2008. Therefore the documentation of the operating theaters of these hospitals were investigated. We compared laparotomy versus laparoscopy in general surgery, urology, and gynecology. The approaches to treat the typical indications in the specialties were also compared. In 2008 a total of 7,963 surgical interventions has been realized in gynecology, urology, and general surgery in the five public hospitals of the Ecuadorian capital.

Almost 80% of all the interventions were conventional surgeries and only 20% minimally invasive surgeries. Comparing the results of the different hospitals the laparoscopic approach reached only 2% of more than 2,000 surgeries in the Hospital Baca Ortiz as a mínimum and 34.7% as a maximum in the Hospital Isidro Ayora. In gynecology 90% of all interventions have been open surgeries. The most frequent gynecologic procedure was hysterectomy with 639 interventions. Only 13 (2%) hysterectomies had been performed by laparoscopic approach in one of the institutions. In the same hospital, 22 of 45 surgeries for ovarian masses had been realized by laparoscopy (Table 2).

In the other 23 cases, a laparotomy was the choice to treat the ovarian tumor. Interestingly in case of infertility, the laparoscopy is the preferred approach in only 12.7% of the cases in three institutions. That means that 87.3% of the patients with infertility had been treated by a laparotomy.

Table 1 Universities with subspecialization in surgery (CONESUP)

Universities with specialization in surgery		
University		Postgraduate
1	Universidad de Cuenca	•General surgery
2	Universidad del Azuay	•Oncologic surgery
3	PUCE Guayaquil	•General surgery •Pediatric surgery •Plastic surgery
4	Universidad de Guayaquil	•General surgery •Pediatric surgery •Oncologic surgery
5	Universidad Nacional de Loja	•General surgery
6	Universidad Central del Ecuador	•General surgery •Oncologic surgery
7	Universidad Internacional	•General surgery
8	Universidad San Francisco de Quito	•General surgery •Cardiothoracic surgery

Table 2 Laparoscopic (LAP) versus conventional (CS) approaches in 2008

Public hospitals in Quito, Ecuador

Hospitals	Specialties											
	Surgery		Urology		Gynecology		Subtotal				Total	Percentage
	LAP	CS	LAP	CS	LAP	CS	LAP		CS			
							No.	Percentage	No.	Percentage		
HEE	325	1,114	4	163	15	136	344	19.57	1,413	80.42	1,757	100.00
HEG	601	1,373	0	91	9	181	610	27.00	1,645	73.00	2,255	100.00
HOIA	0	0	0	0	99	186	99	34.70	186	65.20	285	100.00
HBO	16	953	5	35	21	988	42	2.08	1,976	97.92	2,018	100.00
HPAS	501	668	20	31	30	398	551	33.43	1,097	66.50	1,648	100.00
Subtotal	1,443	4,108	29	320	174	1,889	1,646	20.67	6,317	79.33	7,963	100.00

For simple diagnostic reasons, the laparoscopy is the procedure of first choice. In 77.1% of the cases, the surgeons preferred the minimally invasive surgery for an intraabdominal diagnostic. In one hospital the percentage of laparoscopies reached almost 30% of the interventions. Due to the very rare endoscopic approach in the other hospitals, the total percentage of laparoscopies in the gynecologic departments of the public hospitals in Quito, Ecuador did not reach more than 10% of all surgeries (Table 3).

Interestingly in general surgery, the acceptance of laparoscopy seems to be bigger. After all 25% of 5,614 surgeries have been laparoscopies in the year 2008. The most important laparoscopic procedure is the cholecystectomy with 67% laparoscopic approach of all interventions, while the general surgeons in case of a diagnostic surgery prefer the open approach (98.9%). Only 1.5% of 1,539 apendectomies had been performed by laparoscopy. However the Ecuadorian laparoscopy plays a more important role in general surgery compared with gynecology.

Discussion

Only 9.9% of all gynecologic surgeries in the public sector of the Ecuadorian capital are laparoscopies. That means that 90.1% of all gynecologic surgeries in the five most important public hospitals in the Ecuadorian capital were laparotomies in the year 2008. In gynecology of public hospitals in Ecuador, the laparoscopy still is just an approach in diagnostics and sterilization. As the results reveal, laparoscopy already is the standard procedure in cholecystectomy. Most of the general, gynegological, and urological surgeons working in public hospitals of the Ecuadorian capital Quito obtained basic skills in laparoscopy and participated in one or more workshops of minimally invasive surgery. Anyway their daily practice is not backed up by certifications.

In Ecuador, like in most of the other South American countries, a certification system in laparoscopy is not yet implemented. Neither the medical faculties of Ecuadorian universities nor the societies of gynecologic endoscopy in Ecuador offer a standardized education system or training programs in laparoscopic surgery respectively endoscopic gynecology. A certification of laparoscopic procedures for example by the Ecuadorian society of endoscopic gynecology would be a possible way to control the standards and the quality of the surgery. These certification systems are implemented since various years in Europe and North America. The German association of gynecologic endoscopy differs the individual education in three personal levels of laparoscopic and hysteroscopic procedures (MIC I–MIC III) and a standard for institutions to become a center of excellence in gynecologic endoscopy. Part of the certification process is the participation of the applicant in congresses and workshops of laparoscopy and hysteroscopy. The curriculum of the workshops is standardized by the respective working group [4]. These conditions lead to a controlled continuing education. However the most important part of the application procedure is the presentation of surgery reports. The required number of realized surgeries depends on the respective level. A minimum number of surgeries must be submitted to receive the first national level of endoscopic gynecology. The value of such a certification is undoubtable for the physician, particularly as insurance companies in a few years will demand on it. In the long term, the patients will look for certified surgeons considering the proved quality of their work. The common practice to offer laparoscopy without having the skills to perform it will be stopped by a transparent certification system.

As the results of this evaluation show, 100% of the interviewed surgeons trained themselves in animal models before operating on humans. Anyway 60% of the surgeons realize laparoscopies just occasionally or one to three times

Table 3 Laparoscopy versus conventional surgery in gynecology, 2008

Public hospitals in Quito, Ecuador—gynecology

Hospital	Ovarian mass		Hysterectomy		Endometriosis		Diagnostic		Infertility		Oncology		Subtotal				Total	Percentage
	LAP	CS	LAP	CS	LAP	CS	LAP	CS	LAP	CS	LAP	CS	LAP		CS			
													No.	Percentage	No.	Percentage		
HEE	0	7	0	119	0	0	4	3	1	3	0	4	5	3.5	136	96.5	141	12.7
HEG	0	0	0	181	0	0	0	0	0	0	0	0	0	0	181	100	181	16.4
HGOIA	22	13	13	167	0	0	23	3	13	3	0	0	71	27.6	186	72.4	257	23.2
HPAS	0	25	0	172	0	0	0	2	29	290	0	9	29	5.5	498	94.5	527	47.7
Subtotal	22	45	13	639	0	0	27	8	43	296	0	13	105	9.9	1,001	90.1	1,106	100.0

a month. The quality of laparoscopic surgery, the percentage of complications, and the duration particularly in more complex surgeries depend on the learning curve of the individual surgeons, which depends on the frequency of interventions. Morelli et al. publicated a comparison of vaginal versus laparoscopic hysterectomy, demonstrating the higher level of complications in laparoscopic hysterectomies only in the first year of the learning curve [13]. Boyd et al. showed that the rate of morbidity and mortality after hysterectomy depend on the number of performed procedures per year [3]. The percentage of persistent menstrual bleeding after subtotal laparoscopic hysterectomy is higher in surgeons with few experience [10]. In a prospective evaluation, Kirby et al. demonstrated the positive effect of training programs on the duration of a procedure [7]. Bojahr et al. analyzed 1,000 cases of subtotal laparoscopic hysterectomy, demonstrating an average time benefit of 13 min after a period of 4 years of performing the same procedure with a higher degree of difficulty [2]. The residents and young specialists must given the chance to assist laparoscopic procedures as often as possible under the supervision of a qualified laparoscopist. This could be part of the curriculum of a postgraduate university level education. The interest of all interviewed surgeons to continue their education is very high. Unfortunately the doors of the operating theaters of the private gynecologic institutions with high percentages and wider indications in gynecologic endoscopy are often closed to most of the residents. This is for legal reasons and also for economic reasons.

To educate means to open a lucrative market to competitors. An Australian publication revealed the lack of instruments and materials, training, experience, and the encouragement by colleagues as the main reasons to not perform more complex laparoscopic surgeries like myomectomies or hysterectomies [6]. Marret et al. concluded that skilled surgeons in laparoscopy and in laparoscopic myomectomy must help their trainees during their learning curve in order to decrease laparoconversions [12], respectively, in order to allow them the safe performance of more complex surgeries. In 2007 Kolkman et al. [8] published the current status of the implementation of operative laparoscopy in gynecology in the Netherlands, based on a questionnaire which had been sent to all hospitals (n=102) in 2003. The total number and type of laparoscopic procedures performed in 2002 stratified by level of difficulty was compared to the results from 1993. The diffusion and acceptance of level 2 procedures (adhesiolysis, ectopic pregnancy, laparoscopic treatment of endometriosis, cystectomy, oophorectomy, LAVH) increased significantly. Anyway the diffusion of LAVH was only 58%. The authors concluded that the implementation of operative gynecological laparoscopy in the Netherlands seems to develop at a slow pace. A Canadian survey from 2007 revealed that 24.5% of Canadian gynecologists performed laparoscopic myomectomy. Of the respondents 70.7% felt that lack of training was the main barrier to perform complex laparoscopic procedures [11]. Another recent Canadian study [9] revealed that Canadian residents in obstetrics and gynecology are not receiving adequate training to feel comfortable using the laparoscopic approach as opposed to the vaginal and abdominal routes. The positive effects of training and education in laparoscopy has been shown in various publications. Edelman et al. for example [5] described the impact of the integration of laparoscopic skill training in the medical school curriculum on the final surgical performance of residents. A French prospective study revealed that simulator training provides a more rapid acquisition of competence in surgical technique [1]. Morgan Ortiz et al. described the teaching of total laparoscopic hysterectomy in a Mexican university training program in gynecologic laparoscopy. Eighteen participants received the respective university diploma in the last 2 years [14]. Further national and international educational initiatives are needed to ensure that graduates and specialists are capable of performing more different and complex types of endoscopic surgery in gynecology, but also urology and general surgery.

Conclusion

In the public Ecuadorian health sector, laparoscopy still does not play an important role in general surgery, urology, and particularly in gynecology. The lack of training programs and a frequent access to more complex interventions under supervision of a skilled specialist does not allow the motivated surgeons to develop their skills in laparoscopy. A national concept of resident and specialist training is needed to implement laparoscopy as a frequent procedure in a wider range of indications and to make it a safe and cost-effective alternative to conventional surgery for the population.

Declaration of interest The authors report no conflicts of interest. The authors alone are responsible for the content and writing of the paper.

References

1. Beyer L, Troyer JD, Mancini J, Bladou F, Berdah SV, Karsenty G (2011) Impact of laparoscopy simulator training on the technical skills of future surgeons in the operating room: a prospective study. Am J Surg 202(3):265–272
2. Bojahr B, Tchartchian G, Ohlinger R (2009) Laparoscopic supracervical hysterectomy: a retrospective analysis of 1000 cases. JSLS 13(2):129–134
3. Boyd LR, Novetsky AP, Curtin JP (2010) Effect of surgical volumen on the route of hysterectomy and short-term morbidity. Obstet Gynecol 116(4):909–915
4. DeWilde RL, Hucke J, Kolmorgen K, Tinneberg H (2011) Recommendations by the Gynecologic Endoscopy Working Group of the German Society of Obstetrics and Gynecology for the advancement of training and education in minimal-access surgery. Arch Gynecol Obstet 283(3):509–512
5. Edelman DA, Mattos MA, Bouwman DL (2011) Impact of fundamentals of laparoscopic surgery training during medical school on performance by first year surgical residents. J Surg Res 170(1):6–9
6. Englund M, Robson S (2007) Why has the acceptance of laparoscopic hysterectomy been slow? Results of an anonymous survey of Australian gynecologists. J Minim Invasive Gynecol 14(6):724–728
7. Kirby TO, Numnum TM, Kilgore LC, Straughn JM (2008) A prospective evaluation of a simulator-based laparoscopic training program for gynecology residents. J Am Coll Surg 206(2):343–348
8. Kolkman W, Trimbos-Kemper TC, Jansen FW (2007) Operative laparoscopy in the Netherlands: diffusion and acceptance. Eur J Obstet Gynecol Reprod Biol 130(2):245–248
9. Kroft J, Moody J, Lee P (2011) Canadian hysterectomy educational experience: survey of recent graduates in obstetrics and gynecology. J Minim Invasive Gynecol 18(4):438–444
10. Lieng M, Qvigstad E, Istre O, Langebrekke A, Ballard K (2008) Long-term outcomes following laparoscopic supracervical hysterectomy. BJOG 115(13):1605–1610
11. Liu G, Zolis L, Kung R, Melchior M, Singh S, Cook EF (2010) The laparoscopic myomectomy: a survey of Canadian gynaecologists. J Obstet Gynaecol Can 32(2):139–148
12. Marrett H, Chevillot M, Giraudeau B, Study Group of the French Society of Gynaecology and Obstetrics (Quest Division) (2006) Factors influencing laparoconversions during the learning curve of laparoscopic myomectomy. Acta Obstet Gynecol Scand 85 (3):324–329
13. Morelli M, Caruso M, Noia R, Chiodo D, Cosco C, Lucia E, Biamonte M, Zullo F (2007) Total laparoscopic hysterectomy versus vaginal hysterectomy: a prospective randomized trial. Minerva Ginecol 59(2):99–105
14. Morgan Ortiz F, Lopez Zepeda MA (2011) Teaching of total laparoscopic hysterectomy in a gynecological laparoscopy university diploma course. Ginecol Obstet Mex 79(9):547–552

9

Management of adnexal torsion by laparoscopic approach

Ibrahim Alkatout · Liselotte Mettler · Martin Anlauf · Walter Jonat · Christel Eckmann-Scholz · Thoralf Schollmeyer

Abstract The study aimed to evaluate the effectiveness and safety of laparoscopic management of adnexal torsion. Early minimal invasive surgical management of adnexal torsion with the main emphasis on an organ-preserving procedure can safely be recommended. Although the incidence of adnexal torsions has increased, the morbidity rate has declined due to safer diagnostics and operative strategies. This is a retrospective case–control study (Canadian Task Force classification II-3) of 33 cases of adnexal torsion over an 11-year period (December 1999–September 2010) in a gynecologic endoscopy unit of a university hospital. Interventions include early diagnostic laparoscopy and utmost protection of the surrounding tissue. Thirty-three cases of laparoscopically managed adnexal torsions were analyzed. Fifty-two percent had conservative organ-sparing procedures, while 48 % underwent resection of ovary, tube, or both. The mean operating time was 69.2 min. There were no complications or conversions to laparotomy. The most common predisposing factor was an adnexal mass with symptoms of pain. Torsion on the right tube is more common than on the left. Laparoscopic surgery is an effective, safe, and feasible method in the diagnosis and treatment of adnexal torsion.

I. Alkatout (✉) · L. Mettler · W. Jonat · C. Eckmann-Scholz · T. Schollmeyer
Department of Gynecology and Obstetrics, University Hospitals Schleswig-Holstein, Campus Kiel, Arnold-Heller Strasse 3, House 24, 24105, Kiel, Germany
e-mail: ibrahim.alkatout@uk-sh.de
URL: www.endo-kiel.de

M. Anlauf
Institute of Pathology, University Hospital Düsseldorf, 40225, Düsseldorf, Germany

Keywords Adnexal torsion · Laparoscopy · Pelviscopic treatment · Organ preservation

Introduction

Torsion of the adnexa is the fifth most common gynecologic surgical emergency [1]. The condition is more common in premenarcheal females (children or premenarcheal adolescents) in whom torsion involving previously normal adnexa may constitute up to 15–50 % of adnexal torsion cases [2]. It is difficult to diagnose because although adnexal torsion may present in the form of acute pelvic pain, the symptoms can sometimes be deceptive. When the lesions are asymptomatic, the diagnosis may be made only during the surgical procedure. Doppler evaluation in cases of ovarian torsion can be a useful tool, but it was found to be normal in 60 % of these cases. The absence of Doppler flow was predictive of surgically confirmed cases of ovarian torsion, demonstrating the low sensitivity but high specificity of Doppler studies in the diagnosis of torsion [3, 4].

In the past, adnexal torsion was treated by salpingo-oophorectomy without untwisting the adnexa to avoid potential thromboembolism from ovarian vein thrombosis [5]. However, a significant association between thromboembolism and untwisting an ischemic pedicle has never been established [6]. Recently, a review of literature concluded that the risk of pulmonary embolism after adnexal torsion was 0.2 % and was not increased when the adnexa was untwisted. Over 400 cases managed with untwisting the adnexa have been reported, with no embolic phenomena [4, 6].

The conservative management of torsion with untwisting (detorsion) of the fallopian tube and ovary has proved to be safe and effective in multiple case series in the late 1980s and early 1990s. This type of management, first proposed by

Way in 1946, is highly desirable since torsion occurs most often in women of reproductive age, and ovarian conservation is preferable in this age group.

Progress made in operative laparoscopy now suggests that treatment of adnexal torsion can be carried out laparoscopically which is the procedure of choice. Laparoscopic management of adnexal torsion has been shown to be feasible and preferable to laparotomy. The advantages of laparoscopy include short hospital stay and recovery time, in addition to the fact that conservative procedures, such as detorsion and ovarian cystectomy, can be done laparoscopically [7].

Patients and methods

Data from 33 patients with adnexal torsion who underwent laparoscopic management were collected retrospectively from the computerized operating logs of the Department of Obstetrics and Gynecology, University of Schleswig-Holstein, Campus Kiel, Germany over an 11-year period between December 1999 and September 2010.

All patients underwent a clinical examination, ultrasound scanning, routine blood count, electrolyte analysis, urine analysis, and coagulation profile. In patients diagnosed to have an adnexal cyst, tumor markers, namely, CA125 and CEA, were measured. Other imaging techniques, such as MRI, were done in selected cases according to the sonographic findings. Presence of any predisposing factors such as adhesions, neoplasm, and pregnancy were noted.

Data regarding patient's demographics, intraoperative findings, and the operation performed were obtained from the clinical records. Cases were included in the analysis only if there was evidence of torsion of the ovary, fallopian tube, or entire adnexa at the time of definitive surgical evaluation. The final pathological diagnosis was also documented.

Results

For 33 patients, the diagnosis of adnexal torsion during the study period was confirmed. The mean age of the patients was 34.9 years (range 14–68 years). Of the 33 patients, 4 patients (12 %) were in the premenarcheal age group, 23 patients (70 %) were in the reproductive age group, and 6 patients (18 %) were postmenopausal (Table 1). Four out of 23 patients in the reproductive age group (17 %) were pregnant at the time of the operative intervention. One of them had a singleton pregnancy of 10 weeks gestation and two patients had triplets [in vitro fertilization (IVF)/ICSI cycle] of 7 and 14 weeks gestation, respectively. Both of them had multiple ovarian cysts because of ovarian hyperstimulation syndrome (OHSS). One patient had cornual interstitial ectopic pregnancy of 6 weeks gestation as well as a dermoid cyst on the same side.

All 33 patients had a unilateral torsion. The torsion was more common on the right side (61 %, n=20) than on the left side (39 %, n=13). Fourteen patients (43 %) had only an ovarian torsion, 10 patients (30 %) only a tubal torsion, and 9 patients (27 %) had a torsion of the entire adnexa (Table 2). Multiple predisposing conditions were found in association with torsion. The most common association was adnexal cyst in 24 patients (72 %), adhesions in 10 cases (30 %), pregnancy in 4 cases (12 %), long tube in 3 cases (9 %), OHSS in 3 cases (9 %), endometriosis in 2 cases (6 %), and pelvic inflammatory disease (PID) in only 1 case (3 %). More than one predisposing factor exists in some patients. There was no identifiable cause in 10 cases (30 %) (Table 3).

The size of the adnexal mass was documented in 26 cases (79 %). Measurements were considered accurate only if the removed specimen was intact and measured at pathological examination. The diameter of the cyst ranged from 3 to 15 cm with a median size of 8 cm. There were nine tumors (35 %) which measured less than 5 cm in size and seven tumors (27 %) which measured more than 10 cm. The majority of them, 10 tumors (38 %), measured between 5 and 10 cm.

The categorization of the operations ranged from a conservative procedure, such as laparoscopic detorsion, to an aggressive procedure, such as adnexectomy. There was no conversion to laparotomy. In 17 cases (52 %), the adnexa were preserved by performing detorsion. In two cases (6 %), detorsion alone was performed, in 13 cases, (40 %) detorsion and cyst enucleation, and in another two cases (6 %), detorsion and cyst aspiration were performed (Table 4).

Following detorsion, we waited for about 30 min, if allowed by the operation conditions, for recovery. Meanwhile, the operative field was continuously irrigated with warm saline in order to observe any sign of reperfusion. After torsion, the enlarged and blood-filled tube, ovary, or whole adnexa, with a variable diameter, are usually dark blue to

Table 1 Patient demographics

Age group	No. (%)
Premenarcheal girls	04 (12)
Reproductive age	23 (70)
Postmenopausal	06 (18)

Table 2 Intraoperative data regarding side and site of torsion

Side of torsion	Right, 20 (61%)
	Left, 13 (39%)
Site of torsion	Ovary, 14 (43%)
	Tube, 10 (30%)
	Adnexa, 9 (27%)

Table 3 Conditions associated with adnexal torsion

Condition	No. (%)
Ovarian cyst (functional and organic)	24 (72)
Adhesions	10 (30)
Pregnancy	04 (12)
Long tube	03 (9)
OHSS	03 (9)
Endometriosis	02 (6)
PID	01 (3)
None	10 (30)

OHSS ovarian hyperstimulation syndrome, *PID* pelvic inflammatory disease

black and partly necrotic. After detorsion, the according organ is left atraumatically to wait for any signs of reperfusion. This is a slight change of color towards a pinkish appearance; however, if reperfusion did not occur, the ovary, tube, or both were resected, which occurred in 16 patients (48 %). Unilateral salpingectomy was performed in 5 patients (15 %) and unilateral adnexectomy in 11 patients (33 %), 6 of them (37 %) were postmenopausal. The mean operating time was 69.2 min (range 40–120 min). No patient had serious complications, such as thromboembolic events, blood transfusion, febrile morbidity, or reoperation. The average duration of stay in the hospital was 2.5 days (range 1–3 days).

The histopathological reports revealed functional or developmental adnexal cyst in 15 cases (45 %), dermoid cyst in 4 cases (12 %), endometrioma in 2 cases (6 %), serous cystadenoma in 3 cases (9 %), ovarian fibroma in only 1 case (3 %), hydrosalpinx in 3 cases (9 %), and normal adnexa in 1 case (3 %) (Table 5). All removed tubes and ovaries showed focal necrosis next to hemorrhage in submucosal as well as orthotopic normal ovarian cortical tissue. There was no histopathological specimen in four patients (4 %) who underwent adnexal-sparing procedures.

Discussion

Despite recent progress with the color Doppler techniques [8], preoperative diagnosis is often difficult, and adnexal torsion can be confused with many other gynecological conditions. The surgical evaluation of these patients should be performed by laparoscopy, thereby avoiding unnecessary laparotomies.

Table 4 Operation performed for adnexal torsion

Operation	No. (%)
Only detorsion	2 (6)
Detorsion and cyst enucleation	13 (40)
Detorsion and cyst aspiration	2 (6)
Detorsion and adnexectomy	11 (33)
Detorsion and salpingectomy	5 (15)

Table 5 Pathological diagnosis

Diagnosis	No. (%)
Functional ovarian cyst	7 (21)
Serous cystadenoma	3 (9)
Dermoid cyst	4 (12)
Endometrioma	2 (6)
Paraovarian cyst	7 (21)
Hydrosalpinx	3 (9)
Para tubal hydatid cyst	1 (3)
Ovarian fibroma	1 (3)
Normal adnexa	1 (3)
No histological specimen	4 (12)

Adnexal torsion is a rare condition which predominantly occurs in the reproductive age group although it has also been reported in premenarcheal girls [9, 10]. Unilateral torsion associated with an adnexal mass is seen more commonly although cases of torsion of normal adnexa have been reported [11]. The mechanism of adnexal torsion is not known conclusively; however, various theories, such as the presence of a long tube, sudden valsalva maneuver [12], pelvic congestion [13], and autonomic dysfunction of tubal peristalsis, have been suggested [14]. Factors that could possibly influence the occurrence of fallopian tube torsion are divided into two types: internal and external (Table 5). Taken together, the existing reports indicate that the mechanism underlying tubal torsion is apparently a sequential mechanical event (Table 6).

In our study, the most common predisposing factor was adnexal cyst in 24 patients (72 %). Ten patients (30 %) had no individual predisposing factors; however, an equal number of patients (30 %) had adhesions which may promote torsion. These results correspond with current literature [15]. Four patients (12 %) were pregnant. The presence of

Table 6 Intrinsic and extrinsic causes of fallopian tube torsion

Intrinsic	Extrinsic
Congenital anomalies	Changes in the neighboring organs
Excessive length of tube or spiral course	Neoplasm, adhesions, pregnancy
Acquired pathology	Mechanical factors
Hydrosalpinx, hematosalpinx, neoplasm, surgery	Movement or trauma to the pelvic organs
Autonomic dysfunction and abnormal peristalsis	Pelvic congestion

Table 7 Possible mechanisms for tubal torsion

• Mechanical disturbance
• Venous obstruction
• Lymphatic congestion
• Diffuse edema
• Tubal enlargement
• Tubal torsion

long tube, OHSS, endometriosis, and PID were all associated with less than 10 % of cases.

Adnexal torsion was more common on the right side (61 %) than on the left (39 %) which may be attributed to the protective effect of the sigmoid colon on the left side and subclinical appendicial infection on the right side, as confirmed, e.g., by Nichols [14]. In the present study, we encountered isolated ovarian torsion in 14 (43 %), entire adnexal torsion in 9 (27 %), and isolated fallopian tube torsion in 10 (30 %) patients. However, isolated fallopian tube torsion has been reported as sporadic cases by many authors [9, 16, 17].

The most common pathological diagnosis in our series was benign ovarian neoplasm (24 %). Half of them were dermoid cyst, functional ovarian cyst (21 %), paraovarian and paratubal cyst (24 %), endometrioma (6 %), hydrosalpinx (9 %), and normal adnexa (3 %). There was no case of malignancy in our series. Many studies report organic ovarian pathologies to be the most common pathological finding [1, 4]. Intrinsic and extrinsic causes of fallopian tube torsion and the possible mechanisms for tubal torsion are given in Tables 5 and 7.

Historically, the treatment of choice for adnexal torsion has been laparotomy and unilateral salpingo-oophorectomy. Although, there has been concern about the significant risk of thromboembolic events by detorsion, various reports, starting from as early as 1946 by S. Way, have suggested the safety of ovarian conservation by detorsion. Laparoscopy has been shown to be a favorable option in patients with torsion. There has been a trend towards increased used of laparoscopy and adnexal-sparing procedures in many centers because of its obvious benefits regarding safety, reliability, and preserving fertility [1, 7, 18, 19].

For the whole of our series, we were able to use laparoscopic surgery to treat 100 % of cases (33 patients) because there was no suspicion of neoplastic pathology during the diagnostic part of the laparoscopy. Seventeen cases of adnexal torsion (52 % of patients) benefited from conservative laparoscopic treatment. These patients underwent detorsion only, with or without cyst aspiration or enucleation. The majority of these were young women desiring fertility. In 48 % of cases, detorsion followed by salpingectomy or adnexectomy was performed. More than half of the patients having an adnexectomy were postmenopausal. In the recent literature, the rate of conservative laparoscopic treatment varies from 35 to 93 % [1, 4, 7, 18, 20].

Laparoscopy in early pregnancy provides a better chance for successful continuation of pregnancy. In our study, there were four pregnant women at the time of conservative laparoscopic surgery. One of the pregnant women who underwent laparoscopic detorsion and cyst aspiration during the 10th week of gestation has an ongoing pregnancy of 30 weeks gestation. Two women of 7 and 14 weeks gestation, with triplets after IVF, miscarried at 20 and 22 weeks, respectively, due to cervical incompetence. The last one had an interstitial ectopic pregnancy. Laparoscopy in pregnancy, especially in later pregnancy, is technically difficult owing to the increased risk of perforation and bleeding. Postoperatively, there is an increased risk of miscarriage or preterm delivery [21].

Conclusion

This study confirms that laparoscopy is the preferable approach for diagnosis and treatment of adnexal torsion. Conservative treatment should be considered in women within the reproductive age, still desiring fertility. Adnexectomy should only be considered beyond the reproductive age and really only in cases with extreme pathology on the adnexa.

Conflict of interest The authors report no conflicts of interest. The authors alone are responsible for the content and writing of the paper.

References

1. Balci O, Icen MS, Mahmoud AS, Capar M, Colakoglu MC (2010) Management and outcomes of adnexal torsion: a 5-year experience. Arch Gynecol Obstet 284(3):643–646. doi:10.1007/s00404-010-1702-z
2. Pansky M, Abargil A, Dreazen E, Golan A, Bukovsky I, Herman A (2000) Conservative management of adnexal torsion in premenarchal girls. J Am Assoc Gynecol Laparosc 7(1):121–124
3. Pena JE, Ufberg D, Cooney N, Denis AL (2000) Usefulness of Doppler sonography in the diagnosis of ovarian torsion. Fertil Steril 73(5):1047–1050
4. Erdemoglu M, Kuyumcuoglu U, Guzel AI (2011) Clinical experience of adnexal torsion: evaluation of 143 cases. J Exp Ther Oncol 9(3):171–174
5. Zweizig S, Perron J, Grubb D, Mishell DR Jr (1993) Conservative management of adnexal torsion. Am J Obstet Gynecol 168(6 Pt 1):1791–1795
6. McGovern PG, Noah R, Koenigsberg R, Little AB (1999) Adnexal torsion and pulmonary embolism: case report and review of the literature. Obstet Gynecol Surv 54(9):601–608
7. Oelsner G, Cohen SB, Soriano D, Admon D, Mashiach S, Carp H (2003) Minimal surgery for the twisted ischaemic adnexa can preserve ovarian function. Hum Reprod 18(12):2599–2602
8. Fleischer AC, Brader KR (2001) Sonographic depiction of ovarian vascularity and flow: current improvements and future applications. J Ultrasound Med 20(3):241–250
9. Schollmeyer T, Soyinka AS, Mabrouk M, Jonat W, Mettler L, Meinhold-Heerlein I (2008) Chronic isolated torsion of the left fallopian tube: a diagnostic dilemma. Arch Gynecol Obstet 277 (1):87–90. doi:10.1007/s00404-007-0411-8

10. Breech LL, Hillard PJ (2005) Adnexal torsion in pediatric and adolescent girls. Curr Opin Obstet Gynecol 17(5):483–489. doi:00001703 200510000 00008
11. Bider D, Mashiach S, Dulitzky M, Kokia E, Lipitz S, Ben-Rafael Z (1991) Clinical, surgical and pathologic findings of adnexal torsion in pregnant and nonpregnant women. Surg Gynecol Obstet 173 (5):363–366
12. Rosado WM Jr, Trambert MA, Gosink BB, Pretorius DH (1992) Adnexal torsion: diagnosis by using Doppler sonography. AJR Am J Roentgenol 159(6):1251–1253
13. Stock RJ (1987) Clinicopathologic changes resulting from adnexal torsion. J Reprod Med 32(3):201–207
14. Nichols DH, Julian PJ (1985) Torsion of the adnexa. Clin Obstet Gynecol 28(2):375–380
15. Argenta PA, Yeagley TJ, Ott G, Sondheimer SJ (2000) Torsion of the uterine adnexa. Pathologic correlations and current management trends. J Reprod Med 45(10):831–836
16. Kurzbart E, Mares AJ, Cohen Z, Mordehai J, Finaly R (1994) Isolated torsion of the fallopian tube in premenarcheal girls. J Pediatr Surg 29(10):1384–1385
17. Wong SW, Suen SH, Lao T, Chung KH (2010) Isolated fallopian tube torsion: a series of six cases. Acta Obstet Gynecol Scand 89(10):1354–1356. doi:10.3109/00016349.2010.503870
18. Oelsner G, Bider D, Goldenberg M, Admon D, Mashiach S (1993) Long-term follow-up of the twisted ischemic adnexa managed by detorsion. Fertil Steril 60(6):976–979
19. Way S (1946) Ovarian cystectomy of twisted cysts. Lancet 2 (6411):47
20. Mage G, Canis M, Manhes H, Pouly JL, Bruhat MA (1989) Laparoscopic management of adnexal torsion. A review of 35 cases. J Reprod Med 34(8):520–524
21. Koo YJ, Lee JE, Lim KT, Shim JU, Mok JE, Kim TJ (2011) A 10-year experience of laparoscopic surgery for adnexal masses during pregnancy. Int J Gynaecol Obstet 113(1):36–39

10

Single-port laparoscopic surgery in gynecology

William Kondo • Reitan Ribeiro • Monica Tessmann Zomer

Abstract The objective of this study is to report the current status on single-port laparoscopic surgery in gynecology. A systematic MEDLINE review of the English language literature from 2007 to 2011 was performed using the search term "single-port surgery," which contained information on single-port laparoscopic surgery in gynecology. Overall, 1,152 patients (26 studies) were included in the analysis. The operative time varied according to the type of procedure. The conversion rate to conventional laparoscopy was 1.99 %, and the conversion rate to laparotomy was 0.35 %. Postoperative complications were encountered in 1.48 % of cases. Different gynecologic procedures have been effectively performed by means of single-port laparoscopic surgery. The procedure seems to be feasible, reproducible, and safe. Reduced pain and improved cosmesis are supposed to be the potential advantages of these procedures, but it was not completely confirmed yet! Further studies are still necessary to establish the real benefits of this new surgical approach over the traditional multi-port laparoscopy.

W. Kondo · M. T. Zomer
Sugisawa Medical Center,
Curitiba, Paraná, Brazil

W. Kondo · R. Ribeiro · M. T. Zomer
Red Cross Hospital,
Curitiba, Paraná, Brazil

W. Kondo · R. Ribeiro · M. T. Zomer
Vita Batel Hospital,
Curitiba, Paraná, Brazil

W. Kondo (✉)
Av. Getulio Vargas, 3163 ap 21,
80240-041 Curitiba, Paraná, Brazil
e-mail: williamkondo@yahoo.com
URL: drwilliamkondo.site.med.br

Keywords Single-port surgery · Laparoscopic surgery · Gynecology · Minimally invasive surgery

Background

Laparoscopic surgery has increasingly assumed a central role in the management of benign and malignant conditions in gynecology [1]. In the last years, various efforts have been made to further minimize the invasiveness of traditional laparoscopy reducing the port size and/or the port number [2–6]. As a result of these efforts, single-port transumbilical laparoscopic surgery has been introduced as a further development of conventional laparoscopy. In this technique, the procedure requires only one incision at the umbilicus, reducing the morbidity of additional incisions (epigastric vessels injury, operative wound infection, visceral organ damage) and improving the final cosmetic outcome [2, 7].

Several terms have been used to describe this surgical procedure [8]: single-port surgery, single-incision laparoscopic surgery (SILS), single-port access surgery, transumbilical endoscopic surgery, laparoendoscopic single-site (LESS) surgery, and embryonic natural orifice transumbilical endoscopic surgery. No matter what term is used, the single-incision approach to gynecological diseases is not a new idea. It has been used in gynecology as early as 1969, when a laparoscopic tubal ligation was described by Wheeless [9]. In 1973, Wheeless and Thompson [10] reported on 2,600 cases of one-incision laparoscopic tubal ligation. The first hysterectomy with bilateral salpingo-oophorectomy performed by means of laparoscopic single-incision access was described by Pelosi and Pelosi [11], in 1991.

Despite the technical challenges associated with complex intracorporeal maneuvers, lack of instrument triangulation, limited traction of tissue, and external crowding and clashing [3, 12], single-port laparoscopic surgery has been successfully

Table 1 Twenty-six studies including 1,152 women undergoing single-port laparoscopic surgery for gynecological pathologies

	Type of surgery (disease)	*N*	Time	Conversion to		Complications
				Laparoscopy	Laparotomy	
[14]	Total hysterectomy	105	120	11	2	6
	Subtotal hysterectomy	11	180			
	Oophorectomy	43	60			
	Ovarian cystectomy	31	105			
	Salpingectomy	5	60			
	Myomectomy	2				
	Adhesiolysis	3				
	Total	200	[a]			
[18]	Pelvic and/or para-aortic lymph node sampling or lymphadenectomy (early stage gynecologic malignancies)	21	120	0	0	0
[19]	Risk-reducing salpingo-oophorectomy with and without hysterectomy	58	38.1	0	0	0
[20]	Benign adnexal disease	9	N/A	1	0	0
[21]	Total hysterectomy	100	80	0	0	0
[22][b]	Laparoscopic-assisted vaginal hysterectomy	183	78.8	2	0	0
[23][b]	Salpingo-oophorectomy	17				
	Cystectomy	2				
	Ectopic pregnancy (salpingectomy)	2				
	Myomectomy	5				
	Laparoscopic assisted vaginal hysterectomy	1				
	Hysterectomy	11	199			
	Total	38	[a]	0	0	0
[24]	Adnexal tumors	94	50.33	2	2	0
[25]	Extraperitoneal para-aortic lymphadenectomy (locally advanced cervical cancer)	14	190	0	0	0
[26]	Low-risk early endometrial cancer	20	105	0	0	0
[27]	Myomectomy	12	100	0	0	0
[28]	Salpingoophorectomy (n=9), ovarian cyst enucleation (n=5), and salpingectomy (n=2) (benign adnexal pathologies)	16	42	0	0	0
[29]	Adnexal lesions	86	64.5	2	0	4
[30]	Adnexal tumors	12	79	0	0	0
[31]	Myomectomy with transumbilical morcellation	15	96.7	0	0	0
[32][b]	Salpingectomy	30	52.6	0	0	0
[33][b]	Hand-assisted laparoscopic surgery (large adnexal tumors)	43	75	0	0	0
[34]	Myomectomy	15	81	1	0	0
[35][b]	Laparoscopically assisted vaginal hysterectomy	47	92.4	0	0	2
[36]	Adnexal tumors	100	55	1	0	0
[37]	Ectopic pregnancy	12	48.5	0	0	2
[38]	Pelvic surgeries	19	96	0	0	0
[39]	Abdominal sacral colpopexy	10	162	0	0	0
[40]	Salpingectomies	27	70	1	0	0
	Salpingotomies	5				
[17][b]	Laparoscopic-assisted vaginal hysterectomy	50	122	2	0	1
[12]	Hysterectomy	11	163.3	0	0	2
TOTAL	Different surgical procedures	1152	[a]	23 (1.99 %)	4 (0.35 %)	17 (1.48 %)

[a] Operative time varied according to the type of procedure

[b] Comparative studies between single-port laparoscopic surgery and traditional laparoscopy

performed by experienced groups in gynecologic surgery [1, 12–17].

In this paper, we conducted a MEDLINE literature search of all publications in English language from 2007 to 2011 using the search term "single-port surgery," as well as a review of all references to summarize the existing clinical experience on single-port laparoscopic surgery in gynecology.

Methods

Sources

A systematic MEDLINE review of the English language literature from 2007 To 2011 was performed using the search term "single-port surgery," which contained information on single-port laparoscopic surgery in gynecology.

Study selection

Entrance criteria for the MEDLINE search term "single-port surgery" included: patients undergoing single-port surgery in gynecology. Review articles and case reports were excluded from the analysis. The review of the English language literature identified 995 papers on single-port surgery. A total of 72 papers included gynecologic procedures and 26 studies were selected for further analysis.

Findings

A total of 72 papers were published from 2007 to 2011 on gynecologic single-port surgery. Twenty-six studies were put together in the Table 1. A total of 1,152 women underwent different surgical procedures by means of single-port surgery. The operative time varied according to the type of procedure. Overall, the conversion rate to conventional laparoscopy was 1.99 %, and the conversion rate to laparotomy was 0.35 %. The surgical morbidity was low (1.48 %). Therefore, single-port laparoscopic surgery may be applied to most benign gynecologic surgeries without detrimental effects on clinical outcomes.

The implementation of the single-port surgery in a gynecologic service was evaluated by Lee et al. [41]. They retrospectively evaluated the medical records of 500 consecutive patients undergoing laparotomic or laparoscopic surgery for benign gynecologic diseases. The surgeries included hysterectomy (n=239), adnexal surgery (n=194), myomectomy (n=33), adnexal surgery + myomectomy (n=18), and other procedures (n=16). They divided the patients into five groups of 100 patients each, and they observed an increasing rate of single-port laparoscopic procedures over the period—29 %, 62 %, 72 %, 71 %, and 86 %. In the last group, laparotomy and multiport laparoscopy were required in only 4 % and 10 % of the cases, respectively. They did not notice any differences in the median operative time or complication rate over the study period.

Despite these preliminary optimistic results in the outcomes of single-port surgery, an experienced laparoscopic skill set seems to be essential for the safe and effective completion of surgery [42].

Technique

The procedure may be typically performed by means of two approaches. The first is single-site surgery, in which two or more conventional ports are placed through a single incision (Fig. 1). The second approach is performed by using a single-port multichannel device, through which multiple instruments and the laparoscope are passed [43].

Instruments and devices

Different single-port devices have been developed to try to fulfill the requirements of this new surgical technique:

- SILS port multiple instrument access port (Covidien®, Mansfield, MA) (Fig. 2);
- TriPort (Advanced Surgical Concepts, Wicklow, Ireland);
- GelPOINT system (Applied Medical, Rancho Santa Margarita, CA) (Fig. 3);
- AirSeal DPS (SurgiQuest, Orange, CT);
- R-Port (Advanced Surgical Concepts, Wicklow, Ireland);
- Quadriport (Advanced Surgical Concepts, Wicklow, Ireland);
- Uni-X single-port access laparoscopic system (PNavel systems, Cleveland, OH);
- Single-site laparoscopy access system (Ethicon Endo-surgery, Cincinnati, OH) (Fig. 4);
- SITRACC (Edlo Company, Porto Alegre, Brazil) (Fig. 5).

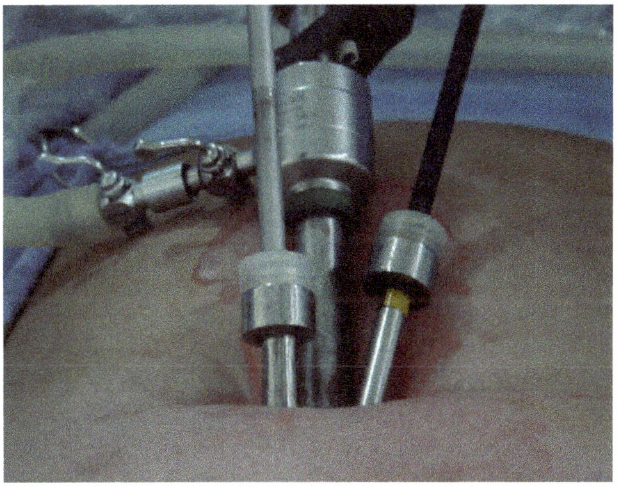

Fig. 1 Right salpingectomy performed by means of three conventional trocars placed inside the umbilicus

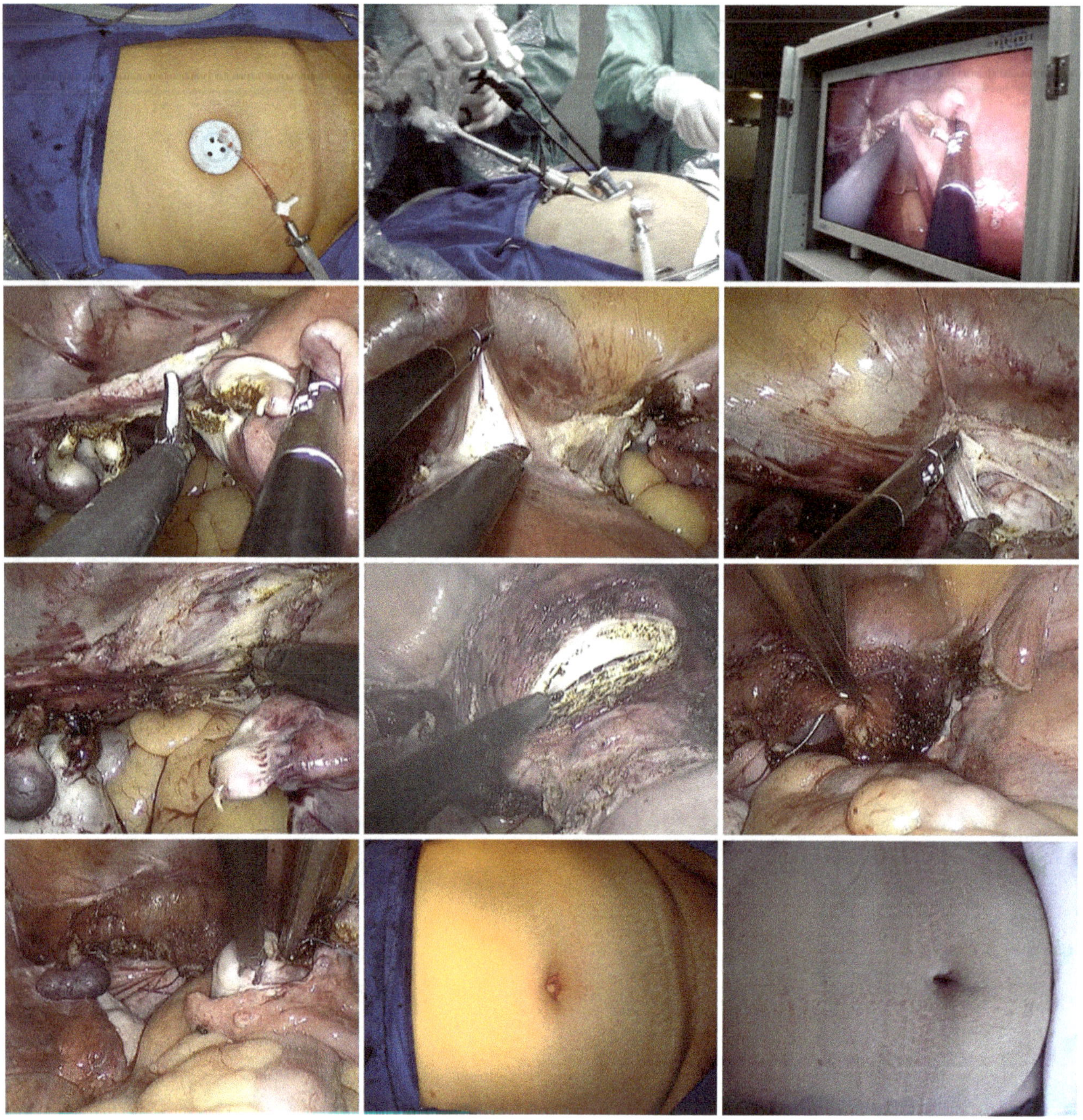

Fig. 2 Single-port total laparoscopic hysterectomy using the SILS device

One study [44] compared the technical performance between conventional laparoscopic and single-port devices (SILS port, the TriPort access system, and the GelPOINT system) in a surgical simulator. Overall, the TriPort was more challenging for novices to use in learning the single-port procedure than either the SILS port or the GelPOINT system. The GelPOINT system offered the most consistent platform for single-port surgery performance and novice skill acquisition. In our preliminary experience using the single-site surgery, the SILS port, the SITRACC device, the GelPoint, and the single-site laparoscopy access system, both the SILS platform and the single-site laparoscopy access system seemed to be the more comfortable devices for pelvic gynecologic procedures.

Also, the development of articulating and bent instrumentation permits triangulation intracorporeally despite the close proximity of several instruments via a single port [42].

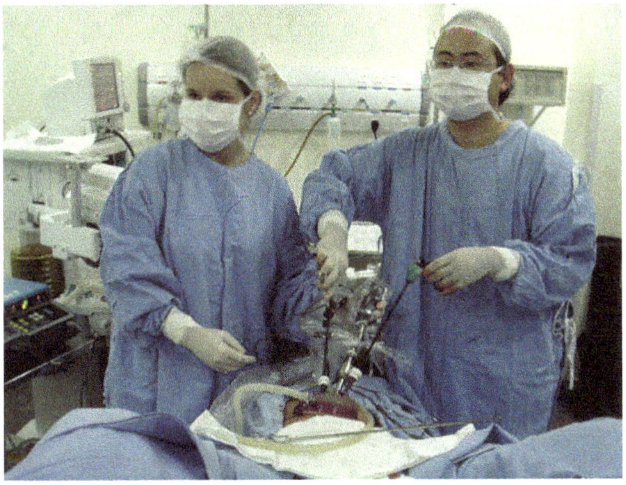

Fig. 3 Single-port laparoscopic salpingectomy using the GelPOINT system

Learning curve

Whenever a new surgical technique is introduced into clinical practice, there is a specific learning curve that surgeons have to manage in order to improve their skills and the safety of the procedure.

Paek et al. [21] evaluated 100 patients who underwent single-port total laparoscopic hysterectomy to define the learning curve for the procedure. The median time until the removal of the specimen was 45 min, and the median time for closure of the vaginal cuff was 18 min. The median total operative time (from skin opening to closure) was 80 min. Proficiency at the procedure was achieved after 40 cases. The time for vaginal closure the decreased significantly from the first 20 cases to the next, and the total operating time decreased significantly from the second 20 cases to the next.

In the experience of Song et al. [45], the proficiency and plateau were determined after approximately 25 and 75 cases of single-port laparoscopic-assisted vaginal hysterectomies, respectively. Conversely, Lee et al. [46] showed a shorter learning curve for such procedure. They observed a tendency toward a decreased operative time after ten cases of single-port laparoscopic-assisted vaginal hysterectomy.

Comparative studies

Prospective randomized studies comparing the outcomes of single-port and traditional laparoscopic surgeries are required to establish the actual benefits and disadvantages of the new minimally invasive technique.

Lee et al. [47] compared the perioperative outcomes between 17 single-port laparoscopic adnexal surgeries and 34 conventional laparoscopic adnexal surgeries. There were no differences between the two groups in median operative time (64 vs. 57.5 min, p=0.252), the number of patients that requested additional parenteral non-steroidal anti-inflammatory drugs (7 patients vs. 19 patients, p=0.597), and the absolute decrease (1.3 mg/dl vs. 1.1 mg/dl, p=0.640) from preoperative hemoglobin to postoperative day 1 measurements. No blood transfusion was required. There were no complications.

From January to June 2009, Yoon et al. [32] conducted a comparative study between single-port laparoscopic salpingectomy (n=30) and conventional laparoscopic salpingectomy (n=30) for the treatment of tubal pregnancy. All operations were completed successfully. No significant difference was observed between the two groups in terms of mean operative time (52.6±16.1 min vs 46.8±16.2 min; p= 0.174), mean difference between pre- and postoperative hemoglobin (1.7±0.8 g/dl vs 1.8±1.0 g/dl; p=0.636), or mean postoperative hospital stay (2.4±0.5 days vs 2.4±

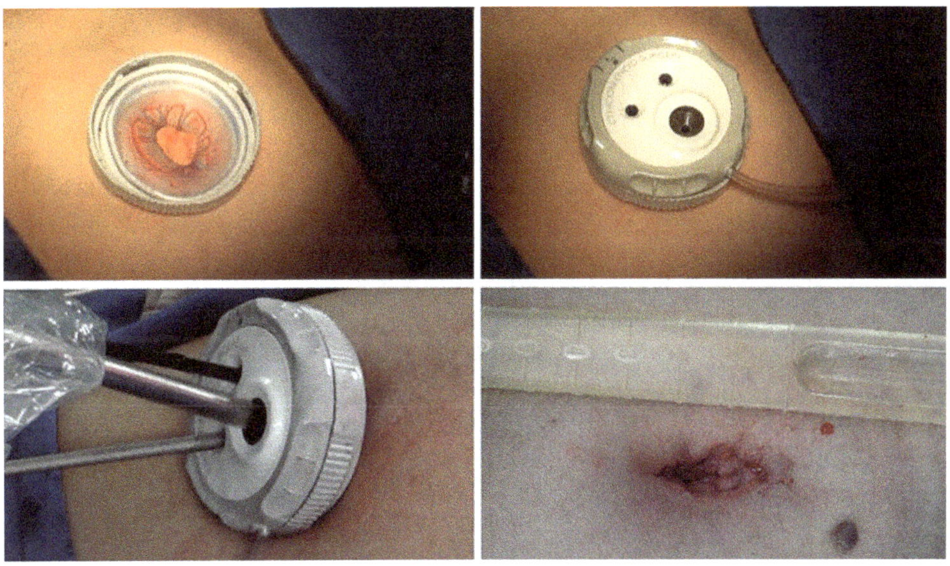

Fig. 4 Single-port total laparoscopic hysterectomy using the single-site laparoscopy access system

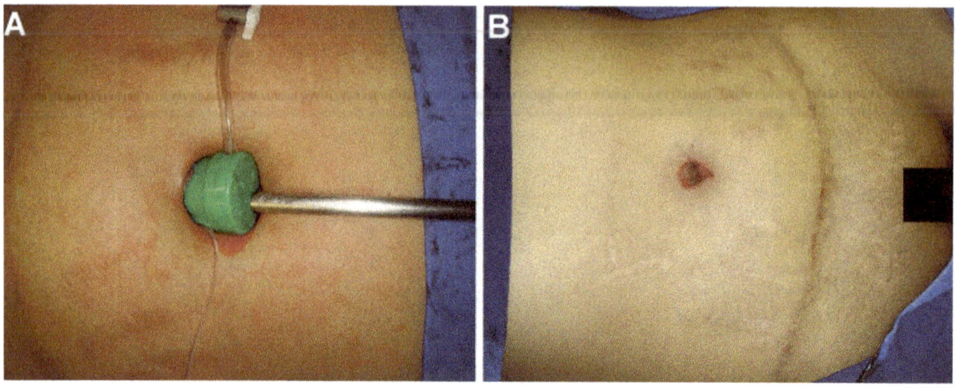

Fig. 5 Single-port total laparoscopic hysterectomy using the SITRACC

0.9 days; $p=1.000$). No complications were encountered in either group, and there was no conversion to conventional laparoscopy in the single-port surgery group.

In a retrospective study, Yim et al. [13] compared surgical outcomes and postoperative pain between single-port total laparoscopic hysterectomy ($n=52$) and conventional four-port total laparoscopic hysterectomy ($n=105$). The single-port group had less intraoperative blood loss ($p<0.001$), shorter hospital stay ($p=0.001$), and earlier diet intake ($p<0.001$) compared with the conventional group. There was no difference in perioperative complications. Immediate postoperative pain score was lower in the single-port group ($p<0.001$). Postoperative pain after 6 and 24 h was lower in single-port group with marginal statistical significance.

Kim et al. [48] retrospectively compared the perioperative outcomes of single-port laparoscopic-assisted vaginal hysterectomy ($n=43$) and conventional laparoscopic-assisted vaginal hysterectomy ($n=43$). There was one conversion to laparotomy in the former group and two in the latter group. Additionally, three patients in the former group needed the placement of additional trocars (conversion to traditional laparoscopy). The operative time (119 vs. 124 min; $p=0.6$), estimated blood loss (369 vs. 378 ml; $p=0.9$), drop in hemoglobin preoperatively to postoperative day 1 (14.6 % vs. 12.1 %; $p=0.2$), and postoperative hospital stay were comparable between both groups (2.8 vs. 2.7 days; $p=0.9$). Single-port laparoscopic-assisted vaginal hysterectomy was associated with reduced postoperative pain. There were no complications, including reoperation, adjacent organ damage, and any postoperative morbidity, in both groups.

Escobar et al. [49] compared the surgical outcomes of single-port laparoscopy for the surgical treatment of presumed early stage endometrial cancer (stage I or occult stage II endometrial cancer) to laparoscopy and robotics. Thirty patients were included in each group. There were no significant differences in median operating time or estimated blood loss between the three groups. The median number of pelvic lymph nodes obtained was significantly higher in the robotic ($n=17$) and single-port group ($n=16$) compared with the laparoscopy group ($n=13$). However, there was no significant difference in the median number of para-aortic nodes obtained between the three groups. There was no significant difference between the groups in length of hospital stay, comorbid conditions, complication rates, or operative times.

Training courses

Training courses allow inexperienced surgeons to learn and improve minimally invasive surgical techniques. They play an important role in the acquisition of specific skills in the single-port approach.

Botden et al. [50] evaluated 15 participants performing three basic tasks (translocation, clip and cut, and tissue dissection, based on the fundamentals of laparoscopic surgery) in the box trainer in laparoscopy and single-port access settings with both (conventional) crossed and curved instruments. Although conventional laparoscopy appeared most effective for proper dissection and tissue exposure, single-port access surgery showed potential. Especially in the tissue dissection task, there was no significant difference in time or errors between conventional laparoscopy and single-port surgery, using especially designed curved instruments.

In the study of Montero et al. [51], single-port laparoscopic surgery was associated with poorer performance and increased surgeon workload compared with standard laparoscopy. It was improved when angulated instruments were used for simulated tasks instead of straight instruments, but it still remained inferior to standard laparoscopy. Therefore, specialized training courses seem to be effective for developing single-port laparoscopic skills [52].

Robotics single-port surgery

Robotics may enhance surgical skills during single-port laparoscopic surgery and decrease the learning curve.

In 2011, Escobar et al. [53] evaluated a novel single-port robotic platform in the cadaver model. They demonstrated that the performance of various procedures in gynecologic oncology using the new da Vinci® single-site robotic platform is feasible and, more importantly, reproducible in the cadaver model.

In the initial series of Nam et al. [54], they operated on seven patients using robotics to perform single-port transumbilical total hysterectomy. Procedures included total hysterectomy due to benign gynecological disease ($n=5$), extra-fascial hysterectomy due to carcinoma in situ of the cervix ($n=1$), and radical hysterectomy due to cervical cancer IB1 ($n=1$). The median total operative time was 109 min (range, 105 to 311 min); the median blood loss was 100 ml (range, 10 to 750 ml), and the median weight of the resected uteri was 200 g (range, 40 to 310 g). One benign case was converted to three-port robotic surgery due to severe pelvic adhesions, and no post-operative complications occurred.

Controversies

Most studies do not show any superiority of the single-port access over conventional laparoscopic procedures [14]. The possible cosmetic advantage was not proved yet. Depending on the shape of the patient's umbilical scar, the skin incision cannot be performed completely inside the umbilicus. Some studies demonstrated a reduction in the postoperative pain using the single-port access [13, 17, 48]; however, one could think that maybe a bigger single incision could be more painful that four smaller incisions and could have an increased risk of incisional hernia.

Chen et al. [17] compared the immediate results of patients undergoing either two-channel single-port laparoscopic-assisted vaginal hysterectomy ($n=50$) or conventional multi-port laparoscopic-assisted vaginal hysterectomy ($n=50$). There were no statistically significant differences in operative time, estimated blood loss, time to first flatus, intraoperative and immediate postoperative complications, shoulder tip pain, or length of hospital stay between the two groups. However, postoperative pain was significantly less in the single-port group compared with the conventional group, as evidenced by lower mean scores on the visual analog scale and less mean accumulated dose of postoperative analgesics. Conversely, a randomized prospective study of single-port and four-port approaches for hysterectomy conducted by Jung et al. [2] did not demonstrate any reduction of the postoperative pain with single-port access. The surgical outcomes were similar for both groups.

Tsimogiannis et al. [55] conducted a randomized study of 20 patients undergoing standard four-port laparoscopic cholecystectomy and 20 patients undergoing LESS. They observed a higher inflammatory reaction in the latter group, demonstrated by the higher levels of postoperative α-defensins in this group. However, pain was statistically significantly less for the LESS group at the 24-h interval, and less pain medication was needed for LESS patients after the sixth postoperative hour.

In the experience of Gunderson et al. [56], the risk of umbilical hernia with laparoendoscopic single-site surgery was 2.4 %. When they excluded some patients ("high risk" subjects for incisional disruption) from the analysis, the umbilical hernia rate was 0.5 %.

Final considerations

Single-port surgery is the latest innovation in minimally invasive surgery and seems to be feasible, reproducible, and safe to perform different gynecologic procedures. Reduced pain and improved cosmesis are supposed to be the potential advantages of these procedures, but it was not completely confirmed yet! Further studies are still necessary to establish the real benefits of this new surgical approach over the traditional multi-port laparoscopy.

Declaration of interest The authors report no conflicts of interest. The authors alone are responsible for the content and writing of the paper.

References

1. Mohd J, Siow A (2011) Single-port access total laparoscopic hysterectomy for stage 1A1 cancer of the cervix. Singapore Med J 52(6):e111–e114
2. Jung YW, Lee M, Yim GW, Lee SH, Paek JH, Kwon HY, Nam EJ, Kim SW, Kim YT (2011) A randomized prospective study of single-port and four-port approaches for hysterectomy in terms of postoperative pain. Surg Endosc 25(8):2462–2469
3. Branco AW, Kondo W, Stunitz LC, Filho AJ, de George MA (2009) Transumbilical laparoscopic urological surgery: are special devices strictly necessary? BJU Int 104(8):1136–1142
4. de George MA, Rangel M, Noda RW, Kondo W (2009) Laparoscopic transumbilical cholecystectomy: surgical technique. JSLS 13(4):536–541
5. Romanelli JR, Earle DB (2009) Single-port laparoscopic surgery: an overview. Surg Endosc 23(7):1419–1427
6. Canes D, Desai MM, Aron M, Haber GP, Goel RK, Stein RJ, Kaouk JH, Gill IS (2008) Transumbilical single-port surgery: evolution and current status. Eur Urol 54(5):1020–1029
7. Fader AN, Escobar PF (2009) Laparoendoscopic single-site surgery (LESS) in gynecologic oncology: technique and initial report. Gynecol Oncol 114(2):157–161
8. Zhu JF (2009) Which term is better: SILS, SPA, LESS, E-NOTES, or TUES? Surg Endosc 23(5):1164–1165
9. Wheeless CR Jr (1969) A rapid, inexpensive, and effective method of surgical sterilization by laparoscopy. J Reprod Med 3:65–69
10. Wheeless CR Jr, Thompson BH (1973) Laparoscopic sterilization. Review of 3600 cases. Obstet Gynecol 42(5):751–758
11. Pelosi MA, Pelosi MA 3rd (1991) Laparoscopic hysterectomy with bilateral salpingo-oophorectomy using a single umbilical puncture. N J Med 88(10):721–726
12. Phongnarisorn C, Chinthakanan O (2011) Transumbilical single-incision laparoscopic hysterectomy with conventional laparoscopic instruments in patients with symptomatic leiomyoma and/or adenomyosis. Arch Gynecol Obstet 284(4):893–900
13. Yim GW, Jung YW, Paek J, Lee SH, Kwon HY, Nam EJ, Kim S, Kim JH, Kim YT, Kim SW (2010) Transumbilical single-port

access versus conventional total laparoscopic hysterectomy: surgical outcomes. Am J Obstet Gynecol 203(1):26.e1–26.e6
14. Park HS, Kim TJ, Song T, Kim MK, Lee YY, Choi CH, Lee JW, Kim BG, Bae DS (2011) Single-port access (SPA) laparoscopic surgery in gynecology: a surgeon's experience with an initial 200 cases. Eur J Obstet Gynecol Reprod Biol 154(1):81–84
15. Paek J, Nam EJ, Kim YT, Kim SW (2011) Overcoming technical difficulties with single-port access laparoscopic surgery in gynecology: using conventional laparoscopic instruments. J Laparoendosc Adv Surg Tech A 21(2):137–141
16. Lee JH, Choi JS, Jeon SW, Son CE, Hong JH, Bae JW (2011) A prospective comparison of single-port laparoscopically assisted vaginal hysterectomy using transumbilical GelPort access and multiport laparoscopically assisted vaginal hysterectomy. Eur J Obstet Gynecol Reprod Biol 158(2):294–297
17. Chen YJ, Wang PH, Ocampo EJ, Twu NF, Yen MS, Chao KC (2011) Single-port compared with conventional laparoscopic-assisted vaginal hysterectomy: a randomized controlled trial. Obstet Gynecol 117(4):906–912
18. Escobar PF, Fader AN, Rasool N, Espalliat LR (2010) Single-port laparoscopic pelvic and para-aortic lymph node sampling or lymphadenectomy: development of a technique and instrumentation. Int J Gynecol Cancer 20(7):1268–1273
19. Escobar PF, Starks DC, Fader AN, Barber M, Rojas-Espalliat L (2010) Single-port risk-reducing salpingo-oophorectomy with and without hysterectomy: surgical outcomes and learning curve analysis. Gynecol Oncol 119(1):43–47
20. Escobar PF, Bedaiwy MA, Fader AN, Falcone T (2010) Laparoendoscopic single-site (LESS) surgery in patients with benign adnexal disease. Fertil Steril 93(6):2074.e7–2074.e10
21. Paek J, Kim SW, Lee SH, Lee M, Yim GW, Nam EJ, Kim YT (2011) Learning curve and surgical outcome for single-port access total laparoscopic hysterectomy in 100 consecutive cases. Gynecol Obstet Invest 72(4):227–233
22. Jung MH, Lee BY (2011) Transumbilical single-port laparoscopic-assisted vaginal hysterectomy via 12-mm trocar incision site. J Laparoendosc Adv Surg Tech A 21(7):599–602
23. Ichikawa M, Akira S, Mine K, Ohuchi N, Iwasaki N, Kurose K, Takeshita T (2011) Evaluation of laparoendoscopic single-site gynecologic surgery with a multitrocar access system. J Nihon Med Sch 78(4):235–240
24. Kim WC, Lee JE, Kwon YS, Koo YJ, Lee IH, Lim KT (2011) Laparoendoscopic single-site surgery (LESS) for adnexal tumors: one surgeon's initial experience over a one-year period. Eur J Obstet Gynecol Reprod Biol 158(2):265–268
25. Gouy S, Kane A, Uzan C, Gauthier T, Gilmore J, Morice P (2011) Single-port laparoscopy and extraperitoneal para-aortic lymphadenectomy: about fourteen consecutive cases. Gynecol Oncol 123 (2):329–332
26. Fanfani F, Rossitto C, Gagliardi ML, Gallotta V, Gueli Alletti S, Scambia G, Fagotti A (2012) Total laparoendoscopic single-site surgery (LESS) hysterectomy in low-risk early endometrial cancer: a pilot study. Surg Endosc 26(1):41–46
27. Yoshiki N, Okawa T, Kubota T (2011) Single-incision laparoscopic myomectomy with intracorporeal suturing. Fertil Steril 95 (7):2426–2428
28. Mereu L, Angioni S, Melis GB, Mencaglia L (2010) Single access laparoscopy for adnexal pathologies using a novel reusable port and curved instruments. Int J Gynaecol Obstet 109(1):78–80
29. Jung YW, Choi YM, Chung CK, Yim GW, Lee M, Lee SH, Paek JH, Nam EJ, Kim YT, Kim SW (2011) Single port transumbilical laparoscopic surgery for adnexal lesions: a single center experience in Korea. Eur J Obstet Gynecol Reprod Biol 155(2):221–224
30. Lim MC, Kim TJ, Kang S, Bae DS, Park SY, Seo SS (2009) Embryonic natural orifice transumbilical endoscopic surgery (E-NOTES) for adnexal tumors. Surg Endosc 23(11):2445–2449
31. Kim YW, Park BJ, Ro DY, Kim TE (2010) Single-port laparoscopic myomectomy using a new single-port transumbilical morcellation system: initial clinical study. J Minim Invasive Gynecol 17(5):587–592
32. Yoon BS, Park H, Seong SJ, Park CT, Jun HS, Kim IH (2011) Single-port versus conventional laparoscopic salpingectomy in tubal pregnancy: a comparison of surgical outcomes. Eur J Obstet Gynecol Reprod Biol 159(1):190–193
33. Roh HJ, Lee SJ, Ahn JW, Kwon YS, Cho HJ, Kim DY (2012) Single-port-access, hand-assisted laparoscopic surgery for benign large adnexal tumors versus single-port pure laparoscopic surgery for adnexal tumors. Surg Endosc 26(3):693–703
34. Lee JH, Choi JS, Jeon SW, Son CE, Lee SJ, Lee YS (2010) Single-port laparoscopic myomectomy using transumbilical GelPort access. Eur J Obstet Gynecol Reprod Biol 153(1):81–84
35. Lee JH, Choi JS, Hong JH, Joo KJ, Kim BY (2011) Does conventional or single port laparoscopically assisted vaginal hysterectomy affect female sexual function? Acta Obstet Gynecol Scand 90 (12):1410–1415
36. Takeda A, Imoto S, Mori M, Nakano T, Nakamura H (2011) Isobaric laparoendoscopic single-site surgery with wound retractor for adnexal tumors: a single center experience with the initial 100 cases. Eur J Obstet Gynecol Reprod Biol 157(2):190–196
37. Takeda A, Imoto S, Mori M, Nakano T, Nakamura H (2011) Early experience with isobaric laparoendoscopic single-site surgery using a wound retractor for the management of ectopic pregnancy. Eur J Obstet Gynecol Reprod Biol 154(2):209–214
38. Rettenmaier MA, Abaid LN, Erwin MR, John CR, Micha JP, Brown JV 3rd, Goldstein BH (2009) A retrospective review of the GelPort system in single-port access pelvic surgery. J Minim Invasive Gynecol 16(6):743–747
39. White WM, Goel RK, Swartz MA, Moore C, Rackley RR, Kaouk JH (2009) Single-port laparoscopic abdominal sacral colpopexy: initial experience and comparative outcomes. Urology 74(5):1008–1012
40. Lamourdedieu C, Rua S, Lazard A, Marcelli M, Cravello L, Gamerre M, Agostini A (2011) Surgical treatment of ectopic pregnancy by single port access with SILS® system: preliminary study. J Gynecol Obstet Biol Reprod (Paris) 40(7):620–625
41. Lee M, Kim SW, Nam EJ, Yim GW, Kim S, Kim YT (2011) Single-port laparoscopic surgery is applicable to most gynecologic surgery: a single surgeon's experience. Surg Endosc (in press)
42. Kommu SS, Rané A (2009) Devices for laparoendoscopic single-site surgery in urology. Expert Rev Med Devices 6(1):95–103
43. Fader AN, Levinson KL, Gunderson CC, Winder AD, Escobar PF (2011) Laparoendoscopic single-site surgery in gynaecology: a new frontier in minimally invasive surgery. J Minim Access Surg 7(1):71–77
44. Brown-Clerk B, de Laveaga AE, LaGrange CA, Wirth LM, Lowndes BR, Hallbeck MS (2011) Laparoendoscopic single site (LESS) surgery versus conventional laparoscopic surgery: comparison of surgical port performance in a surgical simulator with novices. Surg Endosc 25(7):2210–2218
45. Song T, Kim TJ, Lee YY, Choi CH, Lee JW, Kim BG, Bae DS (2011) What is the learning curve for single-port access laparoscopic-assisted vaginal hysterectomy? Eur J Obstet Gynecol Reprod Biol 158(1):93–96
46. Lee YY, Kim TJ, Kim CJ, Kang H, Choi CH, Lee JW, Kim BG, Lee JH, Bae DS (2009) Single-port access laparoscopic-assisted vaginal hysterectomy: a novel method with a wound retractor and a glove. J Minim Invasive Gynecol 16(4):450–453
47. Lee YY, Kim TJ, Kim CJ, Park HS, Choi CH, Lee JW, Lee JH, Bae DS, Kim BG (2010) Single port access laparoscopic adnexal surgery versus conventional laparoscopic adnexal surgery: a comparison of peri-operative outcomes. Eur J Obstet Gynecol Reprod Biol 151(2):181–184
48. Kim TJ, Lee YY, Cha HH, Kim CJ, Choi CH, Lee JW, Bae DS, Lee JH, Kim BG (2010) Single-port-access laparoscopic-assisted

vaginal hysterectomy versus conventional laparoscopic-assisted vaginal hysterectomy: a comparison of perioperative outcomes. Surg Endosc 24(9):2248–2252

49. Escobar PF, Frumovitz M, Soliman PT, Frasure HE, Fader AN, Schmeler KM, Ramirez PT (2011) Comparison of single-port laparoscopy, standard laparoscopy, and robotic surgery in patients with endometrial cancer. Ann Surg Oncol (in press)
50. Botden S, Strijkers R, Fransen S, Stassen L, Bouvy N (2011) The use of curved vs. straight instruments in single port access surgery, on standardized box trainer tasks. Surg Endosc 25(8):2703–2710
51. Montero PN, Acker CE, Heniford BT, Stefanidis D (2011) Single incision laparoscopic surgery (SILS) is associated with poorer performance and increased surgeon workload compared with standard laparoscopy. Am Surg 77(1):73–77
52. Yang B, Xu B, Zeng Q, Altunrende F, Wang H, Xiao L, Wang L, Xu C, Sun Y (2011) A specialized course of basic skills training for single-port laparoscopic surgery. Surgery 149(6):766–775
53. Escobar PF, Kebria M, Falcone T (2011) Evaluation of a novel single-port robotic platform in the cadaver model for the performance of various procedures in gynecologic oncology. Gynecol Oncol 120(3):380–384
54. Nam EJ, Kim SW, Lee M, Yim GW, Paek JH, Lee SH, Kim S, Kim JH, Kim JW, Kim YT (2011) Robotic single-port transumbilical total hysterectomy: a pilot study. J Gynecol Oncol 22(2):120–126
55. Tsimogiannis KE, Tellis CC, Tselepis AD, Pappas-Gogos G, Bakola MS, Tsimoyiannis EC, Simopoulos CE, Pitiakoudis M (2012) α-Defensins and hsCRP levels in inflammatory response of standard and laparoendoscopic single-site cholecystectomy. Surg Endosc 26(3):627–631
56. Gunderson CC, Knight J, Ybanez-Morano J, Ritter C, Escobar PF, Ibeanu O, Grumbine FC, Bedaiwy MA, Hurd WW, Fader AN (2012) The risk of umbilical hernia and other complications with laparoendoscopic single-site surgery. J Minim Invasive Gynecol 19(1):40–45

11

Office microlaparoscopic ovarian drilling versus conventional laparoscopic ovarian drilling for women with polycystic ovary syndrome

Imaduldin Salah

Abstract It is a prospective controlled study to compare the beneficial effects of office microlaparoscopic ovarian drilling (OMLOD) under augmented local anesthesia, as a new modality treatment option, compared to those following ovarian drilling with the conventional traditional 10-mm laparoscope under general anesthesia. The study included 60 anovulatory women with polycystic ovary syndrome (PCOS) who underwent OMLOD (study group) and 60 anovulatory PCOS women, where the conventional laparoscopic ovarian drilling (LOD), using 10-mm laparoscope under general anesthesia, was performed (comparison group). Transvaginal ultrasound scan and blood sampling to measure the serum concentrations of LH, FSH, testosterone, and androstenedione had been performed before and after the procedure. Intra- and postoperative pain score in candidate women had been evaluated during the office microlaparoscopic procedure, in addition to the number of candidates who needed extra analgesia. The women undergoing OMLOD showed a good intra- and postoperative perception pain score. The number of those patients discharged within the first 2 h after office procedure was significantly higher, without the need for postoperative analgesia with most patients. The LH/FSH ratio and mean serum concentrations of LH, testosterone, and free androgen index have decreased significantly after both OMLOD and LOD within a postoperative year follow-up. The mean ovarian volume decreased significantly ($P<0.05$) within the year after both OMLOD and LOD. There were no significant differences in those results after both procedures. Intra- and postoperative augmented local anesthesia allows outpatient bilateral ovarian drilling by microlaparoscopy without general anesthesia. The relatively high pregnancy rate, the simplicity of the method, and the faster discharge time after the operation offer a new modality option for patients with PCOS, who are resistant to clomiphene citrate ovarian induction. Moreover, ovarian drilling could be performed simultaneously during the routine diagnostic microlaparoscopy and integrated in the fertility work-up investigations for those patients.

Keywords Endocrine effects · Office microlaparoscopic ovarian drilling · Long-term follow-up · Polycystic ovary syndrome · Polycystic ovaries

I. Salah (✉)
College of Medicine,
El Minya, Egypt
e-mail: imaduldin69@hotmail.com

Background

Polycystic ovary syndrome (PCOS) is the most frequent etiological cause of anovulation observed in approximately 75 % of infertile women with ovulation disorder. Patients with PCOS have various clinical symptoms and laboratory findings. PCOS presents mainly as a menstrual abnormality and infertility associated with ovulation disorder. A variety of surgical options for the treatment of PCOS have been applied during laparoscopy procedure, such as condemned laparoscopic ovarian wedge resection, electrocoagulation, and laser surgery. Laparoscopic ovarian diathermy represents an effective treatment for clomiphene citrate (CC)-resistant patients and possesses numerous advantages over gonadotropin therapy, including no increased risk of ovarian hyperstimulation or multiple pregnancy and a lower incidence of spontaneous abortion [1, 2].

Ovarian stimulation has been shown to increase the risk of perinatal complications. Even in vitro fertilization-assisted reproductive techniques lead to a higher risk for multiple pregnancies, prematurity, low and very low birth weight, transfer to the neonatal intensive care unit, and various neonatal morbidity parameters. Thus, it has been proposed that ovulation induction by laparoscopic ovarian drilling (LOD) may improve the overall outcomes of pregnancies in PCOS patients. A comparison of pregnancy outcomes of women with PCOS, who had undergone LOD and non-PCOS pregnancy controls, demonstrated a significantly higher risk of hypertensive disorders and gestational diabetes mellitus for the PCOS group [3–7].

Laparoscopic ovarian drilling has been approved as the gold standard second-line treatment for anovulatory infertility due to polycystic ovary syndrome after failure to respond after course of clomiphene citrate. Not only does LOD produce high ovulation and pregnancy rates, but it also corrects the endocrine abnormalities associated with the syndrome [4, 8]. With the development of new, small-diameter laparoscopes that provide an optical view comparable to conventional instruments, microlaparoscopy can now be used routinely for diagnostic laparoscopy [9, 10]. In association with pre- and postoperative local anesthesia [9–12] and new protocols for conscious sedation [4], this new approach can be used for outpatient operative microlaparoscopy without general anesthesia.

Recently, there is a great tendency to use finer laparoscopic instruments which are more suitable for office procedure under local anesthesia instead of the general anesthesia (Fig. 1). Introduction of this new technology has been limited with the narrow scope view of the finer laparoscopic instruments. A newer highly advanced microendscope, using the new fiber optic technology, has solved this great problem, offering a laparoscopic view nearly similar to the traditional 10-mm telescope. This new updated 2-mm telescope has been recently applied for many gynecologic procedures, which were previously performed using the older traditional telescope [9–14].

In this study, a controlled prospective randomized study had been performed, recruiting 60 consenting PCOS-diagnosed patients, as a study group, to evaluate the following: (1) the feasibility of ovarian drilling during the proposed microlaparoscopy under augmented local anesthesia in terms of intraoperative pain control and postoperative analgesic requirements and (2) the efficacy of this technique compared with the conventional laparoscopic approach in another 60 PCOS-diagnosed patients as a control group, in terms of operative and discharge times and subsequent ovulation rates and pregnancy rates (PRs) within a year follow-up.

Materials and methods

Subjects

A total of 60 women with anovulatory infertility associated with PCOS underwent office microlaparoscopic ovarian drilling (OMLOD) under local anesthesia (using 2.2-mm telescope and instruments) in a private specialized fertility care center in Egypt, in addition to another 60 anovulatory women with polycystic ovaries (PCO), who underwent the conventional 10-mm laparoscopic ovarian drilling under general anesthesia. All patients included provided the data for our study. All the women had anovulatory infertility for more than 1-year duration and had been unsuccessfully treated with CC at up to 150 mg/day for 5 days in the early follicular phase of the menstrual cycle prior to OMLOD or LOD sessions.

PCOS diagnosis

The diagnosis of PCOS in both groups of women was based on the Rotterdam criteria. (1) Evidence of hyperandrogenism, early follicular phase (defined as days 2–5 of the menstrual cycle) serum LH/FSH ratio of >2, and/or raised serum androgen concentrations (testosterone 2.5 nmol/l, androstenedione 10 nmol/l, or free androgen index (FAI) >4 (Rotterdam ESHRE/ASRM-sponsored PCOS Consensus Workshop Group, Revised 2003). FAI was calculated using the formula: testosterone 100/sex hormone-binding globulin. (2) Evidence of un- or hypo-ovulation or (3) ultrasonographic evidence of PCO: ovarian stromal hypertrophy and multiple small (6–8 mm) follicles arranged in the periphery [9–11].

OMLOD

The microlaparoscopic system consists of a light source, a high speed pneumoperitoneum device, and a 1CCD video camera. The diameter of the scope was a malleable fiber

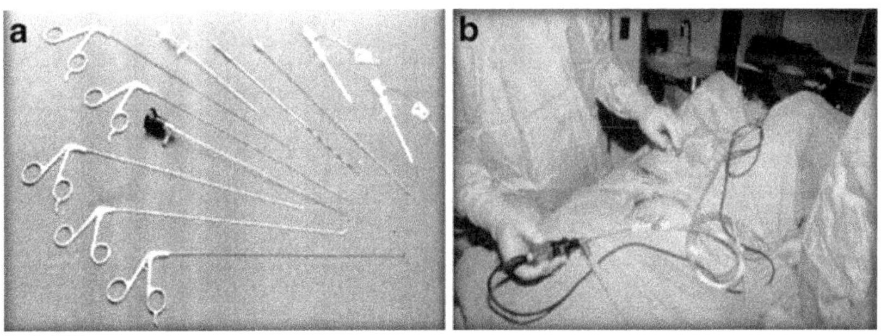

Fig. 1 Microlaparoscopic instruments (**a**) and the setup for the Office microlaparoscopy under augmented local anesthesia (**b**)

optic 2.2 mm, and the grasping forceps, scissors, needle probes, biopsy forceps, and irrigator–aspirator were also 2.2 mm in diameter (all equipment made by Olympus, Tokyo, Japan). The instruments could be used by specially designed trocar (access needle; Ethicon, Cincinnati, OH, USA), which is 12-cm long and 2.5 mm in diameter metal sleeve that fits over the veress needle. Premedication, consisting of 0.5 mg of atropine sulfate and 1 mg/kg of midazolam, was given intramuscularly. Fentanyl (1 mg/kg) followed by 1.5 mg/kg of ketamine was intravenously administered through a drip infusion line.

The patient was placed in a lithotomy position. An access needle (Eticon, Tokyo, Japan) was inserted through a small incision created in the subumbilical region using the closed method, after been locally infiltrated with Xylocaine local anesthesia. Pneumoperitoneum was induced with carbon dioxide gas. Other access needles were then inserted into both sides of the hypogastric region under microlaparoscopy. Four milliliters per port of 0.25 % bupivacaine were locally injected at the trocar insertion sites in advance. All the scopes and forceps used were from the microlaparoscopy set of 2.2 mm in outer diameter (Olympus, Tokyo, Japan). The ovarian ligament was held with holding forceps to fix it (Fig. 2).

Subsequently, the peritoneal cavity was inspected carefully, and a micrograsper was used to expose the fimbrial end of the fallopian tube at the time of chromopertubation. Chromopertubation was performed by injecting 15 ml of methylene blue with 15 ml of 1 % mepivacaine through the uterine manipulator tubing. The ovaries were observed under the microlaparoscope. During microlaparoscopic procedure, the size of the ovary was measured using Maryland forceps. When the forceps are extended, the distance between the two arms is 1.4 cm, and this distance was used to measure the length, width, and depth of the ovary. A high frequency 2.2-m electrocautery probe was used for ovarian drilling. The number of ovarian punctures differs according to the size and the total surface area of the ovary. A number, which ranges from 5–10 punctures, had been used for ovarian drilling. The electrocautery probe is provided with a cool water irrigation channel to rapidly cool the drilled ovary.

At the end of the procedure, a 16-gauge, 36-cm needle was inserted through an ancillary port, and 40 ml of 0.5 % lidocaine was sprayed over the diaphragmatic vault. After the removal of all trocars, the SC tissue of the insertion sites was injected with 5 ml of bupivacaine. Pain control during the procedure was scored on a scale of 1 to 4, indicating excellent, good, sufficient, and poor pain control, respectively. Postoperative analgesics were given when requested by the patient. The analgesics consisted of 100 mg of Dicolfenac Sodium (IM) or 30 mg of ketorolac (IM). No oral postoperative medications were administered, even after hospital discharge. Patients were discharged only when completely free of discomfort.

LOD

Conventional laparoscopic ovarian drilling was performed using a traditional 10-mm endoscope and under general anesthesia. The operation was performed through three ports: a 10-mm laparoscope was inserted through the primary subumbilical trocar, with two additional 5-mm trocars in the lower abdomen. A grasping forceps was used for manipulation of the ovary. The unipolar needle was introduced through the other secondary site of entry. Patients underwent the same procedures as performed in the study group, such as hysteroscopy and chromopertubation, except that they received no local anesthesia. The operative time and the number of patients discharged at 2 h were recorded.

Ultrasound scanning

Patients underwent transvaginal scanning prior to OMLOD and LOD and after surgery. Two ultrasound machines of the same model (Toshiba, model Sonolayer SSA-250A, with a convex 6-MHz transvaginal ultrasound probe) have been used in this center during the year follow-up period. Each ovary was localized in relation to the iliac vessels and scanned from inner to outer margins in longitudinal cross-sections and from upper to lower ends in transverse cross-sections. The characteristic ovarian polycystic ultrasound image (increased in the ovarian stroma, the number of small follicles of more than eight in number, and the characteristic

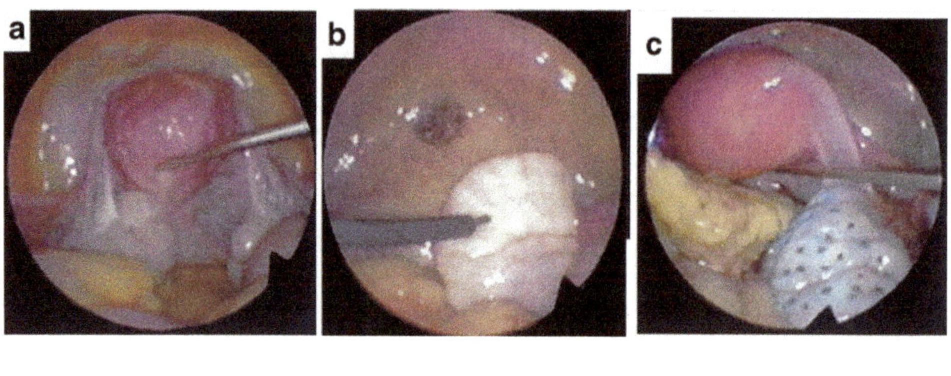

Fig. 2 **a** The microlaparoscopic image of the pelvis before the ovarian drilling procedure, which is apparently similar to the 10-mm laparoscopic view, **b** the microlaparoscopic ovarian drilling, **c** the microlaparoscopic image after the microlaparoscopic ovarian drilling procedure

pathognomonic arrangement of those small follicles—necklace shaped) is diagnosed before the procedure and followed up postoperatively. The three diameters of the ovary were measured (longitudinal, anteroposterior, and transverse). The ovarian volume was calculated using the formula of a prolate ellipsoid: 0.523 × length × width × thickness. The mean volume of the right and left ovaries was calculated for each subject.

Hormonal assays

Blood samples were taken from women in both groups early in the follicular phase (defined as days 2–5 of the menstrual cycle—basal hormonal levels) or at a random time in women with severe oligomenorrhoea or amenorrhoea. The samples were collected from the patients prior to both procedures, and LH, FSH, LH/FSH ratio, testosterone, androstendione, and free androgen index serum hormonal levels are measured. Serum hormonal concentrations were measured using well-established assays, which have been validated in our laboratory at the Department of Clinical Chemistry, in a fertility care center laboratory. Another blood samples for hormonal assays had been taken during the year follow-up after both laparoscopic procedures, to be compared with the preoperative serum hormonal levels, performed in the same lab.

Statistical analysis

For statistical analysis, the data were entered into the Statistical Package for Social Sciences for PC version 10.0.5. Continuous data were compared by Mann–Whitney U and Wilcoxon signed-ranks tests. Comparisons of categorical data were carried out using contingency table analyses. Hormonal values were compared with the postoperative values in each group with a Student's t test for paired data. Ovulation, pregnancy, and miscarriage rates and the number of patients (two) discharged, 2 h after surgery, were evaluated by the x. Significance was assumed if $P<0.05$.

Findings

A total of 60 PCOS-diagnosed patients were included in this part of the study (OMLOD study group), in addition to another PCOS 60 patients (LOD comparison group). The demographic, clinical, and endocrinological characteristics of both groups of subjects had been shown in Table 1. The characteristics of the comparison subjects are also shown in the same table.

The pain score recorded for the study group was as 2.86± 0.7 (Table 2). The operative time required for diagnostic evaluation and ovarian drilling was not significantly different between the groups. The mean discharge time and the need for additional analgesics were significantly lower in the study group than in the control group (Table 2). The proportion of patients discharged 2 h after surgery was significantly higher in the study group (75.8 %) than that in the comparison group (0 %) (Table 2). PRs within 1 year of follow-up were slightly higher in the study group (65.6 %) than that in the comparison group (60 %). The ovulation rate was 86.2 % in the study group and 85.6 % in the comparison group. The incidence of miscarriage was almost similar in both groups.

Endocrine data were reported in Table 3. LH values decreased significantly after surgery in both groups. Similarly, the serum levels showed a statistically significant reduction after surgery in both groups. In contrast, FSH levels did not change significantly after either OMLOD or the conventional laparoscopy. No complications from local anesthetics were observed during the study. The mean serum concentration of androstenedione showed no significant change shortly in both groups, but showed a significant reduction later on. The percentage of women with FAI showed a significant ($P<0.01$) decrease from 69 % prior

Table 1 The characteristics of 60 women with polycystic ovary syndrome, who had office microlaparoscopic ovarian drilling for anovulatory infertility (the study group) and 60 anovulatory PCOS women who had undergone conventional LOD (the comparison group)

Characteristic	Cases group		Comparison group	
	Mean ± SD	Range	Mean ± SD	Range
Age at follow-up (years)	33.3±4.4	21–45	32.2±4.9	20–44
Body mass index (kg/m^2)	26.7±4.9	19–4	29.9±7.9	18–45
Duration of infertility (years)	3.1±2.1	1–12	1.8±1.8	1–10
Serum LH (TU/l)	14.4±7.5	1.8–49.0	13.0±6.2	4.9–31.0
Serum FSH (TU/l)	5.4±1.5	1.2–10.4	5.0±1.6	2.6–10.0
Serum LH/FSH ratio	2.7±1.2	0.4–5.7	2.6±1.4	0.8–7.3
Serum testosterone (nmol/l)	2.6±1.3	0.8–6.1	3.2±1.2	0.8–6.6
Serum androstenedione (TU/l)	9.8±4.0	1.7–27	11.0±3.9	2.5–19.0
Free androgen index	8.6±8.2	1.0–36.9	11.3±7.3	3.6–28.0
Ovarian volume (ml)	11.0±3.7	4.3–20.0	11.5±5.2	5.8–19.5

Table 2 Operative and reproductive data in patients treated by the proposed microlaparoscopy under augmented local anesthesia (study group, n=60) and after conventional 10-mm laparoscopy under general anesthesia (comparison group, n=60)

Variable	Case group	Comparison group
Intraoperative pain score	2.8±0.7	–
Operative time (min)	20.3±9.1	28.4±7.3
Discharge time (h)	2.4±0.7	6.2±2.3
Number of patients discharged		
2 h after surgery (%)	42 (71.8)	0
Number of patients who required		
Additional analgesics (%)	18 (21.8)	34 (53.3)
Ovulation rate (%)	85.2	86.6
PR (%)	65.6	60.0
Miscarriage rate (%)	2.2	3.3

to ovarian drilling to 41 % shortly after surgery in both groups.

The proportion of women with ultrasound evidence of polycystic ovaries (PCO), prior to treatment and postoperatively, is shown. The results showed that the proportion of women with ultrasound evidence of PCO significantly ($P<$ 0.01) decreased after ovarian drilling and remained low during the 1-year follow-up periods in both groups, without a significant difference after the two procedures. The mean ovarian volume decreased significantly ($P<0.05$) after 1-year follow-up after both LOD and OMLOD procedures.

The characteristic phenotypic picture for PCOS, including the androgenic type of obesity involving the suprapubic and waist loss, hirsutism, and acne, had been compared before and after both procedures. Those phenotypic pictures had never shown significant changes after both procedures, but with minimal improvement of both acne and the androgenic type of obesity. There was no increase in the hirsutism score; moreover, the extra hair picture had shown a slight improvement.

Other gynecologic problems had been diagnosed during both procedures. Pelvic endometriosis was confirmed in 10 women with OMLOD and 12 during LOD; all had been managed laparoscopically. Pelvic adhesions, affecting the free mobility of both tubes and ovaries, had been managed in seven women during OMLOD and in ten during LOD. Abnormally situated ovaries with disturbed tubo-ovarian relationship had been diagnosed in two cases during OMLOD and in three women during LOD. All the gynecologic problems had been laparoscopically managed without a difference between the two procedures. All those case with other problems rather than anovulation (PCOS), who had been diagnosed during both procedures, had been excluded from the study.

Discussion

The laparoscopic approach to PCOS has been described extensively [1–14]. Local anesthesia has been used for many gynecologic procedures and has been reported to reduce the postoperative pain after day-surgery diagnostic laparoscopy. Previous studies documented the implementation of microlaparoscopy without general anesthesia in terms of both diagnostic efficacy [6] and pain control during and after the procedure [10, 15–17]. The recent development of small-diameter fiber optic microlaparoscopy allows an optical resolution comparable to that obtained with traditional 10-mm laparoscopes [18, 19]. In addition, improvements in sedation and local anesthesia protocols [3, 4] may allow microlaparoscopy to become a routine outpatient procedure.

The aim of the present study was to evaluate the feasibility and efficacy of microlaparoscopic ovarian drilling under local anesthesia and conscious sedation in terms of ovulation rates and PRs after the procedure as compared with the traditional 10-mm laparoscopic approach under general anesthesia. This technique represents a new option for gynecologists, which allows a significant reduction of androgen levels comparable to those observed after laparoscopic ovarian resection or laparoscopic electrocauterization, with the additional benefit of being a less invasive technique that can be performed as an outpatient procedure without the need for general anesthesia.

Table 3 Hormonal profile before and immediately after 1-year follow-up of ovarian drilling in patients treated by microlaparoscopy under augmented local anesthesia (study group), compared to the results after the conventional 10-mm laparoscopic ovarian drilling under general anesthesia

Hormone	Study group		Comparison group	
	Before surgery	After surgery	Before surgery	After surgery
LH (IU/l)	17.4±3.6	14.4±2.9	18.3±3.9	14.7±3.1
FSH (IU/l)	7.1±0.7	7.7±1.2	6.8±0.9	7.2±1.1
LH/FSH ratio	2.7±0.3	2.1±0.1	2.7±1.2	2.2±0.3
FAI (nmol/l)	8.1±0.9	6.2±0.6	8.9±1.2	6.9±1.2
T (nmol/l)	3.1±1.0	2.3±0.7	3.3±0.8	2.3±1.0
Androstendione (IU/l)	9.4±1.3	7.1±0.5	9.8±1.9	7.6±2.3
Ovarian volume (ml)	11.5±2.2	9.9±1.3	11.7±1.7	10. 1±0.5

Moreover, the high PRs and ovulation rates in the follow-up period should encourage this approach especially in patients with PCOS, who require a diagnostic evaluation for tubal patency. The low degree of invasiveness and the modified conscious–sedation protocol of this new approach, with the use of increasing but low doses of midazolam, allow an outpatient procedure with a quick patient discharge [3, 4]. This simple procedure appears to be particularly useful for outpatient microlaparoscopies, in which the average discharge time is 2 to 3 h after the operation. The effect of local anesthesia is temporary; however, this approach allows the possibility of a quicker discharge at 2 h after surgery [19–24].

The good intraoperative pain control reported in this study demonstrates the feasibility of operative microlaparoscopy. Even though only a small volume of CO_2 is needed during the technique, the surgeon performs maneuvers to remove air from the abdomen at the end of the procedure because residual gas can accumulate under the diaphragm and cause peritoneal irritation, especially when an upright position is maintained at the time of hospital discharge. For this reason, it is useful to spray lidocaine at the end of the procedure. Moreover, reduced exposure to CO during 2-mm microlaparoscopy may decrease the rate of adhesion formation as compared with conventional 10-mm laparoscopy.

It had been also showed that serum testosterone concentrations decreased after both LOD and OMLOD. The proportion of women with high LH concentrations (>10 IU/l) decreased significantly from 70 to 33 % shortly after OMLOD and LOD as well. There was a trend toward a decrease of serum androgen levels with the increasing post-operative duration after both OMLOD and LOD, possibly due to the effect of advancing age or due to increased loss of the cauterized ovarian stroma, the main source of the ovarian androgens. A similar trend toward a decrease of androgen levels was also observed in the comparison group, in particular, the significant reduction of serum androstenedione concentrations.

Felemban et al. [10] reported that LOD reduced both blood LH and androgens, and that, among androgens, dehydroepiandrosterone sulfate (DHEA-S) derived from the adrenal gland was significantly reduced. In this passed study, testosterone and androstenedione, probably derived from the ovary, were significantly reduced, but DHEA-S was not. Considering the fact that either OMLOD or LOD is a local procedure targeting the ovary, LOD or OMLOD is unlikely to reduce DHEA-S derived from the adrenal gland. LOD may exert their effect through a reduction of ovary-derived androgens. Amar et al. and Rossmanith et al. Also reported similar results, regarding the post drilling effects on serum androgens [24, 25].

The current work had shown nearly similar results to a previous research work performed in 2000, where minilaparoscope of 3.5-mm rigid lens system telescope and instruments, in contrast to the fiber optic malleable 2-mm telescope and instruments. The limited narrow telescope view was one of the problems which faced of the minilaparoscope work [26]. The fiberoptic 2-mm telescope used in the current work offers a relatively similar image to the 10-mm telescope. Moreover, the malleable 2-mm soft telescope and instruments have never shown any complications, with a remote possibility to injure any abdominal viscera, as they are like needle punctures, without the need for an extra repair of those needle punctures. The finer telescopic and other laparoscopic instruments had gone smoothly within the abdominal wall with the least discomfort and almost without augmented sedation, but only with local anesthetic filtration of those microlaparoscopic entries.

Ovarian drilling resulted in a significant reduction in the ovarian volume after 1-year follow-up. In one study, it had been reported on the short-term effect of ovarian drilling on the ovarian volume as measured by three-dimensional (3D) ultrasound [1–14]. They found that ovarian drilling resulted in a transient increase followed by a significant reduction in ovarian volume from a preoperative mean value of 12.2 to 6.9 ml 3 weeks after surgery. The mechanism of this reduction of the ovarian volume by ovarian drilling is not clear. In a previous study, the volume of ovarian tissue destroyed by the needle electrode in an excised ovary using a 3D projection of colored serial microscopic images [25–28]. They found that a single drilling would destroy an average of 0.4 ml of stromal tissue. They concluded that 10–15 drillings in an ovary would result in a total tissue destruction of 4–6 ml. This could account for the observed reduction of the ovarian volume.

Conclusion

In conclusion, laparoscopic ovarian drilling has been approved after extensive and prolonged research works to be the gold standard treatment tool for clomiphene citrate-resistant PCOS infertile women. Technical improvements, such as smaller optical fiberoptic systems, ancillary instruments, and improved anesthetic procedures, allow these drilling procedures to be performed using microlaparoscopy under local anesthesia. OMLOD normalizes ovarian function and morphology in women with PCOS, efficiently as after conventional LOD. The question is the long-term outcome and prognosis of OMLOD, compared with those after LOD. Another question is that the patients' compliance to face the office microlaparoscopic procedure for different gynecologic and obstetric indications. The answers for those questions would appear after follow-up of the long-term outcome after OMLOD; another ongoing study and the forthcoming results might appear sooner.

Acknowledgment I have to thank all colleagues in the university obstetrics and gynecology department for their great and kind support to this work. I am also quite grateful for Mr. Amer et al. and his colleagues for their very nice work which has added a lot to this work. I should also express my thankful feelings to all women included in the work for their patience to be followed up after the procedure and for more than 3 years. Finally, there is still an effort to be made for further implementations of this proposed microlaparoscopic procedure in another gynecologic and obstetric indications

References

1. Mercorio F, Mercorio A, Di Spiezio Sardo A, Barba GV, Pellicano M, Nappi C (2008) Evaluation of ovarian adhesion formation after laparoscopic ovarian drilling by second-look minilaparoscopy. Fertil Steril 89:1229–1233
2. Almeida OD Jr, Val-Gallas JM (1998) Office microlaparoscopy under local anesthesia in the diagnosis and treatment of chronic pelvic pain. J Am Assoc Gynecol Laparosc 5(4):407–410
3. Amer SAKS, Gopalan V, Li TC, Ledger WL, Cooke ID (2002) Long-term follow-up of patients with polycystic ovary syndrome after laparoscopic ovarian drilling: clinical outcome. Hum Reprod 17:2035–2042
4. Bayram N, vanWely M, Kaaijk EM, Bossuyt PM, van der Veen F (2004) Using an electrocautery strategy or recombinant follicle stimulating hormone to induce ovulation in polycystic ovary syndrome: randomised controlled trial. BMJ 328:192
5. Armar NA, McGarrigle HHG, Honour J, Holownia P, Jacobs HS, Lachelin GCL (1990) Laparoscopic ovarian diathermy in the management of anovulatory infertility in women with polycystic ovaries: endocrine changes and clinical outcome. Fertil Steril 53:45–49
6. Malkawi HY, Qublan HS (2005) Laparoscopic ovarian drilling in the treatment of polycystic ovary syndrome: how many punctures per ovary are needed to improve the reproductive outcome? J Obstet Gynaecol Res 31:115–119
7. Risquez F, Pennehouat G, Mc Corvey R (1997) Diagnostic and operative microlaparoscopy: a preliminary multicentre report. Hum Reprod 12(8):1645–1648
8. Dahlgren E, Johansson S, Lindstedt G, Knutsson F, Oden A, Janson PO, Mattson LA, Crona N, Lundsberg PA (1992) Women with polycystic ovary syndrome wedge resected in 1956 to 1965: a long-term follow-up focusing on natural history and circulating hormones. Fertil Steril 57:505–513
9. Kaya H, Sezik M, Ozkaya O (2005) Evaluation of a new surgical approach for the treatment of clomiphene citrate-resistant infertility in polycystic ovary syndrome: laparoscopic ovarian multi-needle intervention. J Minim Invasive Gynecol 12:355–358
10. Felemban A, Tan SL, Tulandi T (2000) Laparoscopic treatment of polycystic ovaries with insulated needle cautery: a reappraisal. Fertil Steril 73:266–269
11. Barber TM, Wass JA, McCarthy MI, Franks S (2007) Metabolic characteristics of women with polycystic ovaries and oligo-amenorrhoea but normal androgen levels: implications for the management of polycystic ovary syndrome. Clin Endocrinol (Oxf) 66(4):513–517
12. Gjonnaess H (1994) Ovarian electrocautery in the treatment of women with polycystic ovary syndrome (PCOS). Factors affecting the results. Acta Obstet Gynecol Scand 73:407–412
13. Gjonnaess H (1998) Late endocrine effects of ovarian electrocautery in women with polycystic ovary syndrome. Fertl Steril 69;697–701
14. Jedel E, Labrie F, Odén A et al (2011) Impact of electro-acupuncture and exercise on hyperandrogenism and oligo/amenorrhea in women with polycystic ovary syndrome: a randomized controlled trial. Am J Physiol Endocrinol Metab 300:E37–45, Epub 2010 Oct 13
15. Rotterdam ESHRE/ASRM-Sponsored PCOS Consensus Workshop Group (2004) Revised 2003 consensus on diagnostic criteria and long-term health risks related to polycystic ovary syndrome (PCOS). Hum Reprod 19:41–47
16. Palomba S, Orio F Jr, Zullo F (2007) What is the best first-step therapeutic approach in treating anovulatory infertility in patients with polycystic ovary syndrome? Questions that are still unanswered. Gynecol Endocrinol 23(5):245–247
17. The Rotterdam ESHRE/ASRM-sponsored PCOS Consensus Workshop Group (2004) Revised consensus on diagnostic criteria and long-term health risks related to polycystic ovary syndrome. Fertil Steril 81:19–25
18. Keckstein G, Rossmanith W, Spatzier K, Schneider V, Borchers K, Steiner R (1990) The effect of laparoscopic treatment of polycystic ovary disease by CO_2-laser or Nd:YAG laser. Surg Endosc 4:103–107
19. Kovacs G, Buckler H, Bangah M, Outch K, Burger H, Healy D, Baker G, Phillips S (1991) Treatment of anovulation due to polycystic ovary syndrome by laparoscopic ovarian electrocautery. Br J Obstet Gynaecl 98:30–35
20. Li TC, Saravelos H, Chow MS, Chisabingo R, Cooke ID (1998) Factors affecting the outcome of laparoscopic ovarian drilling for polycystic ovary syndrome in women with anovulatory infertility. Br J Obstet Gynaecol 105:338–344
21. Zullo F, Pellicano M, Nappi C (2000) Minilaparoscopic ovarian drilling under local anesthesia in patients with polycystic ovary syndrome. Fertil Steril 74:376–379
22. Naether OGJ, Baukloh V, Fischer R, Kowalczyk T (1994) Long-term follow-up in 206 infertility patients with polycystic ovary syndrome after laparoscopic electrocautery of the ovarian surface. Hum Reprod 9:2342–2349
23. Takeuchi H, Jinushi M (1999) Comparison of anesthetic methods for microlaparoscopy in women with unexplained infertility. J Am Assoc Gynecol Laparosc 6:453–457
24. Seow KM, Juan CC, Hwang JL, Ho LT (2008) Laparoscopic surgery in polycystic ovary syndrome: reproductive and metabolic effects. Semin Reprod Med 26:101–110
25. Palomba S, Zullo F, Diamanti-Kandarakis E, Orio F Jr (2007) Surgery and laser diathermy. In: Diamanti-Kandarakis E, Nestler JE, Panidis D, Pasquali R (eds) Insulin resistance and polycystic ovarian syndrome. Humana, Totowa, pp 461–477
26. Fulvio Zullo MD, Massimiliano Pellicano MD, Errico Zupi MD, Maurizio Guida MD, Pasquale Mastrantonio MD, Carmine Nappi MD (2000) Minilaparoscopic ovarian drilling under local anesthesia in patients with polycystic ovary syndrome. Fertil Steril 74:376–79
27. Taskin O, Yalcinoglu AI, Kafkasli A, Burak F, Ozekici U (1996) Comparison of the effects of ovarian cauterization and gonadotropin-releasing hormone agonist and oral contraceptive therapy combination on endocrine changes in women with polycystic ovary disease. Fertil Steril 65:1115–1118
28. Tulandi T, Watkin K, Tan SL (1997) Reproductive performance and three-dimensional ultrasound volume determination of polycystic ovaries following laparoscopic ovarian drilling. Int J Infertil 42:436–440

12

Deep rectovaginal endometriotic nodules: perioperative complications from a series of 3,298 patients operated on by the shaving technique

Jacques Donnez · Pascale Jadoul · Sébastien Colette · Mathieu Luyckx · Jean Squifflet · Olivier Donnez

Abstract The purpose of this study was to analyze complication and recurrence rates after deep endometriotic nodule surgery. A total of 3,298 cases of deep endometriotic nodules were analyzed. The shaving technique was used, avoiding bowel resection. Laparoscopic nodule resection was performed successfully in all cases. Major complications included: (1) rectal perforation in 42 cases (1.3 %), (2) ureteral retention (<5 days) in 21 cases (0.64 %), (3) ureteral injury in 10 cases (0.3 %), and (4) fecal peritonitis in 1 case (0.04 %). This complication rate is much lower than that observed after bowel resection. In the same period, bowel resection was only required in 1.1 % (n=37) of cases. Histology revealed circumscribed nodular aggregates of smooth muscle, endometrial glands, and scanty endometrial stroma. Lesions were found to be invaded by nerve fibers. Endometriosis is not cancer and does not require the same treatment approach. In young women, conservative surgery using the shaving technique means preservation of organs, nerves, and the vascular blood supply. The shaving technique yields low complication and recurrence rates and should be considered the first line in surgical approach in the case of deep endometriotic lesions.

Keywords Deep endometriosis · Nodules · Shaving technique · Bowel resection

J. Donnez · P. Jadoul · S. Colette · M. Luyckx · J. Squifflet
Pôle de Recherche en Gynécologie, Institut de Recherche Expérimentale et Clinique (IREC),
Université Catholique de Louvain (UCL),
1200 Brussels, Belgium

J. Donnez · P. Jadoul · S. Colette · M. Luyckx · J. Squifflet
Department of Gynecology, Cliniques Universitaires Saint-Luc,
1200 Brussels, Belgium

O. Donnez
Gynecology, CHU Mont-Godinne,
Université Catholique de Louvain,
5530 Yvoir, Belgium

J. Donnez (✉)
Department of Gynecology, Université Catholique de Louvain,
Cliniques Universitaires St Luc,
Avenue Hippocrate 10,
1200 Brussels, Belgium
e-mail: jacques.donnez@uclouvain.be

Introduction

In 1996, we were the first to publish the concept of three different forms of endometriosis: (1) peritoneal endometriosis, (2) ovarian endometriosis, and (3) deep rectovaginal endometriosis [1, 2]. The third form of the disease has been defined as deep endometriosis, rectovaginal endometriosis, or adenomyosis of the rectovaginal septum. In the literature, it is also called deep-infiltrating endometriosis or posterior deep-infiltrating endometriosis.

Many different surgical approaches have been proposed. The first study reporting the shaving technique and data from a series of 231 cases of laparoscopic management of deep endometriosis was published in *Human Reproduction* in 1995 [3], followed by a second study (n=500 patients) published in *BJOG* in 1997 [4] and a third one (n=1,942 patients) published in 2004 [5]. But surprisingly, the number of manuscripts advocating bowel resection has dramatically increased over recent years [6–15]. Koninckx et al. (see [16]) and Donnez et al. [17], firm advocates of the shaving technique, are increasingly confounded by this rapidly growing prevalence of bowel resection in the case of deep endometriosis with rectal muscularis involvement. During meetings on this topic, there is often heated debate between advocates of the two respective techniques.

The goals of this manuscript are to present data from a consecutive series of 3,298 cases and discuss perioperative complications and recurrence rates by analyzing the existing literature and our own data.

Patients and methods

Three thousand, two hundred and ninety-eight patients operated on for deep endometriotic nodules were included in this study.

Symptoms and diagnosis

In this series of 3,298 patients, the main symptoms were pelvic pain and/or dysmenorrhea in 95 % of cases, deep dyspareunia in 87 % of cases, and rectal dyschezia in 44 % of cases. About 45 % of patients were suffering from pelvic pain associated with infertility. In all cases of infertility, evaluation of ovulation, cervical mucus–sperm interaction (postcoital test), and male factor (defined as <15 million sperm/ml using a Makler counting chamber) were undertaken.

Careful clinical examination [18], transrectal ultrasonography (TRUS) [19], rectal endoscopic sonography [20], transvaginal sonography, barium enema, and magnetic resonance imaging (MRI) [21] have all been recommended to identify deep rectovaginal endometriotic lesions [22]. In our series, examination with a speculum revealed either a normal vaginal mucosa or a protruded bluish nodule in the posterior fornix. By palpation, the diameter of the lesion could be evaluated. Palpation is very often painful, and the presence of a nodule accounts for symptoms like deep dyspareunia and dysmenorrhea.

Preoperative radiography of the colon (barium enema) was systematically carried out in order to assess the involvement of the rectal surface. Profile radiography allows the best evaluation of infiltration of the anterior rectal wall. In our series, MRI and TRUS have also been systematically performed preoperatively since 1997, and Squifflet et al. [21] distinguished three types of deep lesions by analyzing their location, as precisely defined by the above procedures.

Surgery: the shaving technique

The shaving technique was already reported in a recent publication [17]. The principal steps involve (1) separation of the anterior rectum from the posterior vagina, (2) excision or ablation of deep endometriosis after complete dissection of the nodule from the posterior part of the cervix, and (3) resection of the posterior vaginal fornix and vaginal closure (Fig. 1).

Care must always be taken to preserve the pelvic autonomic nerves, as they are the pathway for the neurogenic control of rectal, bladder, and sexual arousal function [23–27]. The shaving technique allows preservation of the nerves by avoiding deep lateral rectal dissection (necessary for rectosigmoid resection). Indeed, lateral dissection is mandatory only in the case of lateral extension of the disease with ureteral involvement [17, 28] and, even in this case, rarely involves dissection of the posterolateral compartment of the rectum.

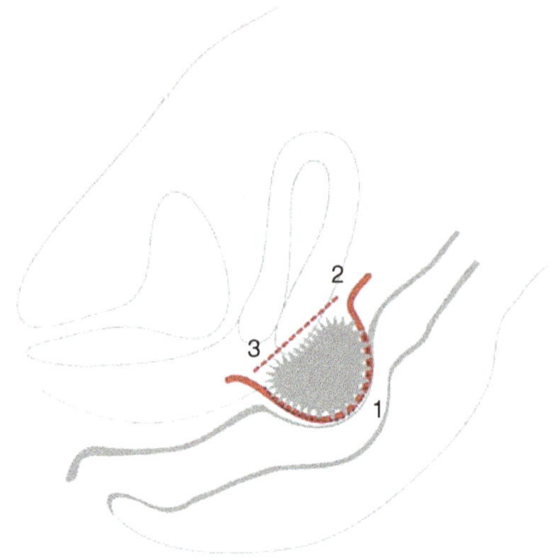

Fig. 1 *1* Shaving to free the rectum, *2* resection of the nodule from the cervix, *3* resection of the posterior vaginal fornix

Histology

All biopsies were dissected by an expert gynecologist, fixed in 4 % formaldehyde, embedded in paraffin, and serially sectioned (5 μm) for histological confirmation of endometriosis (presence of glands and stroma).

More recently, immunohistochemistry (IHC) was also performed using a standard immunoperoxidase method [29] to evaluate the expression of PGP9.5 (nerve marker). Briefly, endogenous peroxidase activity quenching, heat epitope retrieval, and blocking of nonspecific staining were carried out. The specimens were then incubated for 1 h at room temperature with rabbit polyclonal antihuman PGP9.5 (1/1,000, Dako, CA, USA), followed by incubation with secondary antibody conjugated to peroxidase (EnVision +™, Dako). The presence of peroxidase was revealed using 3,3′-diaminobenzidine (Dako), and specimens were counterstained with Mayer's hemalum solution (Merck, Darmstadt, Germany).

Human intestinal tissue was used as a positive control for PGP9.5 expression. Negative controls were processed using nonspecific IgG or omitting the specific primary antibodies.

Every fifth slide of each lesion was stained with hematoxylin–eosin to identify the section with the largest surface area of endometriotic glands and stroma, and the following serial section was immunostained with PGP9.5. Stromal surface area was delimited and measured using the MIRAX Viewer (MIRAX Viewer 1.12.22.0, Carl Zeiss MicroImaging GmbH, Germany). Nerve fiber density was then determined in this stromal area, as well as in the area neighboring the lesion (up to 1.5 mm away).

Results

There is a big difference in symptoms and evolution between sigmoid and deep rectovaginal lesions. Symptoms of sigmoid endometriosis are mainly related to bowel stenosis and include cramps, constipation, and abdominal distension, while symptoms of deep rectovaginal lesions are dysmenorrhea, deep dyspareunia, and dyschezia.

Their pathogenesis is also different. Sigmoid lesions may be due to lymphatic or nervous system dissemination, while rectovaginal lesions are due either to metaplasia of Mülleri-an rests or to retrocervical extension of metaplastic nodules originating from either the cervix or the attachment area between the cervix and posterior vaginal fornix. Our manuscript focuses only on deep rectovaginal endometriosis and not sigmoid lesions.

Our series of 3,298 cases of deep rectovaginal endometriotic nodules treated by laparoscopy is presented in Table 1. All patients were operated on between 1989 and 2010. Operating time ranged from 31 to 238 min (median, 78 min), and median lesion size was 2.8 cm (range, 1–6 cm). In the same period, 37 patients (1.1 %, not included in the series of 3,298) underwent rectosigmoid bowel resection by laparotomy or laparoscopy–mini laparotomy, because of bowel lumen stenosis of more than 80 % with circular stenosis (not only anterior involvement), as well as mucosal involvement visible on colonoscopy and confirmed by biopsy and histological evaluation. These three criteria (stenosis of the lumen >80 %, circular stenosis, and mucosal involvement) are, in our view, indications for bowel resection, but they are infrequently encountered. Indeed, in our series, bowel resection was only required in 1.1 % of cases.

In this series of 3,298 patients, laparoscopic dissection was performed successfully in all cases, even when radiography of the colon showed anterior bowel involvement of up to 5 cm or more.

Table 1 A series of 3,298 cases of deep endometriosis treated by the laparoscopic shaving technique without segmental resection

Laparoscopic shaving surgery (n=3,298)	
Lesion size (cm)	2.8 (1–6)
Duration of surgery (min)	70 (31–238)
Hospitalization (days)	2.7 (2–7)
Complications	
•Rectal perforation during shaving	42 (1.3 %)
•Fecal peritonitis requiring colostomy	1 (0.03 %)
•Rectovaginal fistula	2 (0.06)
•Delayed hemorrhage (<24 h postoperatively)	3 (0.09 %)
•Ureteral injury (transection)	4 (0.12 %)
•Ureteral fistula (thermal damage)	6 (0.18 %)
•Urinary retention (temporary, <5 days)	21 (0.64 %)

In 37 cases, bowel resection was carried out by laparotomy because of bowel stenosis with mucosal involvement (not included in the series of 3,298 patients). In this series of 37 cases, 27 were for recurrence of severe pain after shaving

1. Lesion types according to MRI

   According to MRI, there are three types of lesions. These three types are: (a) type I, rectovaginal septum lesions; (b) type II, posterior vaginal fornix lesions; and (c) type III, hourglass-shaped lesions. Their prevalence is, respectively, 10, 58, and 32 % of all deep nodular lesions [21].

   The source of debate is the type III nodule. Indeed, these nodules occur when posterior fornix lesions extend cranially to the anterior rectal wall. As stated above, their prevalence is 32 %. Clinical evaluation usually reveals a larger lesion (more than 3 cm) (mean, 4.2 cm; range, 3–6 cm), and barium enema always shows infiltration and retraction of the rectal muscularis, known as perivisceritis. This continuum between the rectal muscularis and the cervix is found to obliterate the rectovaginal septum cranially. A clearly defined continuum exists between these two parts of the lesion. This is why we termed these lesions diabolo-like or hourglass-shaped (Fig. 2).

   These lesions always occur under the peritoneal fold of the recto-uterine pouch of Douglas. Infiltration of the rectal muscularis is systematically observed in this subtype, as demonstrated by barium enema (profile image) and TRUS, but infiltration is generally limited to the muscularis without mucosal involvement (Fig. 3). They may also extend laterally and involve the ureter [17, 28, 30, 31].

   It is essentially the treatment of these type III nodules that causes such contention and debate among surgeons.
2. Peri- and postoperative complications (Table 1)

   In our series of 3,298 cases, laparoscopic rectal perforation occurred in 42 cases (1.3 %). All perforations were diagnosed at the time of laparoscopy. In the first three cases (in the early 1990s), the rectum was repaired by laparotomy and, in all others, by laparoscopy. Laparoscopic suture was carried out through a full-thickness layer using Vicryl 2.0 (Ethicon, Johnson and Johnson, USA) with separate stitches. The area was finally covered with fibrin glue (Tissucol, Johnson and Johnson,

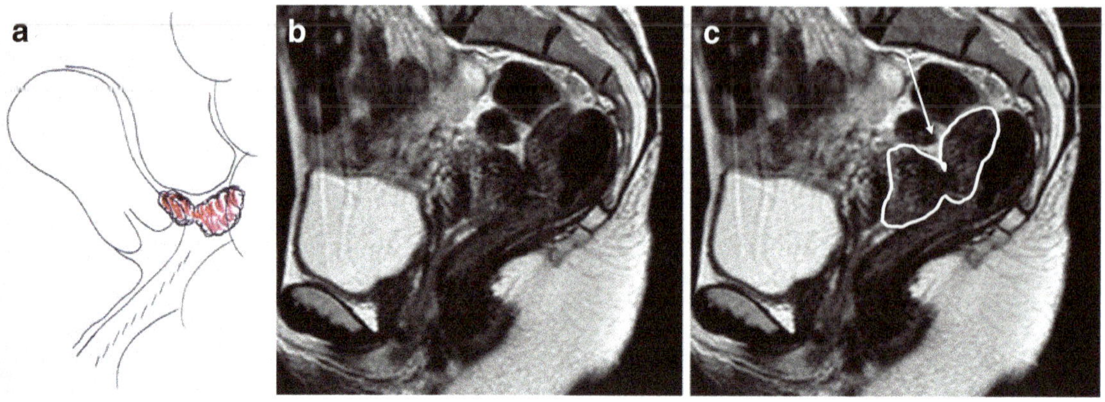

Fig. 2 **a** Type III nodule; **b** and **c** MRI: type III nodule; the nodule extends from the posterior part of the cervix to the anterior rectal wall and an "hourglass" shape can be seen

USA). Among the 42 cases, neither fistula nor any other complications were observed.

Rectal muscle defects frequently arise during the shaving procedure and are repaired by suturing. If the rectal lumen is not entered, it is not considered a complication, just part of the procedure. It should be noted, however, that in the early years of shaving practice, rectal muscularis defects were not closed, and that two cases (0.06 %) of rectovaginal fistula occurred 6 to 8 days after surgery. Both cases were treated conservatively by antibiotics and diet for 10 days.

One case of fecal peritonitis occurred 7 days after surgery. During surgery, bleeding at the site of lateral dissection of the rectum required extensive bipolar coagulation. At the end of surgery, bowel integrity was checked by CO_2 intrarectal insufflation and the blue test. No rectal defect was diagnosed. Seven days later, a hole of 2.5 cm in size was detected. Extensive coagulation probably provoked thermal rectal injury, with subsequent necrosis and a fistula. A colostomy was therefore carried out. Three months later, the colostomy was closed.

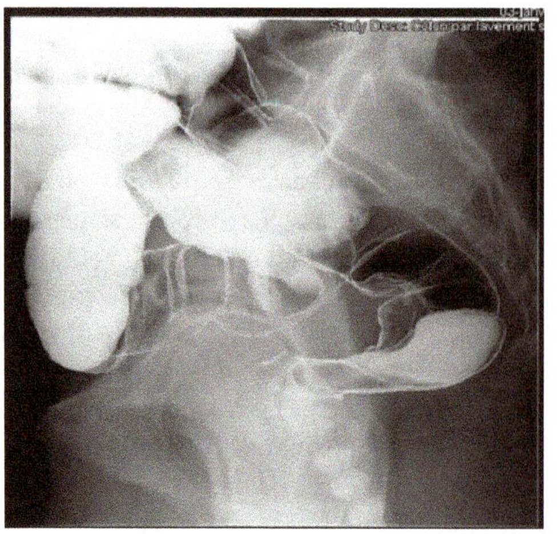

Fig. 3 Barium enema: infiltration of the muscularis of the anterior rectal wall

Ten cases (0.3 %) of ureteral injury were noted in our patients. Four cases (0.1 %) of ureteral transection were diagnosed on the first postoperative day by the presence of abundant fluid in the peritoneal cavity. High levels of urea and creatinine in the "peritoneal" fluid and intravenous pyelography (IVP) confirmed the diagnosis. Nephrostomy was carried out. One case resolved spontaneously with complete healing of the ureter 2 months later. The other three cases required vesico-ureteral reimplantation.

The remaining six cases (0.2 %) of ureteral injury were due to thermal damage (bipolar coagulation) and were treated by insertion of a JJ stent, which was removed 3 months later. Among these six patients, four recovered completely. Two women needed vesico-ureteral reimplantation for hydronephrosis due to stenosis of the lower ureteral segment (fibrosis). In these cases, hydronephrosis was detected approximately 1 month after removal of the JJ stent. This is why, in the case of large nodules with possible ureteral involvement (suspected by MRI or IVP), a JJ stent is inserted before starting the laparoscopic procedure, and ureterolysis is then performed [17, 28]. The usefulness of JJ stents in preventing subsequent complications was recently confirmed by Weingertner et al. [32]. The group of Koninckx also published a large series of ureteral injuries [16]. They demonstrated that ureteral repair was often possible by laparoscopy with excellent outcomes.

Urinary retention occurred in 21 cases (0.64 %). All were patients with large nodules (>4 cm) and bilateral extension, requiring extensive lateral dissection. A Foley catheter was inserted for 2 days, and all but two cases resolved spontaneously. These last two cases required bladder catheterization for 5 days, then resolved.

3. Recurrence and pregnancy rates

   Recurrence and pregnancy rates could only be analyzed in a prospective study. This was done in a prospective series of 500 patients operated on by the shaving technique for deep rectovaginal endometriotic nodules (types II and III). This series was recently published [17].

   In case of type I nodules, recurrence was shown to be well under 5 % [5]. In types II and III, recurrence of severe pelvic pain was 7 % (36 of 500) [17] and was found to be significantly lower ($p<0.05$) in women who became pregnant after surgery (3.6 %) than those who did not (14 %).
4. Histology

   Deep endometriosis associated or not with pelvic endometriosis can take the form of nodular masses involving the posterior vaginal fornix. They have been called "adenomyotic nodules of the rectovaginal septum" [5]. An adenomyoma is a circumscribed nodular aggregate of smooth muscle, endometrial glands and, usually, endometrial stroma (Fig. 4). This type of lesion is a specific form called adenomyosis, characterized by the presence of abundant muscular tissue invaded by glandular epithelium, covered with scanty stroma [4]. Nodular lesions exhibit a varied functional response to ovarian hormones. They may not respond to physiologic levels of progesterone, and secretory changes are frequently absent or incomplete during the second half of the cycle [1, 2]. In our study, endometriotic glands and stroma were often found by serial section up to the vaginal mucosa (Fig. 4), which was sometimes replaced by endometrial epithelium, confirming the need to remove the posterior vaginal fornix, as already suggested in our first series of publications.

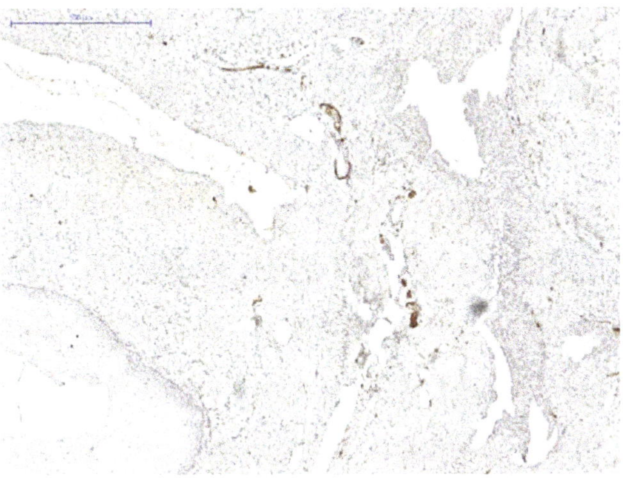

Fig. 4 Type III nodule (histology): aggregate of smooth muscle, endometrial glands, and scanty stroma. The vaginal mucosa is clearly visible (on the left side)

In a preliminary study, mentioned in the methods, we were able to demonstrate the presence of nerve fibers (PGP9.5-positive) in deep endometriotic lesions. All deep-infiltrating endometriosis (affecting the rectovaginal septum or rectal muscularis) was found to be invaded by nerve fibers, especially around intestinal tissue. The closer the lesion was to the digestive tract, the higher the nerve fiber density (data not shown) (Fig. 5).

Discussion

The first two large series including 231 and 500 women undergoing surgery for deep rectovaginal endometriosis were published in 1995 and 1997, respectively [3, 4]. The conclusion, already back in 1997, was that it is prudent to curtail rather than encourage the widespread use of an aggressive and potentially morbid procedure. Nevertheless, increasingly aggressive surgery, including bowel resection, is still systematically proposed in the case of deep endometriosis with muscularis involvement, even in the absence of mucosal involvement [6–11, 14, 15, 20, 33, 34].

The debate is not new. In a paper by Hudelist et al. [35], different past series and theories on the etiology of adenomyosis and endometriosis are described, and we are shown a specimen of deep endometriosis involving the rectum (a typical hourglass-shaped nodule). Back in 1903, Füth reported a case of rectal shaving for a hard mass between the uterus and the rectum [36] (Fig. 6a). In 1912, Renish performed resection of the anterior rectal wall (the first "disk resection") (Fig. 6b) together with hysterectomy [37], while Lockyer performed hysterectomy and bowel resection over a length of 20 cm for the same type of lesion (drawing by Lockyer from 1918) [38].

Almost 100 years later, the debate still rages on, not only rearing its head during the World Congress on Endometriosis in Melbourne [39], but also in the literature, with two

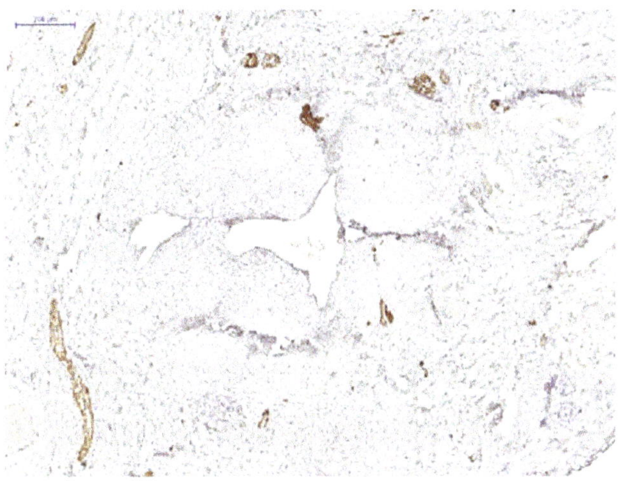

Fig. 5 Deep rectovaginal nodule. IHC: sections were immunostained with PGP9.5; abundant nerve fibers are visible

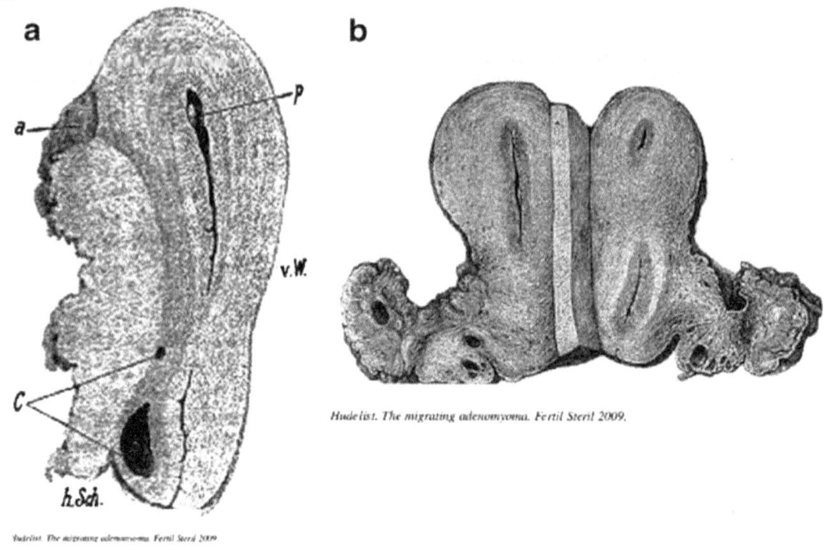

Fig. 6 **a** First case of rectal shaving published by Füth, who performed total hysterectomy revealing a hard thick mass fixed to the rectum, which was removed "to a major extent leaving the rectum behind". **b** First case of disk resection by Renish [37], showing deep endometriotic nodule (hourglass-shaped) with rectal mucosal involvement

conflicting articles recently appearing in the same journal: "Should we operate for deep-infiltrating endometriosis?—No. Choose realism instead of idealism!" by Fernandez et al. [40] and: "Yes, patients with deep-infiltrating endometriosis should be operated! Prefer optimistic will to pessimistic intelligence!" by Canis et al. [41].

Complications

We conducted a review of complication rates encountered after bowel resection for deep nodular endometriosis [6–15, 42] (Table 2.). Unfortunately, much of the recent literature appears to encourage very invasive techniques, including bowel resection in case of rectal muscularis involvement. Our review of recent publications reporting the results and complications of laparoscopy-assisted bowel resection for deep endometriotic nodules reveals a relatively high complication rate compared to the shaving technique ([17 and present data). Indeed, rates of urinary retention (3–10 %), ureteral lesions (2–4 %), fecal peritonitis (3–5 %), severe anastomotic stenosis (3 %), rectovaginal fistulas (6–9 %), and pelvic abscesses (2–4 %) were found to be significantly higher than with the shaving technique. A possible bias could have been the relatively small number of patients involved in some series, but it should be pointed out that, even in very experienced hands [12, 42], the rate of severe complications (rectovaginal fistulas, abscesses, stenosis, fecal peritonitis) can be more than 10 %.

In 2009, Meuleman et al. reported an 11 % rate of severe complications, some of which were due to the duration of surgery (mean over 7 h) [14]. Indeed, lower leg compartment syndrome was observed in three cases (3 of 56),

Table 2 Complication rate after the shaving technique compared to bowel resection (meta-analysis)

	Shaving technique (personal data), n=3,298	Rectal resection (meta-analysis) (Redwine and Wright [6], Chapron et al. [7], Daraï et al. [8, 42], Emmanuel and Davis [9], Fleisch et al. [10], Ford et al. [11]; Keckstein and Wiesinger [12]; Mereu et al. [13], Meuleman et al. [14, 15])
Repeat surgery	<0.1 %	10 %
Urinary retention	0.64 %	3–10 %
Ureteral lesions (uroperitoneum)	0.3 %	2–4 %
Severe anastomotic stenosis	–	3 %
Sepsis (pelvic abscess)	0.03 %	2–4 %
Rectal perforation upon shaving (diagnosed and repaired during surgery, no further complications)	1.3 %	–
Rectovaginal fistula	0.06 %	6–9 %
Fecal peritonitis, anastomotic leakage	0.06 %	3–5 %

requiring a fasciotomy. It is important to note that there was no mucosal infiltration of the rectum in this series. This relatively high rate of severe complications was encountered despite a multidisciplinary approach including a urologist and digestive surgeon. In this series, the median operating time was 7 h and 56 min (range, 180–780 min). The duration is also related to costs for the hospital (operating room, nurses, anesthesist…).

In our series, the median operating time (including laparoscopy) was just 78 min (range, 31–248 min). Surgery only exceeds 3 h when nodules are removed from the bladder, ureter, and bowel, sometimes including laparoscopic nephrectomy during the same procedure, as described by Jadoul et al. [30].

It should also be pointed out that colorectal segmental resection is a complex procedure, sometimes resulting in pelvic nerve damage and unpleasant urinary and digestive symptoms [26, 27, 43–46]. Indeed, urinary retention is quite frequent (3–10 %) after bowel resection, as often this type of surgery cannot preserve the pelvic autonomic nerves, which are the pathway for the neurogenic control of bladder function. Interestingly, the shaving technique provokes a very low rate of urinary retention because the dissection usually respects, at least on one side, the sympathetic nerves passing laterally to the rectum, which are frequently cut during extensive rectal or rectosigmoidal resection.

In our view, removing part of the rectum is simply not justified, since we know that this technique increases the risk of complications. Furthermore, no randomized studies performed to date have been able to prove that it is any more effective than the shaving technique. The recent review by Meuleman et al. [15] fails to give arguments in favor of bowel resection because of the absence of any real classification of the lesions (e.g., level of lesion, type of infiltration…) or surgery (e.g., rectal, sigmoid, rectosigmoid resection, length…). Landi et al. [25] reported that full-thickness disk excision using a circular stapler could prevent potential morbidity associated with low anastomosis. As only a few months earlier the same group [13] reported a major complication rate that required repeat operations in 20 out of 192 cases (10.4 %), they are now probably evaluating a less aggressive surgical technique than bowel resection [25]. The same trend away from bowel resection toward a less aggressive approach has recently been described by Slack et al. and Roman et al. [43, 47].

The shaving approach is often more than adequate. For type I and II lesions, there is a general consensus that in the absence (or virtual absence) of muscularis infiltration, there is no need for bowel resection. But the controversy arises when muscularis infiltration is present. This infiltration, observed in all cases of type III lesions, may usually be left in place, at least partially, since the shaving technique already removes what is necessary. Residual lesions in the muscularis of the rectum do not evolve and remain constant for a long time [5]. The argument used by some gynecologists and surgeons to defend bowel resection is that this procedure is more "radical." This is simply not true. Indeed, even with bowel resection, the margins are not free of disease in more than 10 % of cases [47, 48], so their argument is not borne out. Moreover, we should bear in mind that radical bowel surgery is associated with long-term morbidity, and as previously reported in a Cochrane Review [49], quality of life is significantly impaired following anterior resection.

Recurrence

The recurrence rate of symptoms (severe dysmenorrhea, severe dyspareunia, and severe pelvic pain) evaluated prospectively was 7 % after shaving surgery in a recent study of 500 cases of type II and III nodules [17]. The rate of recurrent pain observed in this large series was therefore no higher than that encountered after more aggressive surgery, including bowel resection. In the majority of series reporting data on bowel resection, the recurrence rate of severe pelvic pain is evaluated to be 6–20 % [6–14, 42]. However, in these studies, it is difficult to gauge the proportion of women suffering from pelvic pain due to a genuine recurrence of endometriosis and those with postoperative adhesions related to severe complications, such as pelvic abscesses or peritonitis.

The favorable results observed in our study [17] in terms of pelvic pain recurrence may be explained by the almost complete resection of deep nodular endometriosis, which is innervated abundantly by sensory C chlorogenic and adrenergic nerve fibers, as recently demonstrated by Wang [50].

Nerve fibers were identified not only in the eutopic endometrium of endometriosis patients [51, 52], but also in endometriotic lesions themselves. This was especially true of deep-infiltrating endometriosis [50, 53] and, to a lesser extent, peritoneal lesions [54], while it was more controversial in the case of ovarian endometriomas [53–56].

Our preliminary investigations confirm high nerve fiber density in deep-infiltrating lesions. Moreover, it was shown that this high density was mainly observed in deep lesions located near the intestinal lining. Some studies have suggested a correlation between nerve fiber density and pain in endometriosis patients [53, 54]. However, since pain is a suggestive feeling, larger patient populations suffering from different forms of endometriosis should be examined and compared with a disease-free population to conclusively establish a correlation between nerve fiber presence and pain felt by patients. Nevertheless, the present results, associated with previous findings, could explain the painful symptoms encountered by patients suffering from deep-infiltrating endometriosis and the good results in terms of improvement in symptoms after almost complete resection of deep nodules by the shaving technique.

On the other hand, as previously stated, even when bowel resection is carried out, the margins are not free of disease in around 10 % of cases [48, 57]. During the study period, 37 patients underwent bowel resection because of bowel stenosis (>80 %) with mucosal involvement. Among these 37 women, 27 were operated on for recurrence of severe pain with bowel stenosis after shaving (among the 3,298 cases). The fact that only 27 women underwent surgery (bowel resection) for recurrence is an important argument to consider, indicating that bowel resection should not be undertaken as first-line therapy but as a second-line approach in the case of recurrence with stenosis >80 %.

As we have stressed since 1997 and as vigorously discussed at the WES Congress in Melbourne [39], it is time to discourage very aggressive surgery under the false pretenses that a more radical approach is more effective. It is certainly not true of endometriosis, which is a benign disease. Women want to be free of symptoms, have normal bladder and digestive function, and enjoy a normal sex life. They do not necessarily want to be completely free of endometriosis. Indeed, as stated by Vercellini et al. [58, 59], the overall extent of disease correlates neither with the frequency or severity of symptoms, nor with the long-term prognosis in terms of conception or pain recurrence. The question raised by Koninckx and Ussia [60] "Do we need centers of excellence in endometriosis surgery or centers of excellence in endometriosis?" is still pertinent.

Conclusion

Endometriosis is not cancer and does not require the same treatment approach. Conservative surgery for deep endometriosis in young women means preservation of organs, nerves, and the vascular blood supply. There is therefore a need for further strong and energetic debate to weigh up the benefits of shaving (debulking surgery) versus rectal resection (radical surgery). Feasibility is not always synonymous with efficacy. As already pointed out, in the early twentieth century, Füth [36] carried out the first rectal shaving procedure and Renish [37] the first disk resection, while Lockyer [38] performed bowel resection for deep endometriosis involving the anterior rectal wall. One century later, the debate still rages on….

Conflict of interest This study was supported by grants to the institution from the Fonds de la Recherche Scientifique–FNRS, Belgium (no. 1.5015.11), la Région Wallonne, Vicomte Philippe de Spoelberch, Baron Frère and Mr. Pietro Ferrero.

References

1. Donnez J, Nisolle M, Smoes P, Gillet N, Beguin S, Casanas-Roux F (1996) Peritoneal endometriosis and "endometriotic" nodules of the rectovaginal septum are two different entities. Fertil Steril 66:362–368
2. Nisolle M, Donnez J (1997) Peritoneal endometriosis, ovarian endometriosis, and adenomyotic nodules of the rectovaginal septum are three different entities. Fertil Steril 68:585–596
3. Donnez J, Nisolle M, Casanas-Roux F, Bassil S, Anaf V (1995) Rectovaginal septum endometriosis or adenomyosis: laparoscopic management in a series of 231 patients. Hum Reprod 10:630–635
4. Donnez J, Nisolle M, Gillerot S, Smets M, Bassil S, Casanas-Roux F (1997) Rectovaginal septum adenomyotic nodules: a series of 500 cases. Br J Obstet Gynaecol 104:1014–1018
5. Donnez J, Squifflet J (2004) Laparoscopic excision of deep endometriosis. Obst Gynecol Clinics N Am 31:567–580
6. Redwine DB, Wright JT (2001) Laparoscopic treatment of complete obliteration of the cul-de-sac associated with endometriosis: long-term follow-up of en bloc resection. Feril Steril 76:358–365
7. Chapron C, Chopin N, Borghese B, Malartic C, Decuypere F, Foulot H (2004) Surgical management of deeply infiltrating endometriosis: an update. Ann NY Acad Sci 1034:326–337
8. Daraï E, Marpeau O, Thomassin I, Dubernard G, Barranger E, Bazot M (2005) Fertility after laparoscopic colorectal resection for endometriosis: preliminary results. Fertil Steril 84:945–950
9. Emmanuel KR, Davis C (2005) Outcomes and treatment options in rectovaginal endometriosis. Curr Opin Obstet Gynecol 17:399–402
10. Fleisch MC, Xafis D, Bruyne FD, Hucke J, Bender HG, Dall P (2005) Radical resection of invasive endometriosis with bowel or bladder involvement—long-term results. Eur J Obstet Gynecol Reprod Biol 123:224–229
11. Ford J, English J, Miles WF, Giannopoulos T (2005) A new technique for laparoscopic anterior resection for rectal endometriosis. JSLS 9:73–77
12. Keckstein J, Wiesinger H (2006) The laparoscopic treatment of intestinal endometriosis. In: Sutton C, Jones K, David Adamson G (eds) Endometriosis. Taylor & Francis, U.K., pp 177–187
13. Mereu L, Gagliardi ML, Clarizia R, Mainardi P, Landi S, Minelli L (2010) Laparoscopic management of ureteral endometriosis in case of moderate-severe hydroureteronephrosis. Fertil Steril 93:46–51
14. Meuleman C, D'Hoore A, Van Cleynenbreugel B, Beks N, D'Hooghe T (2009) Outcome after multidisciplinary CO_2 laser laparoscopic excision of deep infiltrating colorectal endometriosis. Reprod BioMed Online 18:282–289
15. Meuleman C, Tomasseti C, D'Hoore A, Buyens A, Van Cleynenbreugel B, Fieuws S, Penninckx F, Vergote I, D'Hooghe T (2011) Clinical outcome after CO_2 laser laparoscopic radical excision of endometriosis with colorectal wall invasion combined with laparoscopic segmental bowel resection and reanastomosis. Hum Reprod 26:2336–2343
16. De Cicco C, Schonman R, Craessaerts M, Van Cleynenbreugel B, Ussia A, Koninckx PR (2009) Laparoscopic management of ureteral lesions in gynecology. Fertil Steril 92:1424–1427
17. Donnez J, Squifflet J (2010) Complications, pregnancy and recurrence in a prospective series of 500 patients operated on by the shaving technique for deep rectovaginal endometriotic nodules. Hum Reprod 25:1949–1958
18. Koninckx PR, Meuleman C, Oosterlynck D, Cornillie FJ (1996) Diagnosis of deep endometriosis by clinical examination during menstruation and plasma CA-125 concentration. Fertil Steril 65:280–287
19. Ohba T, Mizutani H, Matsuura K, Ito M, Okamura H (1992) Transrectal ultrasonographic detection of uterosacral ligaments-

preliminary study for ultrasonographic evaluation of endometriosis. Nippon Sanka Fujinka Gakkai Zasshi 44:1187–1188

20. Abrao MS, Gonçalves MO, Dias JA Jr, Podgaec S, Chamie LP, Blasbalg R (2007) Comparison between clinical examination, transvaginal sonography and magnetic resonance imaging for the diagnosis of deep endometriosis. Hum Reprod 22:3092–3097
21. Squifflet J, Feger C, Donnez J (2002) Diagnosis and imaging of adenomyotic disease of the retroperitoneal space. Gynecol Obstet Invest 54:43–51
22. Nightingale AL, Ballard KD, Wright JT (2010) Evidence-based gynaecological practice: clinical review 3. The use of imaging for pre-operative planning in deep infiltrating endometriosis involving the rectum. Gynecol Surg 7:407–415
23. Maas K, Moriya Y, Kenter G, Trimbos B, van de Velde C (1999) A plea for preservation of the pelvic automatic nerves. Lancet 354:772–773
24. Possover M, Diebolder H, Plaut K, Schneider A (2000) Laparoscopically assisted vaginal resection of rectovaginal endometriosis. Obstet Gynecol 96:304–307
25. Landi S, Ceccaroni M, Perutelli A, Allodi C, Barbieri F, Fiaccavento A et al (2006) Laparoscopic nerve-sparing complete excision of deep endometriosis: is it feasible? Hum Reprod 21:774–781
26. Roman H, Vassilieff M, Gourcerol G, Savoye G, Leroi AM, Marpeau L et al (2011) Surgical management of deep infiltrating endometriosis of the rectum: pleading for a symptom-guided approach. Hum Reprod 26:274–281
27. Vassilieff M, Suaud O, Collet-Savoye C, Da Costa C, Marouteau-Pasquier N, Belhiba H, Tuech JJ, Marpeau L, Roman H (2011) Computed tomography-based virtual colonoscopy: an examination useful for the choice of the surgical management of colorectal endometriosis. Gynecol Obstet Fertil 39:339–345
28. Donnez J, Nisolle M, Squifflet J (2002) Ureteral endometriosis: a complication of rectovaginal endometriotic (adenomyotic) nodules. Fertil Steril 77:32–37
29. Colette S, Defrère S, Lousse JC, Van Langendonckt A, Gotteland JP, Loumaye E, Donnez J (2011) Inhibition of steroid sulfatase decreases endometriosis in an in vivo murine model. Hum Reprod 26(6):1362–1370
30. Jadoul P, Feyaerts A, Squifflet J, Donnez J (2007) Combined laparoscopic and vaginal approach for nephrectomy, ureterectomy, and removal of a large rectovaginal endometriotic nodule causing loss of renal function. J Minim Invasive Gynecol 14:256–259
31. Koninckx P, Ussia A, Adamyan L, Wattiez A (2011) An endometriosis classification, designed to be validated. Gynecol Surg 8:1–6
32. Weingertner AS, Rodriguez B, Ziane A, Gibon E, Thoma V, Osario F et al (2008) The use of JJ stent in the management of deep endometriosis lesion, affecting or potentially affecting the ureter: a review of our practice. BJOG 115:1159–1164
33. Chapron C, Liaras E, Fayet P, Hoeffel C, Fauconnier A, Vieira M et al (2002) Magnetic resonance imaging and endometriosis: deeply infiltrating endometriosis does not originate from the rectovaginal septum. Gynecol Obstet Invest 53:204–208
34. Chapron C, Chopin N, Borghese B, Foulot H, Dousset B, Vacher-Lavenu MC et al (2006) Deeply infiltrating endometriosis: pathogenetic implications of the anatomical distribution. Hum Reprod 21:1839–1845
35. Hudelist G, Keckstein J, Wright JT (2009) The migrating adenomyoma: past views on the etiology of adenomyosis and endometriosis. Fertil Steril 92:1536–1543
36. Füth H (1903) Beitrag zur Kasuistik der Adenomyome des Uterus. Zentralblatt für Gynaekologie 26:626
37. Renish N (1912) Ein Beitrag zur Adenomyositis uteri et recti. Zeischrift fuer Geburtshilfe und Gynaekologie. 70:585
38. Lockyer C (1918) Fibroids and allied tumours (myoma and adenomyoma). Macmillan and Co., Ltd, London
39. Donnez J (2008) Is accreditation for surgery necessary? World Endometriosis Society e-journal 10:6–7
40. Fernandez H, Deffieux X, Faivre E, Gervaise A (2008) Should we operate deep infiltrating endometriosis? No. "Choose realism instead of idealism". Gynecol Obstet Fertil 36:214–217
41. Canis M, Matsuzaki S, Jardon K, Rivoire C, Cotte B, Tamburro S et al (2008) Yes, patients with deep infiltrating endometriosis should be operated! "Prefer optimistic will to pessimistic intelligence!". Gynécol Obstet Fertil 36:218–221
42. Daraï E, Thomassin I, Barranger E, Detchev R, Cortez A, Houry S et al (2005) Feasibility and technical outcome of laparoscopic colorectal resection for endometriosis. Am J Obstet Gynecol 192:394–400
43. Slack A, Child T, Lindsey I, Kennedy S, Cunningham C, Mortensen N, Koninckx P, McVeigh E (2007) Urological and colorectal complications following surgery for rectovaginal endometriosis. BJOG 14:1278–1282
44. Roman H, Bourdel N (2009) Against the systematic use of segmental resection in colorectal endometriosis: do not replace the pain by unpleasant digestive symptoms! Gynecol Obstet Fertil 37:358–362
45. Vercellini P, Crosignani PG, Abbiati A, Somigliani E, Viagano P, Fedele L (2009) The effect of surgery for symptomatic endometriosis: the other side of the story. Hum Reprod Update 15:177–178
46. Payá V, Hidalgo-Mora JJ, Diaz-Garcia C, Pellicer A (2011) Surgical treatment of rectovaginal endometriosis with rectal involvement. Gynecol Surg 8:269–277
47. Roman H, Loisel C, Resch B, Tuech JJ, Hochain P, Marpeau L (2010) Delayed functional outcomes associated with surgical management of rectal endometriosis: giving our patients an informed choice. Hum Reprod 25:890–899
48. Anaf V, El Nakadi I, De Moor V, Coppens E, Zaeleman M, Noel JC (2009) Anatomic significance of a positive barium enema in deep infiltrating endometriosis of the large bowel. World J Surg 33:822–827
49. Pachler J, Wille-Jørgensen P (2005) Quality of life after rectal resection for cancer, with or without permanent colostomy. Cochrane Database Syst Rev 18(2):CD004323, Review
50. Wang G (2009) Rich innervation of deep infiltrating endometriosis. Hum Reprod 24:827–834
51. Al-Jefout M, Dezarnaulds G, Cooper M, Tokushige N, Luscombe GM, Markham R, Fraser IS (2009) Diagnosis of endometriosis by detection of nerve fibres in an endometrial biopsy: a double blind study. Hum Reprod 24:3019–3024
52. Bokor A, Kyama CM, Vercruysse L, Fassbender A, Gevaert O, Vodolazkaia A, De Moor B, Fülöp V, D'Hooghe T (2009) Density of small diameter sensory nerve fibres in endometrium: a semi-invasive diagnostic test for minimal to mild endometriosis. Hum Reprod 24:3025–3032
53. McKinnon B, Bersinger NA, Wotzkow C, Mueller MD (2012) Endometriosis-associatednerve fibers, peritoneal fluid cytokine concentrations, and pain in endometriotic lesions from different locations. Fertil Steril 97(2):373–380
54. Mechsner S, Grum B, Gericke C, Loddenkemper C, Dudenhausen JW, Ebert AD (2010) Possible roles of oxytocin receptor and vasopressin-1α receptor in the pathomechanism of dysperistalsis and dysmenorrhea in patients with adenomyosis uteri. Fertil Steril 94(7):2541–2546
55. Tokushige N, Russell P, Black K, Barrera H, Dubinovsky S, Markham R et al (2010) Nerve fibers in ovarian endometriomas. Fertil Steril 94:1944–1947
56. Zhang X, Yao H, Huang X, Lu B, Xu H, Zhou C (2010) Nerve fibres in ovarian endometriotic lesions in women with ovarian endometriosis. Hum Reprod 25:392–397

57. Roman H, Puscasiu L, Kouteich K, Gromez A, Resch B, Marouteau-Pasquier N, Hochain P, Tuech JJ, Scotte M, Marpeau L (2007) Laparoscopic management of deep endometriosis with rectal affect. Chirurgia 102:421–428
58. Vercellini P, Fedele L, Pietropaolo G, Frontino G, Somigliana E, Crosignani PG (2003) Progestogens for endometriosis: forward to the past. Hum Reprod Update 9:387–396
59. Vercellini P, Pietropaolo G, De Giorgi O, Pasin R, Chiodini A, Crosignani PG (2005) Treatment of symptomatic rectovaginal endometriosis with an estrogen-progestogen combination versus low-dose norethindrone acetate. Fertil Steril 84:1375–1387
60. Koninckx PR, Ussia A (2010) Centers of excellence in endometriosis surgery" or "centers of excellence in endometriosis. Gynecol Surg 7:109–111

13

Pain reduction by continuous intraperitoneal nebulization of ropivacaine during gynecological laparoscopic surgery

Y. Kaufman · L. Ostrovsky · O. Klein · I. Hirsh · R. Auslander · R. Pizov · A. Lissak

Abstract The objective of this study was to examine the analgesic effect of intraperitoneal nebulization of ropivacaine during gynecological laparoscopic procedures for patients anesthetized with an ultrashort-acting opiate. The study was a double-blinded placebo-controlled randomized trial (Canadian Task Force classification I) and involved 40 patients (20 patients in each arm) undergoing elective gynecological same-day outpatient laparoscopic surgery including unilateral/bilateral salpingo-oophorectomy or unilateral/bilateral ovarian cystectomy at the University Hospital Ambulatory Gynecological Endoscopic Unit. The study group received 10 ml of 1 % ropivacaine, and the control group received 10 ml of sterile water by intraperitoneal nebulization. Vital signs were recorded and summarized. Postoperatively, patients were followed up for 24 h including visual analogue scale (VAS) scores and analgesic usage. Results showed no significant differences between the two groups in terms of patient characteristics and surgical data. There were no significant differences between the groups in postoperative VAS scores at rest at the different time intervals. VAS scores during strain showed significantly decreased pain at the postoperative 2-h interval ($p<0.05$). Postoperative opiate and nonopiate analgesia consumption was similar for both groups. Patients in the study groups required more antiemetic agents compared to the control group patients ($p<0.05$). There were no reported side effects related to ropivacaine. Intraperitoneal nebulization of 100 mg of ropivacaine during gynecological laparoscopy under general anesthesia with an ultrashort-acting opiate does not reduce postoperative pain and it does not reduce postoperative opiate and nonopiate analgesia consumption.

Keywords Pain · Intraperitoneal · Nebulization · Ropivacaine · Gynecology · Laparoscopy · Visual analog scale (VAS) score · Opiates · Remifentanil

Background

Laparoscopic surgery has been clearly proven to have significant advantages over open surgery in many aspects including decreased postoperative pain. This has allowed many of the laparoscopic procedures to be performed on an outpatient basis. Pain control and reduction of postoperative nausea and vomiting (PONV) are essential for the patient's well-being and adamant for ambulatory surgery. Good postoperative pain relief has been advocated by the Joint Commission on Accreditation of Healthcare Organizations as a patient's right [1].

Pain during and after laparoscopy is multifactorial. This includes factors related to the procedure such as the type and duration of the procedure; factors related to the CO_2 gas including the total volume, pressure, and humidity of the delivered gas as well as the amount of residual gas within the peritoneum at the end of the procedure; and factors related to the intraoperative anesthetic protocol and the postoperative pain control protocol [2–4]. Improvements in postoperative pain may be achieved by reducing the CO_2 pressure, increasing humidity of the gas, and changing the

Y. Kaufman (✉) · L. Ostrovsky · O. Klein · I. Hirsh ·
R. Auslander · A. Lissak
Department of Obstetrics and Gynecology,
The Lady Davis Carmel Medical Center,
Technion Institute of Technology Medical School,
7 Michal Street,
Haifa 34362, Israel
e-mail: mdykaufman@013.net.il

R. Pizov
Department of Anesthesiology and Critical Care,
The Lady Davis Carmel Medical Center,
Technion Institute of Technology Medical School,
Haifa, Israel

intraoperative as well as postoperative use of anesthetics and analgesics.

Postoperative pain is mostly visceral [5]. Pain control is usually done using opiates and opiate derivatives as well as local anesthetics (LA) and nonsteroidal anti-inflammatory drugs. Opiates are effective in pain control but at the price of causing PONV and drowsiness which are counterproductive for outpatient treatment. Reducing the negative effects of the opiates can be done by using short-acting opiates and intraperitoneal local anesthetics during laparoscopy. There are conflicting results regarding the effectiveness of intraperitoneal local anesthetics. Studies on this subject vary in terms of the timing for administration of the local anesthetic in relation to the procedure (i.e., beginning of insufflation, end of insufflation, end of the procedure), location of distribution within the peritoneal cavity, dosage, and the addition of adrenaline, which lowers peak plasma volume of the anesthetic [3]. Previously, we have published a study on continuous intraperitoneal nebulization of ropivacaine throughout gynecological laparoscopic procedures [6]. Ropivacaine pharmacodynamics depend on the method of administration. An animal study has shown that ropivacaine reaches peak concentrations after 1 h from administration, has a half-life of 2 h, and is excreted after approximately 6 h [7]. Our results showed no significant reduction in postoperative pain or in the use of postoperative analgesics. We assumed that residual effects of opiates given during the laparoscopic procedure have a prolonged postoperative effect which might be masking a possible potential pain-decreasing benefit of ropivacaine after surgery. Therefore, we decided to perform a follow-up study using the same technique of intraperitoneal nebulization but with a different anesthetic protocol which is based on ultrashort-acting opiates. Remifentanil is an ultrashort-acting opiate with an onset of action around 1 min and a half-life of 2–3 min which is rapidly eliminated from the body [8].

The objective of our study was to examine the effect of intraperitoneal nebulization of ropivacaine during gynecological laparoscopic procedures under an ultrashort-acting opiate anesthetic protocol on postoperative pain and analgesic consumption.

Methods

The study was a double-blinded placebo-controlled randomized trial approved by the Carmel Medical Center Helsinki Ethics Committee. We included 40 patients (20 patients in each arm), ages 18–70, with an American Society of Anesthesiologists physical status grade I or II, undergoing elective gynecological laparoscopic surgery at our Ambulatory Gynecoendoscopic Unit. All operations were performed by two senior consultants. After signing a consent form, patients who were candidates for a same-day outpatient laparoscopy including unilateral/bilateral salpingo-oophorectomy or unilateral/bilateral ovarian cystectomy randomly received either 10 ml of 1 % ropivacaine to a total of 100 mg (Naropin, 100 mg/10 ml, AstraZeneca, UK) or 10 ml of sterile water. The ampoules were prepared according to a double-blind design with the contents of the ampoules known only to the hospital pharmacy. Patients were randomly assigned to the study and control groups by a computer-generated algorithm.

All patients received the same standard anesthetic technique and standard monitoring including ECG, noninvasive blood pressure, end tidal CO_2, oxygen saturation, and temperature. Anesthesia was induced with a loading dose of remifentanil 1 μg/kg in 10 cc of saline given within a minute. This was followed by propofol 2 mg/kg and droperidol 0.5 mg. Rocuronium 0.6 mg/kg was given to facilitate intubation of the trachea. Anesthesia was maintained with isoflurane at one minimum alveolar concentration, N_2O 60 %, and O_2 40 %. Continuous remifentanil was administered at an initial dose of 0.5 μg/kg/min at the beginning of the procedure and was decreased to 0.2–0.4 μg/kg/min until 5 min before the estimated termination of the operation at which point the remifentanil was stopped. Minute ventilation was controlled and adjusted to keep the end-tidal CO_2 around 40 mmHg.

During laparoscopy, intra-abdominal CO_2 pressure was maintained at 13–15 mmHg throughout filling and maintenance. Nebulization was done using a specially designed nebulizer called Aeroneb Pro® (Aerogen, Ireland) which is an autoclavable Food and Drug Administration-approved device that produces a fine particle aerosol (2.1 μm mass median aerodynamic diameter, 83 % fine particle fraction <5 μm) without heating or degrading medications. The Aeroneb nebulizer can deliver 10 ml of fluid within 30 min regardless of the gas flow. The contents of the blinded ampoule were injected into the Aeroneb reservoir and nebulized along with the CO_2 at a maximal flow rate of 15 l/min. The nebulizer was located proximal to the entry trocar at a distance not exceeding 30 cm to avoid major condensation of the fluid within the tubing. A closed entry

Table 1 Patient characteristics

	Control (*n*=20)	Study (*n*=20)	*p* value
Mean age (SD, 95 % CI)	47 (16.2, 23–77)	45.7 (13.4, 25–69)	0.79
Body mass index	26.5 (5.2, 19.5–43.7)	26.3 (7.2, 16.9–43.7)	0.90

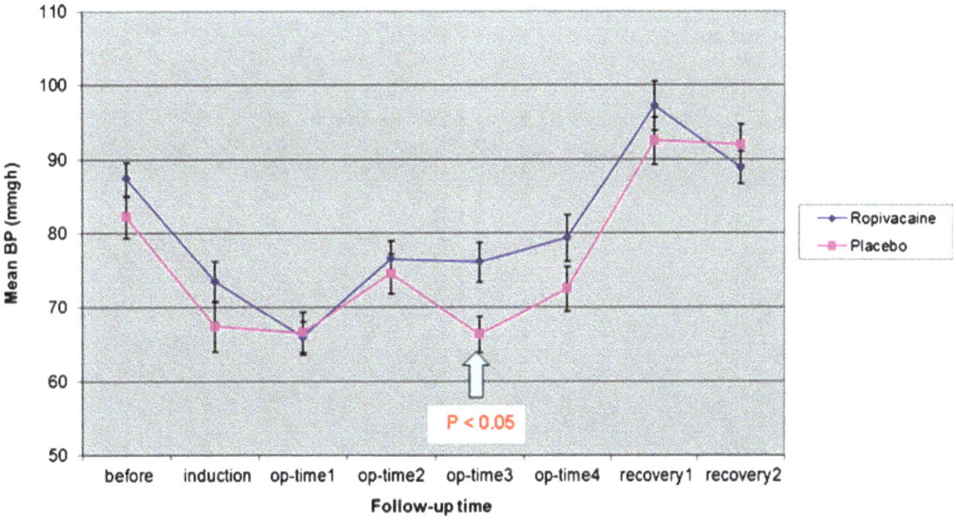

Fig. 1 Mean arterial blood pressure (MAP) during surgery presented as mean and SE

technique was used. Insufflation of CO_2 through the nebulizer system delivered ropivacaine or sterile water into the peritoneal cavity. Mean arterial blood pressure (MAP) and heart rate were recorded before surgery, during induction, and at time intervals during the procedure and at the recovery unit. Intraoperative pain was evaluated by changes in MAP and heart rate. Surgery duration and blood loss were recorded at the end of the procedure. Following the procedure, visual analog scale (VAS) scoring was used to assess pain severity at rest and during strain (cough). This was done in the recovery room postoperatively at 30 min, 1 h, and 2 h from completion of surgery. Intravenous morphine 0.05 mg/kg was administered when the VAS score exceeded 4. Additional doses of morphine were given till the VAS score dropped below 4. Patients with shivers were given 15 mg of IV pethidine. Nausea and vomiting were treated with IV 4 mg ondansetron.

After discharge, patients were interviewed at home by phone at 6 h and 24 h after surgery for VAS scores. Patients were asked whether they required analgesia. The type, dosage, and frequency of analgesic consumption were recorded.

Statistical analysis was performed by using the SPSS 15 software. The continuous variables were presented by mean ± std or median, as appropriate. The categorical variables were presented in percentages.

Comparisons between the two groups regarding patient characteristics and surgical data were done by using independent t test or Mann–Whitney, as appropriate, for the continuous variables. Chi-square test was performed for the categorical variables.

The VAS score analysis comparing the two groups at each point of time was done by using the nonparametric Mann–Whitney test with Bonferroni correction for multiple statistical comparisons. A p value <0.05 was determined as statistically significant.

Findings

Our results show no significant differences between the two groups in terms of patient characteristics and surgical data

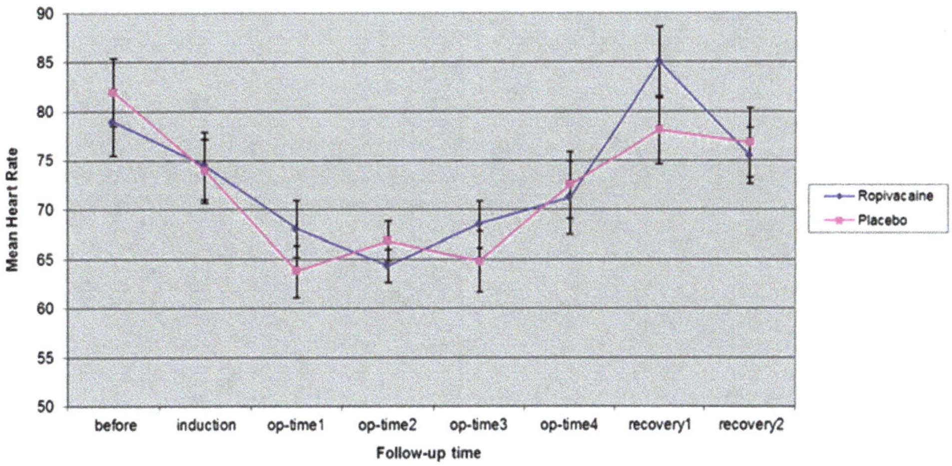

Fig. 2 Heart rate (HR) during surgery presented as mean and SE

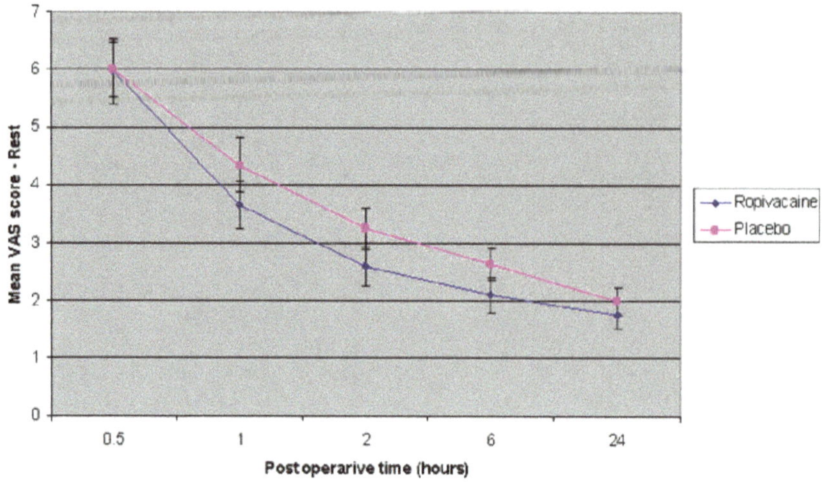

Fig. 3 Visceral visual analog scale (VAS) scores at rest during 24 postoperative hours

(Table 1). This includes mean age, BMI, surgery duration, blood loss, number and size of trocars, total insufflated gas, and type of procedure.

There were no significant differences between the groups at each time interval in terms of mean arterial blood pressure except for operating time interval 3 ($p<0.05$, Fig. 1). No significant changes were found between the groups in terms of heart rate (Fig. 2).

There were no significant differences between the groups in postoperative VAS scores at rest at the different time intervals (Fig. 3). Analysis of VAS scores during strain (cough) showed significantly decreased pain between study and control groups at the postoperative 2-h interval in favor of the study group patients ($p<0.05$, Fig. 4).

Postoperative opiate and nonopiate analgesia consumption was similar for both groups (p=n.s., Table 2). Patients in the study groups required more antiemetics compared to the control group patients ($p<0.05$).

There were no reported side effects related to ropivacaine and no intraoperative or postoperative complications for any of the patients in both the study and control groups (Table 3).

Discussion

The efficacy of intraperitoneal administration of LA for pain relief after laparoscopic surgery has been a subject of many studies. Interpretation of overall results in a meta-analysis is difficult due to the large heterogeneity in methodology. Studies differ with regard to the type of LA, dosage, method and timing of administration, intraoperative and postoperative pain control protocol, and follow-up parameters. Long-acting local anesthetics have been shown to be efficient for postoperative pain relief in different types of laparoscopic procedures such as cholecystectomy [9] and appendectomy [10]. There are several studies showing conflicting results on the effect of LA instillation following gynecological laparoscopic procedures [10–16].

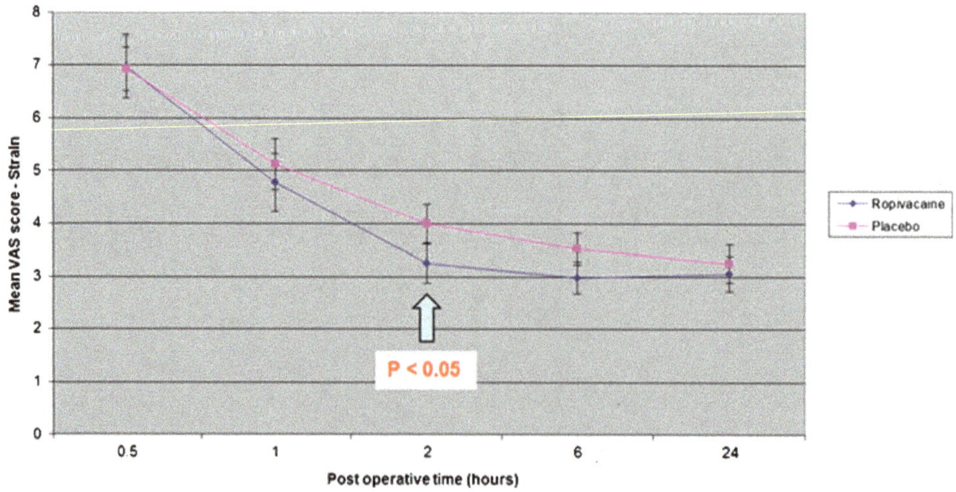

Fig. 4 Visceral visual analog scale (VAS) scores at cough during 24 postoperative hours

Table 2 Surgical data

	Control (n=20)	Study (n=20)	p value
Mean surgery duration (SD, 95 % CI)	56.4 (27.6, 30–135)	56.5 (25.5, 30-110)	0.95
Mean blood loss (SD, 95 % CI)	32.8	36.4	0.11
Trocars (×1, ×2, ×3)			
5 mm	10, 9, 1	14, 6, 0	0.33
10–12 mm	1, 19	0, 20	>0.99
Mean gas insufflation (l), (SD, 95 % CI)	109 (74.2, 36–319)	100 (57.4, 30–289)	0.97
Procedure, total (%)			
Ovarian cystectomy	10 (50)	8 (40)	
Unilateral salpingo-oopherectomy (left/right)	1 (5)	4 (20)	
Bilateral salpingo-oophorectomy (left/right)	9 (45)	8 (40)	
Total	20 (100)	20 (100)	0.461

Timing of administration is of importance. In a meta-analysis on the use of intraperitoneal LA during laparoscopic cholecystectomy, Kahokehr and colleagues have shown that for most studies, the LA was administered at the end of laparoscopy [9]. They advocate that LA should be given just before exsufflation of the gas from the pneumoperitoneum. Other studies argue for the importance of administration from the beginning of the procedure in order to gain a potential preemptive analgesic effect. Coughlin and colleagues performed a meta-analysis of studies comparing preemptive intraperitoneal administration of LA with post-operative instillation [17]. They showed that preemptive administration significantly reduces pain following laparoscopy. Another study showed that postoperative pain and anesthetic consumption were significantly reduced when bupivacaine was instilled prior to CO_2 insufflation as compared to following creation of pneumoperitoneum [18]. The authors concluded this difference can be attributed to the preemptive analgesia effect.

Our current study is a follow-up to two previous studies that were published by our group [6, 19]. All three studies analyzed the effect of continuous nebulization of local anesthetics throughout the laparoscopic procedure, from initiation of CO_2 insufflation. To the best of our knowledge, our studies are the only ones using nebulization instead on instillation of a LA for gynecological laparoscopic procedures. Our first study showed that nebulization of lidocaine significantly decreased postoperative pain but for a limited duration [19]. For the second study, we opted to use a long-acting LA [6]. We chose ropivacaine since it has previously been shown to have a good effect with less toxicity when compared to bupivacaine [20]. The results of our second study showed no significant decrease in postoperative pain or analgesic consumption. The intraoperative anesthetic protocol included fentanyl, a long-acting opiate which can have a prolonged postoperative effect. We concluded that the potential benefit of ropivacaine might be masked by the use of fentanyl. Therefore, we decided to perform our current follow-up study using a different anesthetic protocol which includes remifentanil, a short-acting opiate, instead of fentanyl and to discontinue its administration 5 min prior to termination of surgery. Our decision to nebulize 100 mg of ropivacaine, the same dose that was used during the second study, was based on a study by Labaille and colleagues [21]. They performed a study during which ropivacaine was instilled at the start and end of laparoscopic cholecystectomy. They showed that administering a total dose of 100 mg gives similar results in terms of postoperative analgesic effect, morphine consumption, and side effects when compared to 300 mg of ropivacaine. But patients receiving the larger dose had significantly elevated plasma concentrations of ropivacaine, and for some of the patients, the level exceeded 4 μg/ml, which is the limit for potential toxicity. Based on this study, we decided to maintain a total dosage of 100 mg ropivacaine for the follow-up study.

Table 3 Postoperative analgesia (opiate and nonopiate) and antiemetic consumption

	Study (n=20)	Control (n=20)	p value
Opiate consumption	17 (85 %)	18 (90 %)	0.99
Nonopiate analgesia consumption	14 (70 %)	15 (75 %)	0.72
Antiemetic consumption	11 (55 %)	17 (85 %)	**<0.05**

Bold show less antiemetic consumption within the study group pateints than control group patients

Nebulization of a LA is intended for equal distribution within the peritoneal cavity in order to overcome pain that is transmitted not only from the surgical site but also from other areas of the peritoneum. It is possible that when nebulizing 100 mg of ropivacaine, the total amount of LA that reaches the surgical site is insufficient. Therefore, when remifentanil is discontinued before the end of the procedure, the patient feels pain from the surgical site. As a result, postoperative morphine consumption is relatively high, further masking potential analgesic effects of ropivacaine at later postoperative time intervals.

Our results showed a no significant decrease in postoperative pain after nebulization of ropivacaine. Furthermore, most patients, in both study and control groups, required morphine and ondansetron after surgery.

Unfortunately, there are no other studies for comparison that used nebulization of a long-acting LA during gynecological laparoscopy. Nevertheless, nebulization of a long-acting LA did decrease postoperative pain following laparoscopic cholecystectomy [22].

Further studies are needed to conclude whether nebulization of LA can decrease postoperative pain. A follow-up study should possibly include a higher dose of long-acting LA while monitoring blood levels. Adrenaline can be used to decrease systemic absorption of ropivacaine by half [7]. An addition of intraperitoneal fentanyl can also be beneficial. Most importantly, nebulization should be done using a nebulizing device that is guaranteed to deliver the total amount of substance without losing some of medication along the tubing.

Conclusion

In summary, our current and previous studies show that intraperitoneal nebulization of 100 mg of ropivacaine or lidocaine during gynecological laparoscopy, under ultrashort- and short-acting opiates, does not significantly reduce postoperative pain.

Conflict of interest The authors report no conflicts of interest. The authors alone are responsible for the content and writing of the paper.

References

1. Phillips DM (2000) JCAHO pain management standards are unveiled. Joint commission on accreditation of healthcare organizations. JAMA 284:428–429
2. Coşkun F, Salman MA (2001) Anesthesia for operative endoscopy. Cur Opin Obstet Gynecol 13:371–376
3. Wills VL, Hunt DR (2000) Pain after laparoscopic cholecystectomy. Br J Surg 87(3):273–284
4. Ott DE, Reich H, Love B et al (1998) Reduction of laparoscopic-induced hypothermia, postoperative pain and recovery room length of stay by pre-conditioning gas with the Insuflow device: a prospective randomized controlled multi-center study. J Soc Lap Surg 2:321–329
5. Joris J, Thiry E, Paris P et al (1995) Pain after laparoscopic cholecystectomy: characteristics and effect of intraperitoneal bupivacaine. Anesth Analg 81:379–384
6. Kaufman Y, Hirsch I, Ostrovsky L et al (2008) Pain relief by continuous intraperitoneal nebulization of ropivacaine during gynecologic laparoscopic surgery—a randomized study and review of the literature. J Min Invasive Gynecol 15:554–558
7. Betton D, Greib N, Schlotterbeck H et al (2010) The pharmacokinetics of ropivacaine after intraperitoneal administration: instillation versus nebulization. Anesth Analg 111(5):1140–1145
8. Breen D, Wilmer A, Bodenham A et al (2004) Offset of pharmacodynamic effects and safety of remifentanil in intensive care unit patients with various degrees of renal impairment. Crit Care 8:R21–R30
9. Kahokehr A, Sammour T, Soop M, Hill A (2010) Intraperitoneal use of local anesthetic in laparoscopic cholecystectomy: systematic review and metaanalysis of randomized controlled trials. J Hepatobiliary Pancreat Sci 17:637–656
10. Kang H, Kim BG (2010) Intraperitoneal ropivacaine for effective pain relief after laparoscopic appendectomy: a prospective, randomized, double-blind, placebo-controlled study. J Int Med Res 38 (3):821–832
11. Ceyhar T, Tekosoz E, Gungor S, Goktolg U, Pabuccu R (2005) Effect of bupivacaine after operative gynaecological procedures. J Min Invasive Gynecol 12(4):326–329
12. Ozer Y, Tanriverdi HA, Ozkocak I, Attunkaya H, Demirel CB, Bayan U, Barut A (2005) Evaluation of local anaesthesia regimen using subphrenic catheter after gynaecologic laparoscopy. Eur J Anaesthesiol 22(6):442–446
13. Shaw IC, Stevens J, Krishnamurthy S (2001) The influence of intraperitoneal bupivacaine on pain following major laparoscopic gynaecological procedures. Anaesthesia 56:1041–1044
14. Goldstein A, Patrick G, Henique a, Keller M, Fortin a, Dorai E (2000) Preventing postoperative pain by local anesthetic instillation after gynecologic surgery: a placebo-controlled comparison of bupivacaine and ropivacaine. Anaesth Analg 91:403–407
15. El-Sherbiny W, Saber W, Askalany A, El-Daly A, Abdel-aziz Sleem A (2009) Effect of intra-abdominal instillation of lidocaine during minor laparoscopic procedures. Int J Gyn Obs 106:213–215
16. Savarisa R, Chicarb L, Cristovamc R, Moraesc G, Miguel O (2010) Does bupivacaine in laparoscopic ports reduce postsurgery pain in tubal ligation by electrocoagulation? A randomized controlled trial. Contraception 81:542–546
17. Coughlin S, Karanicolas P, Emmerton-Coughlin H et al (2010) Better late than never? Impact of local analgesia timing on postoperative pain in laparoscopic surgery: a systematic review and metaanalysis. Surg Endosc 24:3167–3176
18. Barczyński M, Konturek A, Herman RM (2006) Superiority of preemptive analgesia with intraperitoneal instillation of bupivacaine before rather than after the creation of pneumoperitoneum for laparoscopic cholecystectomy: a randomized, double-blind, placebo-controlled study. Surg Endosc 20 (7):1088–1093
19. Sharon A, Hirsh I, Kaufman Y et al (2008) The effect of continuous intraabdominal nebulization of lidocaine during gynecological laparoscopic procedures—a pilot study. Surg Endosc 5(3):221–225
20. Knudsen K, Beckman NS, Blomberg S et al (1997) Central nervous system and cardiovascular effects of i.v. infusions of ropivacaine, bupivacaine and placebo in volunteers. Br J Anaesth 78:507–514
21. Labaille T, Mazoit JX, Paqueron X et al (2002) The clinical efficacy and pharmacokinetics of intraperitoneal ropivacaine for laparoscopic cholecystectomy. Anesth Analg 94:100–105
22. Alkhamesi NA, Peck DH, Lomax D, Darzi AW (2007) Intraperitoneal aerosolization of bupivacaine reduces postoperative pain in laparoscopic surgery: a randomized prospective controlled double blinded clinical trial. Surg Endosc 21:602–606

14

3D laparoscopy: technique and initial experience in 451 cases

Rakesh Sinha · Meenakshi Sundaram · Shweta Raje · Gayatri Rao · Manju Sinha · Rushindra Sinha

Abstract This study aims to show that 3D technology in laparoscopy promises to be an indispensable tool. The feasibility and safety of this surgical innovation has been shown. Our objective is to evaluate our initial experience performing 3D laparoscopic surgeries and determine if there is any benefit with respect to the time of surgery, time of morcellation, complications, and blood loss. Study design includes prospective analysis of 451 cases of 3D laparoscopy between September 2011 and August 2012 for total laparoscopic hysterectomy (TLH), laparoscopic myomectomy (LM), and other advanced surgeries. The setting of the study is in a tertiary endoscopic referral center. Between September 2011 and August 2012, 451 laparoscopic surgeries were performed using 3D HD camera and Einstein Vision telescope (Schoelly-Fibreoptic GMBH, Germany) (Fig. 1). An analysis was done showing various indications; the average time taken for surgery and morcellation (whenever indicated), the average blood loss, and the learning curve were determined. 3D TLH was done in 200 cases and was compared to the 200 cases in which 2D was used previously. The weights of specimens were comparable in both groups. The duration of surgery in 3D was less than 60 min in 132 cases, while only 110 cases with 2D took less than 60 min. This difference was statistically significant (p= 0.0316). Similarly, during laparoscopic myomectomy of 97 cases with 3D, 12 cases were done in less than 45 min, while only two cases were done in less than 45 min with the 2D system (p=0.0101). This was statistically significant. The weights of specimens in both groups were comparable. The total blood loss during surgery with 2D and 3D was comparable and not statistically significant in both groups of TLH and LM. We had two conversions to conventional laparoscopy: one ureteric injury (patient with 2.1 kg uterus with anatomical distortion) and one relook after 12 h for hematoma evacuation. The largest uterus removed was 4.87 kg. 3D HD laparoscopy is a quantum leap in minimally invasive gynecology. The tactile feedback is retained; the precision, accuracy, and depth perception are remarkable. The learning curve is short (less than five cases). The initial investment and recurring cost are low compared to robotic-assisted laparoscopies. The time taken for surgery as well as morcellation is less than in 2D HD laparoscopy. The possibility of complications may be less also.

Keywords 3D laparoscopy · Laparoscopic hysterectomy · Laparoscopic myomectomy · Gynecological surgery · Einstein Vision system · Minimally invasive · Depth perception

Background

Despite the introduction of laparoscopic surgeries for two decades, most surgeons globally still perform conventional laparotomies for hysterectomies and myomectomies. Several reasons have been cited, e.g., lack of adequate training in residential programs, lack of adequate training opportunities outside the medical colleges, lack of teachers and mentors, and lack of desire to learn newer skills. However, perhaps the most important reason is that the 2D view on flat screen-laparoscopy is cerebrally intensive (Fig. 1).

The last two decades have been a glorious era for endoscopy in gynecology. The technological advances that have taken place in the last few years were unimaginable and have added to the safety, efficacy, and precision of laparoscopic

R. Sinha · M. Sundaram (✉) · S. Raje · G. Rao · M. Sinha · R. Sinha
Gynaecological Endoscopy, Bombay Endoscopy Academy and Centre for Minimally Invasive Surgery (BEAMS), 674, 16th Cross Road Khar, West Mumbai,
Mumbai, Maharashtra 400052, India
e-mail: drmeena25@yahoo.com

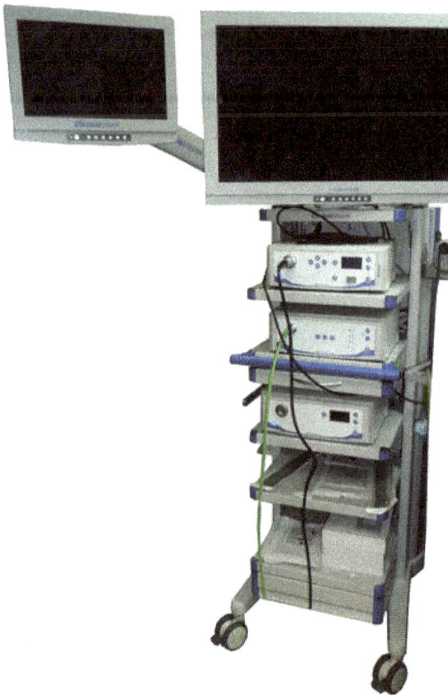

Fig. 1 3D Laparoscope system 65×86 mm (300×300 DPI)

procedures. The innovative advances including high-definition (HD) cameras, vessel sealing devices, the Harmonic Ultracision, electrical morcellator for solid organ tissue retrieval, and articulating instruments for single incision laparoscopy were all brilliant. But every once in a while, innovative technology takes a quantum leap.

Robotic-assisted laparoscopy and three-dimensional (3D) HD laparoscopy are a quantum leap and have taken laparoscopic surgery to a new orbit. In April 2005, the Food and Drug Administration approved the use of the da Vinci Surgical System for use in gynecological procedures.

The major limitation in laparoscopy was its 2D image. This resulted in the lack of depth perception thus increasing the strain for the surgeon and compromise on the safety of laparoscopy. The 3D HD technology is amazing. The precision, accuracy, and depth perception are incredible. It now seems like laparoscopic surgeons were operating with one eye closed! The 3D technology can enhance the skills of talented surgeons.

The question we need to answer is "Is it the use of robotics that can improve the quality of surgery and improve the learning curve?" or "Is it the 3D view on the screen that will enhance the skills of surgeons and improve the quality of advanced surgery?"

Although laparotomy may seem advantageous for the surgeon at first, with depth perception and tactile feedback from the tissue, the large abdominal incision, prolonged hospitalization, increased postoperative analgesic requirements, and higher morbidity are the disadvantages for the patient. Laparoscopic surgery enables faster recovery with shorter hospitalization, improved cosmesis, decreased blood loss, and less postoperative pain [1, 2].

The da Vinci Surgical System has some advantages compared to the conventional laparoscopic surgery, such as the three-dimensional vision, better ergonomics, higher degree of freedom of the robotic instruments, and reduction of tremor interference.

In recent years robotic surgery has been introduced in urological surgery, general surgery, cardiac surgery, and gynecological surgery. The da Vinci Surgical System (Intuitive Surgical, Inc., Sunnyvale, CA, USA) provides robotic control of the laparoscope and all instrumentation. The system employs a 3D vision system and endowrist technology. Endowrist technology facilitates instrument rotation through tiny incisions. The robotic instruments replicate the surgeon's hand, wrist, and finger movements. This allows for extended range of motion and improved manipulation while conducting laparoscopic procedures [3].

Several publications describe safety and feasibility of this approach. After the first excitement over the innovative and sophisticated technology has settled, there should also be some consideration for a critical assessment of the technique and costs, ideally with recommendations for further improvements by experienced laparoscopic surgeons [4]. It was demonstrated that it took approximately 50 robotic cases to develop consistent operative times and predictable outcomes [5]. Whereas when we used 3D HD laparoscopy, it took us about five cases to get absolutely used to the 3D image, i.e., two operative days.

The learning curve for established laparoscopic surgeons to adapt to 3D HD image on a 32-in. monitor is therefore approximately five cases. All the conventional straight instruments used in laparoscopy can be utilized. There is no recurring cost, and newer instruments can be used instantly.

Methods

All surgeries are performed under general anesthesia using laryngeal mask airway with the patient in modified lithotomy position [6]. The Veress needle is inserted at the Palmer's point (a point 3 cm below the left costal margin in the midclavicular line) after ruling out splenomegaly.

The first blind 5-mm trocar–cannula is inserted in the left upper lumbar zone [7] lateral to the inferior epigastric vessels at the level of or above the upper limit of the uterus. A 5-mm telescope (2D HD system) is introduced through this port; and the peritoneal cavity, uterus, and adnexa are evaluated. A 10-mm port is inserted under vision at the supra-umbilical site or higher depending on the size of the uterus. Entry under vision avoids damage to major vessels directly beneath the insertion site. The 3D HD telescope with a fore-oblique 30° view is then attached to the 3D HD camera and inserted through the 10-mm cannula.

Two additional accessory 5-mm trocar–cannulas are inserted—one in the left lateral lower quadrant and one in the right lateral upper quadrant. An optional robotic arm with a remote control is available to attach the camera for prolonged surgeries or for tremor-free camera stabilization. The surgeon and the entire operation theater team wear polarized glasses to appreciate the depth perception on a 3D medical grade 32-in. monitor (Fig. 2).

The 30° fore-oblique view can give a directional view from anterior to posterior or from posterior to anterior. Most of the surgeries can be completed with the antero-posterior view. Only deep posterior uterine wall surgeries or abdominal wall surgeries need the postero-anterior view. All complex surgeries can be done using straight stick; powered endowrist type of instruments is now available for conventional laparoscopies. We have not needed them so far.

Findings

A total of 451 patients were treated using 3D HD laparoscopic system. Out of these, 260 patients had total laparoscopic hysterectomy (TLH), 105 patients had laparoscopic myomectomy, and the remaining surgeries were ovarian cysts, endometriosis, and colpo-suspensions.

3D TLH was done in 200 cases and was compared to the 200 cases in which 2D was used previously. The weights of specimens were comparable in both groups. The duration of surgery in 3D was less than 60 min in 132 cases, while only 110 cases with 2D took less than 60 min. This difference was statistically significant (p=0.0316; Table 1).

Similarly, during laparoscopic myomectomy of 97 cases with 3D, 12 cases were done in less than 45 min, while only two cases were done in less than 45 min with 2D system (p= 0.0101; Table 2). This was statistically significant. The weights of specimens in both groups were comparable. The total blood loss during surgery with 2D and 3D was comparable and not statistically significant in both groups of total laparoscopic hysterectomy and laparoscopic myomectomy. Two patients had to be converted to 2D laparoscopy for angulated views that was difficult with 3D.

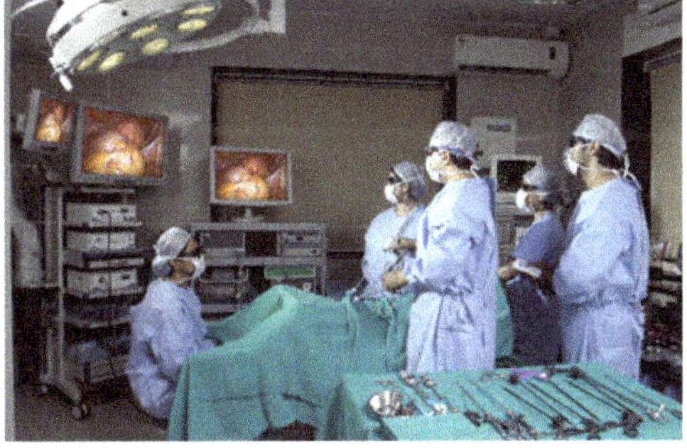

Fig. 2 Theatre set up with 3D glasses 108×72 mm (300×300 DPI)

Table 1 Duration of surgery in total laparoscopic hysterectomy and corresponding number of cases

System	Number of cases	
	Less than 1 h	More than 1 h
2D	110	90
3D	132	68

The p value 0.0316 was statistically significant

Discussion

The incidence of laparoscopy in advanced gynecological procedures is increasing although not dramatically. One of the reasons for this slow progress is the perceived long learning curves. The 3D view technology of conventional laparoscopy and robotic surgery promises to shorten this learning curve.

Physics of 3D

Principles of depth perception

Depth perception is the visual ability to judge the relative distance of objects and the spatial relationship of objects at different distances. As the three-dimensional world projects onto a two-dimensional retina, this projection on its own cannot provide depth information. The brain has to combine various monocular and binocular cues given by the eyes to recover the depth, distance, and three-dimensional shape of objects.

Stereopsis is the most important cue for depth perception. It is the consequence of interpapillary separation between the two eyes, 6 cm, which causes each eye to have a slightly different view of the same scene. This is called "retinal disparity". The brain is then able to combine the two views into a single 3D image—the process is called stereopsis. Stereoscopy (Greek, to look at a solid object) is the technique of creating or enhancing the illusion of depth in an image—by presenting two offset images separately to the left and right eye of the

Table 2 Duration of surgery in laparoscopic myomectomy and corresponding number of cases

System	Number of cases	
	Less than 45 min	More than 45 min
2D	2	98
3D	12	88

The p value 0.0101 was statistically significant

viewer. Both the 2D offset images are then combined in the brain to give the perception of depth.

All laparoscopic surgeons using 2D images actually are operating with one eye closed. This is the reason that 2D laparoscopy is cerebrally intensive.

The 3D HD system by Schoelly has two cameras and two optical lens systems, which transmit two offset images on the medical 3D monitor (Figs. 3, 4, and 5). When the surgeon wears circular, polarized 3D glasses, the two images are merged by the brain into one and this gives the perception of depth. This also provides a clearer visualization of the relationship of organs in the peritoneal cavity in real-time suturing—especially making intra-corporeal stitching very comfortable. 3D HD is the way to go for all laparoscopic surgeons. Consider the fact that currently there are 30,000 three-dimensional screens internationally.

In the last few years, 3D movies grossed US$8.36 billion; six out of ten top hits were 3D movies. Avatar took 10 years to make. It is an audacious, awe-inspiring work of modern art blowing our minds out. 3D HD laparoscopy is audacious, awe-inspiring work of modern surgery which increases safety unbelievably.

Learning curve

A learning curve is defined both by the time (quickness) as well as the number of cases (trials) necessary to attain proficiency. The advent of new technology has brought new challenges and issues. The introduction of laparoscopy had posed the challenge of 2D images on a flat screen i.e., as if viewing with one eye closed. Hence, laparoscopy was considered cerebrally intensive. For the last decade, robotic surgery with its 3D view revolutionized laparoscopic surgery. Several publications discussed the benefits of 3D HD view and improved surgeon performance.

Change and technology are the key words in surgery today; where is the future of surgery headed? Since the "lap hysterectomy" revolution in 1989, no breakthrough has changed modern surgery more rapidly, definitively, or irrevocably than robotic and 3D laparoscopic surgery. A preliminary testing has suggested that the new generation, 3D system, used will be helpful for developing skills in laparoscopy for the novice surgeon [8]

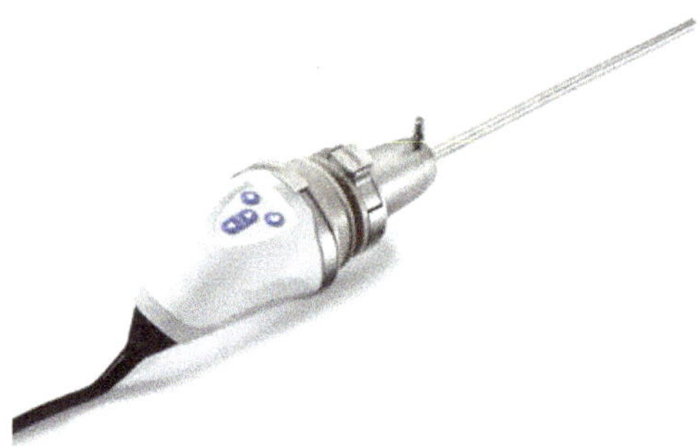

Fig. 3 3D camera head with telescope attached 108×72 mm (300×300 DPI)

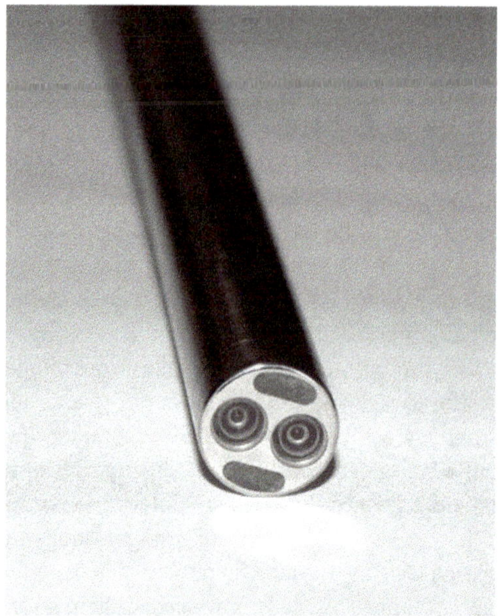

Fig. 4 3D telescope 71×86 mm (300×300 DPI)

The learning curve for some gynecologists was approximately 50 cases to develop consistent operative times and predictable outcomes. These learning curves were dramatically less than those reported for general surgeons and urologists who report learning curves for robotic-assisted laparoscopic prostatectomy to be 150–200 cases [9–11].

We experienced much shorter learning curves with the new Einstein Vision 3D HD system. We took approximately five cases i.e., two OR days to get used to the 3D vision on a 32-in. monitor using conventional instruments. This may also be due to the fact that our center is a dedicated gynecological endoscopy center with about 600 procedures being done every year. We have been operating for about 6 years now with 2D HD system. But, our belief is that the learning curve for 3D HD system will be very short for all laparoscopic surgeons and this system will enhance the skills of good surgeons. What we need to determine in the near

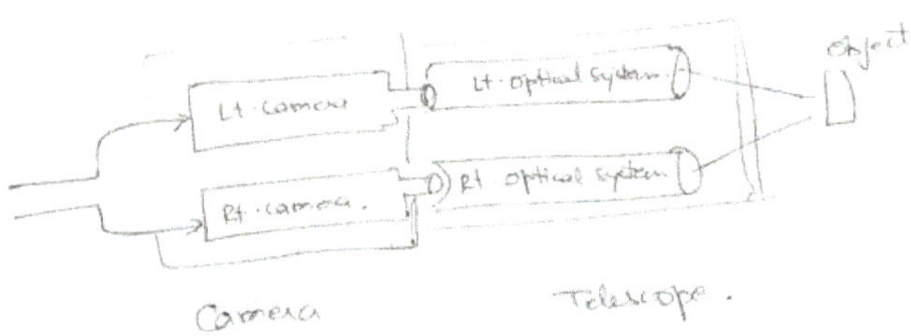

Fig. 5 Physics of a 3D telescope 108×40 mm (300×300 DPI)

future is how long it will take for a postgraduate surgeon who is beginning laparoscopy. Will the 3D HD system shorten his learning curve as compared to conventional laparoscopy and to what degree?

Although some authors suggest that robotics can be a useful method for shortening the learning curve in physicians performing minimally invasive gynecologic surgery, another study suggested that robotic surgery should not serve as a wholesale substitute for a skilled laparoscopic surgeon, especially in procedures where standard laparoscopy is routine [12].

Costs

Another important consideration is that the higher hospital costs associated with robotic surgery is specific to perioperative and postoperative costs (US$1,446 more than conventional laparoscopy) [13] and did not account for the acquisition costs.

The robotic unit costs between US$1 million and US$2.3 million and is associated with annual maintenance costs of US$180,000 a year (Intuitive Surgical Investor presentation Q4-2009). In comparison, the total cost of the 3D HD system, Einstein Vision, and the acquiring costs is about US$250,000 and the annual maintenance cost is US $25,000, while there is no recurring cost per patient.

Medicolegal issues

The advances in robotic-assisted surgery in gynecology evolved after most practicing gynecologists have already completed residency training. Postgraduate training of the new technology for gynecologists in practice is limited.

Therefore, gynecologists with insufficient training who perform robot-assisted surgery may potentially be at risk for liability. In addition to traditional medical negligence claims, plaintiff attorneys are seeking causes of actions for lack of informed consent and negligent credentialing. Thus, it is essential that gynecologists are aware of these potential liability claims that arise in a robot-assisted malpractice suit [14]. Surgical robotics instructors provide an essential service in improving the competency of novice gynecological surgeons in learning robotic surgery and advancing surgical skills on behalf of patients.

The role of a robotics instructor ranges from involving only pure verbal instruction to direct physical guidance during surgery of cases. Despite the degree of involvement, crossing over from a purely observational role to a more active involvement in teaching exposes the surgical robotics instructor to medical malpractice liability in the event of a surgical complication [15].

Limitations of robotic-assisted surgery

Other disadvantages of robotic-assisted surgery are lack of tactile feedback to the surgeon, inability to move the surgical table once the arms of the robot are fixed, and expenses related to the robot and its semi-disposable instruments [16].

Surgeons benefit from using the "robot" by sitting and from 3D view; in addition, the robot makes suturing faster to learn. It does not appear to make a significant difference in the outcome of the patient [17]. Women prefer both single-site and traditional laparoscopic incisions over robotic procedures. In as aesthetics are an important consideration for many women and clinical outcomes are similar, during the informed consent procedure, location and length of incisions should be included in the discussion of risks, benefits, and alternatives [18].

Complexity of surgery

We normally use the 30° telescope for our 3D HD surgeries. It is far more versatile than 0° telescope. The 30° telescope cannot be rotated while it is attached to the 3D HD camera. The standard view is anterior to posterior. However, the telescope can be detached, rotated at 180°, and refixed to the camera, giving a posterior to anterior view. This view is helpful when operating on the deep posterior aspect of the uterus or the anterior abdominal view.

Using the 30° telescope and the 3D HD system does not have a limitation to operate on complex pelvic surgeries. We have done a total laparoscopic hysterectomy where the uterus weighed 4.87 kg (10.71 lb) and performed all kinds of complex endometriotic surgeries. We had only two cases where we converted to 2D HD camera since we needed to view the uterus at odd angles, and the ability to rotate the telescope in the camera coupler helped us. The 3D HD telescope provided a brilliant view for suturing in most oddly located areas.

Benefits of 3D high-definition laparoscopy

- Depth perception
- Tactile feedback retained
- Accuracy
- Safety
- Surgical precision
- Improves hand–eye coordination
- Low capital expenditure
- Low maintenance recurring cost
- Conventional and new straight stick instruments can be used
- Shorter learning curve

Conclusions

Robotic-assisted laparoscopy is new to the field of surgery. Since its introduction, surgeons have been intrigued by it, and each discipline is trying to find its appropriate role. It appears to assist the less skilled laparoscopist in performing surgery that one might have not attempted. It might be the answer to the shortcomings of laparoscopy since it is being adopted by more surgeons. Robotic surgery simply acts as a bridge between laparotomy and advanced operative laparoscopy. It provides 3D vision and easier suture capability without tremor. Its disadvantages are the enormous cost, bulkiness, added time to assemble, and a new learning curve. It is acknowledged that the robot offers a potential advancement in minimally invasive procedures, particularly in complex or highly technical cases such as laparoscopic prostatectomy or certain cardiac cases. It is also acknowledged that robotic surgery is exciting because it is an innovative and cutting-edge technology. However, research indicates that this value proposition tends to be offset when robotics is used in cases where traditional laparoscopic approaches can achieve the same clinical outcomes, but at far less cost to the hospital.

Although subsequent generations of robots may represent the future, it is difficult economically to justify the exuberate uptake of robotic surgery for routine hysterectomies. The evolving literature on robot-assisted surgery in gynecology suggests that the surgical limitations of conventional laparoscopy can be overcome and that the skill level of the surgeon may be enhanced. At present, this seems to be the result of improved instrument, precision and dexterity, and 3D imaging [19]. "There's never been a study showing clinical superiority of the robotic surgery," says Dr. Marty Makary, a surgeon at the Johns Hopkins University School of Medicine in Baltimore. "The benefits of robotic surgery are due more to the laparoscopic approach than to the robot itself," Makary says. In our experience it is the 3D HD view with great depth perception and tactile feedback that will make laparoscopic surgery more acceptable, safe, and cost-effective. It improves surgical precision and hand–eye coordination, conventional and all straight stick instruments can be used, capital expenditure is less, and recurring cost and annual maintenance cost are less. In addition it will enhance the skills of a good surgeon and shorten the learning curve of a novice surgeon.

Conflict of interest The authors report no conflicts of interest. The authors alone are responsible for the content and writing of the paper.

References

1. Yuen PM, Yu KM, Yip SK, Lau WC, Rogers MC, Chang A (1997) A randomized prospective study of laparoscopy and laparotomy in the management of benign ovarian masses. Am J Obstet Gynecol 177:109–114
2. Lo L, Pun TC, Chan S (1999) Tubal ectopic pregnancy: an evaluation of laparoscopic surgery versus laparotomy in 614 patients. Aust N Z J Obstet Gynecol 39:185–187
3. Diaz-Arrastia C, Jurnalov C, Gomez G, Townsend C Jr (2002) Laparoscopic hysterectomy using a computer enhanced surgical robot. Surg Endosc 16:1271–1273
4. Sarlos D, Kots L, Stevanovic N, Schaer G (2010) Robotic hysterectomy versus conventional laparoscopic hysterectomy: outcome and cost analyses of a matched case–control study. Eur J Obstet Gynecol Reprod Biol 150(1):92–96
5. Lerihan JP Jr, Kovanda C, Sestadri-Kreaden U (2008) What is the learning curve for robotic assisted gynecologic surgery? J Minim Invasive Gynecol 15(5):589–594
6. Reich H, Roberts L (2003) Laparoscopic hysterectomy in current gynaecological practice. Rev Gynecol Pract 3:32–40
7. Sinha R, Hegde A (2005) Safe entry techniques during laparoscopy. J Minim Invasive Gynecol 12:463–465
8. Patel HR, Ribal MJ, Arya M, Nauth-Misir R, Joseph JV (2007) Is it worth revisiting laparoscopic three dimensional visualization? A validated assessment. Urology 70(1):47–49
9. Sarle R, Tewari A, Shrivastva A, Peabody J, Menon M (2004) Surgical robotics and laparoscopy drills. J Endourol 18:63–67
10. Giulianotti PC, Coratti A, Angelini M et al (2003) Personal experience in a large community hospital. Arch Surg 138:777–784
11. Talamini MA, Chapman S, Horgan S, Melvin W (2003) A prospective analysis on 211 robotic assisted surgical procedure. Surg Endosc 17:1521–1524
12. Wexner SD, Bergamschi R, Lacy A et al (2009) The current status of robotic pelvic surgery: results of a multidisciplinary consensus conference. Surg Endosc 23:438–443
13. Pasic RP, Rizzo JA, Fang H, Ross S, Moore M, Gunnarsson C. Comparing robotic-assisted with conventional laparoscopic hysterectomy: impact on cost and clinical outcome. JMIG 17:730–738
14. Lee YL, Kilic GS, Phelps JY (2011) Medico legal review of liability risks for gynecologists stemming from lack of training in robot assisted surgery. J Minim Invasive Gynecol 18:512–515
15. Lee YL, Kilic G, Phelps JY (2012) Liability exposure for surgical robotics instructors. J Minim Invasive Gynecol 19:376–379
16. Nezhat et al (2009) Robotic assisted laparoscopic surgery in gynecology: scientific dream or reality? Fertil Steril 91:2620–2622
17. Nezhat C, Watson J, Lemyre M, Hsu S, Barnett O, Lavie O (2009) Robotic assisted laparoscopic myomectomy compared with standard laparoscopic myomectomy—a retrospective matched control study. Fertil Steril 91:556–559
18. Bush AJ, Morris SN, Millham FH, Isacson KB (2011) Women's preferences for minimally invasive incisions. J Minim Invasive Gynecol 18:640–643
19. Advincula AP, Wang K (2009) Evolving role and current state of robotics in minimally invasive gynecologic surgery. J Minim Invasive Gynecol 16:291–301

15

Laparoscopic sacral colpopexy versus total vaginal mesh for vault prolapse; comparison of cohorts

Mariëlla I. J. Withagen · Mark E. Vierhout · Alfredo L. Milani · Guido H. H. Mannaerts · Kirsten B. Kluivers · Robin M. F. van der Weiden

Abstract The surgical treatment of vaginal vault prolapse can either be performed by the vaginal or the abdominal (laparoscopic) route. The objective of this study was to compare the laparoscopic sacral colpopexy (LSC) and total vaginal mesh (TVM) for vaginal vault prolapse. This study compared a prospective cohort of LSC with bone-anchor fixation and mesh limited to the apex to a prospective cohort of TVM as treatment modalities in patients with a symptomatic vaginal vault prolapse (pelvic organ prolapse-quantification (POP-Q) point C≥−3). Primary outcome was failure in the apical compartment after 6 month follow-up, defined as POP-Q stage≥II with prolapse complaints or re-treatment in apical compartment. Based on an overall failure in all compartments of 23 % in the LSC group and 57 % in the TVM group, 29 patients would be needed in each group with a power of 80 % and alpha 0.05. Ninety-seven women were included, 45 LSC and 52 TVM. The failure rate of symptomatic vault prolapse was 1 (2 %) in each group (p=0.99). The failure rate (POP stage≥II) in any compartment was 23 (51 %) in the LSC group and 11 (21 %) in the TVM group (p=0.002). Each technique had its own type of complications. Short-term failure rates in the apical compartment after TVM and LSC were similar. In case of anterior or posterior prolapsed, additional mesh insertion or additional vaginal colporrhaphy is indicated in LSC surgery.

Keywords Bone anchor · Laparoscopic sacral colpopexy · Pelvic organ prolapse · Vaginal mesh · Vaginal vault

M. I. J. Withagen · M. E. Vierhout · K. B. Kluivers
Department of Obstetrics and Gynaecology, Radboud University Nijmegen Medical Centre, Nijmegen, The Netherlands

A. L. Milani
Department of Obstetrics and Gynaecology, Reinier de Graaf Group, Delft, The Netherlands

G. H. H. Mannaerts
Department of Surgery, Sint Franciscus Gasthuis, Rotterdam, The Netherlands

R. M. F. van der Weiden (✉)
Department of Obstetrics and Gynaecology, Sint Franciscus Gasthuis, 3045 PM,
Rotterdam, The Netherlands
e-mail: rmfvdwei@knmg.nl

Introduction

The incidence of post-hysterectomy vaginal vault prolapse that requires surgery has been estimated at 1.3 per 1,000 women-years [1]. The risk of pelvic organ prolapse surgery was 4.7 times higher in women whose initial hysterectomy was indicated by prolapsed [1]. The surgical treatment of vaginal vault prolapse can either be performed by the vaginal (e.g., vaginal sacrospinous colpopexy and total vaginal mesh (TVM), involving mesh placement in the anterior, and apical and posterior compartments) or the abdominal route (e.g., sacral colpopexy). A Cochrane systematic review and meta-analysis on the topic has shown that for the treatment of vaginal vault prolapse the abdominal sacral colpopexy was the superior procedure compared with vaginal sacrospinous colpopexy in terms of a lower rate of recurrent vault prolapse and less dyspareunia [2]. Vaginal sacrospinous colpopexy was, however, quicker and cheaper to perform and women returned earlier to activities of daily living. Laparoscopic sacral colpopexy (LSC) provides the potential to combine the success rate of an abdominal approach with the faster recovery associated with a minimally invasive technique. The success rate of LSC has been reported to be 90–100 % for the apical compartment [3–8].

TVM aims at suspension of the apical compartment by means of a bilateral sacrospinous ligament fixation. The success rate of a TVM has been reported to be 96 to 99 % for the apical compartment and 91 % for all the compartments [9, 10].

Since the recent publication of the update of the FDA notification on complications of surgical mesh for transvaginal repair of POP, it is even more important to consider which treatment of apical compartment prolapse should be used in the individual patient [11]. Both abdominal and vaginal techniques treat the apical compartment, but the techniques are very different and not many gynecologists perform both procedures. As a result, only limited data are available that compare these two techniques. In a recent randomized controlled trial, success rate in all vaginal compartments was 77 % for LSC as compared with 43 % in the TVM group [12].

The aim of this study was to compare LSC and TVM with regard to the management of vaginal vault prolapse in centers with special expertise in either LSC or TVM.

Methods

This study compared two prospective observational cohorts of consecutive women with symptomatic vault prolapse referred to three centers: Sint Franciscus Gasthuis (SFG), Rotterdam, Radboud University Nijmegen Medical Centre (RUNMC), and Reinier de Graaf Group (RdGG) Delft, the Netherlands. SFG is specialized in LSC with bone-anchor fixation and at the time of the inclusion TVM was not an available therapy in this centre. Both RdGG and RUNMC are specialized in pelvic organ prolapse surgery, including TVM technique. At the time of the inclusion, LSC was not an available therapy in these centers.

Patients with a symptomatic vaginal vault prolapse with point C of the Pelvic Organ Prolapse Quantification (POP-Q) examination≥ -3 were included in the study [13]. Exclusion criteria were the inability to understand Dutch, pregnancy or the consideration of pregnancy in the future, a compromised immune system, and treatment for malignancy in the past. Additional exclusion criteria for the LSC were a former rectosigmoid resection, extensive intra-abdominal/pelvic adhesions and a body mass index of >40 kg/m^2.

Approval from the Central Medical Ethics Committee in Rotterdam, the Netherlands was obtained for the LSC cohort study on 22 of December 2004. The data concerning the TVM patients were collected as part of an ongoing outcome registration project, which was approved by the CME/IRB on 19th April 2006. All patients provided written informed consent before participation and were recruited between July 2004 and November 2009.

Baseline as well as postoperative evaluation after 6 weeks and 6 months included a medical history, a gynecologic investigation including a POP-Q examination, and a validated urogynecological questionnaire, which contains the Dutch validated Urogenital Distress Inventory (UDI), Defecatory Distress Inventory (DDI), and the Incontinence Impact Questionnaire (IIQ) [14, 15].

In both groups the patients received, a single prophylactic dose of antibiotics. All LSC were performed by two of the authors together (RW and GM) using bone anchor fixation [16]. The operative procedure can be summarized as follows: after developing the presacral avascular plane, the cortical bone of the sacral segment 3 is penetrated in the midline with the laparoscopic bone anchor. Fixation to the sacrum is performed with a selftapping titanium Corkscrew Suture or with flat headed titanium screws. A 4.0×3.0-cm piece of monofilament knitted polypropylene mesh (Gynemesh Soft, Ethicon, Norderstedt, Germany) was sutured to the apical part of the posterior vaginal wall with four mersilene 1–0 sutures (Ethicon, Norderstedt, Germany) and was subsequently sutured to the polyester-2 ligatures attached to the bone anchor. The mesh was covered with peritoneum placing it in a retroperitoneal position. Since the rate of vaginal mesh exposure is significantly higher when abdominal surgery is combined with vaginal surgery [17] and placement of a posterior mesh might increase the risk of postoperative complications in patients without a patent posterior prolapse [18], additional prolapse procedures were not performed concomitantly. We anticipated on a low rate of postoperative cystocele and rectocele since fixation of the vaginal apex to sacral segment 3 restores the natural axis of the vagina [19–21].

All TVM procedures were performed by four gynecologists who were formally trained for the tension-free vaginal mesh procedure as described in the paper by Fatton et al. prior to the start of this study [22]. As recommended, a full thickness midline incision was made through the fibromuscular wall of the vagina in order to reduce the known risk of mesh exposure. The TVM was placed as one sheet and not divided, as described by Milani et al. [9]. The TVM procedure was in principle not combined with continence surgery to avoid complications [23]; however, in one case the protocol was ignored.

Primary outcome was failure in the apical compartment, defined as apical POP-Q stage≥II with prolapse complaints or re-treatment in the apical compartment (failure outcome I). For secondary outcomes four different definitions for failure were tested:

- Failure outcome II: POP-Q stage≥II in one or more compartment(s).
- Failure outcome III: POP-Q stage≥II in one or more compartment(s) with prolapse complaints or re-treatment.
- Failure outcome IV: POP-Q at or beyond hymen in one or more compartment(s) with prolapse complaints or re-treatment.
- Failure outcome V: prolapse complaints or re-treatment.

Prolapse complaints were considered present if patients responded affirmative to the questions of the UDI referring to seeing or feeling a vaginal bulge and the experience of at least a little bother from either of these symptoms [14]. Data on symptom scores of the UDI, DDI, and IIQ questionnaires, duration of surgery, blood loss, length of hospitalization, and complications were collected. Pain was a secondary outcome as well and considered significant in case a patient responded "yes, moderately to quite a bit" to the question "Do you experience pain in the lower abdomen or genital region?" Dyspareunia was considered significant in case a patient responded "yes; moderately to quite a bit" to the question "Do you experience pain during intercourse?" Stress urinary incontinence was considered significant in case a patient responded "yes, moderately to quite a bit" to the UDI question "Do you experience urinary leakage during physical activity, coughing, or sneezing?"

Sample size calculation prior to the comparison study was performed as follows: given the success rates for the apical compartment in literature of 90–100 % [3–7] after LSC and 96 % after TVM [9, 10], we hypothesized that we would not find a significant difference in primary outcome. Based on an overall failure in all compartments of 23 % in the LSC group and 57 % in the TVM group [12], 29 patients would be needed in each group to detect a difference of 34 % in failure rate with a power of 80 % and alpha 0.05.

Continuous variables were analyzed using the independent-samples *t* test to compare means, the Mann–Whitney *U* test to compare independent medians and the Wilcoxon signed-rank test to compare related medians. Categorical variables were compared using the Chi-square test and the Fisher exact test in case of small numbers. Related samples were compared using the paired-samples *t* test to compare means. A p value of <0.05 was considered statistically significant. After using the Bonferroni correction for multiple testing for the eight different POP-Q points, the p value for statistical significance regarding these points was lowered from 0.05 to 0.006 (alpha 0.05). Statistical analysis was performed using Statistical Package for the Social Sciences, version 18.0 (SPSS inc., Chicago, IL).

Findings

Forty-five women were included in the LSC group and 52 women were included in the TVM group. A flow-chart of the two groups is presented in Fig. 1. All women undergoing LSC and 20 out of 52 (38 %) undergoing TVM have previously been described [9, 24]. Baseline characteristics are shown in Table 1. The TVM group had significantly more patients with overall a higher stage of POP; however, the apical compartment prolapse was similar in the two groups (point C, Table 1). The 2 patients with a POP-Q stage I and point $C \geq -3$ in the LSC group both experienced bulging symptoms.

Peri- and postoperative data are shown in Table 2. POP-Q measurements are shown in Table 3. Improvement was found for each compartment in both groups. No difference was found in the improvement of the apical compartment between the two cohorts.

In Table 4, failure rates for various failure definitions are shown. The failure rate of symptomatic vault prolapse (failure I: apical compartment POP stage≥II with prolapse complaints or apical re-treatment) was 2 % in de LSC group and 2 % in de TVM group (p=0.99). Definitions considering the apical compartment with or without prolapse complaints (I, II apical) showed similar failure rates between the groups. However, when definitions of failure included other compartments or prolapse complaints alone (II–V), the LSC group had a significant higher failure rate compared with the TVM group.

Effect of surgery on symptom bother and health related quality of life scores is shown in Table 5. UDI domain score of genital prolapse, overactive bladder, obstructive micturition, and pain improved significantly after surgery in both groups. The domain score of genital prolapse 6 months after TVM was significantly lower (less bother) compared with the score of de the LSC group.

Fig. 1 Patient enrollment and follow-up

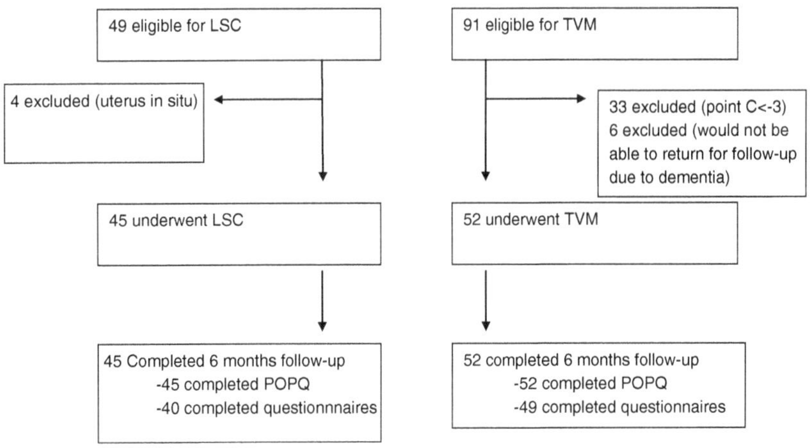

Table 1 Patient characteristics

Characteristics	LSC (n=45)	TVM (n=52)	p value
Age (years)[a]	65.6 (9.7)	69.1 (11.6)	0.12
Parity (number)[b]	2 (0–6)	3 (0–6)	0.12
BMI (kg/m^2)[a]	25.6 (3.1)	26.2 (3.6)	0.33
Comorbidity[c]	5 (11 %)	25 (48 %)	<0.001
Previous surgery[c]			
Abdominal hysterectomy	18 (40 %)	13 (25 %)	0.15
Vaginal hysterectomy	27 (60 %)	39 (75 %)	0.11
Anterior colporraphy	24 (53 %)	23 (44 %)	0.54
Anterior mesh procedure	0 (0 %)	1 (2 %)	0.54
Posterior colporrhaphy	24 (53 %)	18 (35 %)	0.11
Sacrospinous ligament fixation	0 (0 %)	2 (4 %)	0.12
Sacrocolpopexy	0 (0 %)	2 (4 %)	0.17
Colpocleisis	0 (0 %)	2 (4 %)	0.17
Previous POP procedure	29 (64 %)	28 (54 %)	0.29
More than one POP procedure	2 (4 %)	6 (12 %)	0.14
Previous incontinence surgery[c]	9 (20 %)	4 (8 %)	0.08
Overall POP-Q stage[c]			
I[d]	2 (4 %)	0 (0 %)	0.21
II	31 (69 %)	5 (10 %)	<0.001
III	12 (27 %)	43 (83 %)	<0.001
IV	0 (0 %)	4 (7 %)	0.08
Point C[b]	0 (−3 to 4)	1 (−3 to 9)	0.41

POP pelvic organ prolapse, *POP-Q* pelvic organ prolapse quantification, *LSC* laparoscopic sacral colpopexy, *TVM* total vaginal mesh

[a]Data presented as mean (standard deviation), and p value calculated with independent sample t test

[b]Data presented as median (range), and p value calculated with Mann–Whitney U test

[c]Data presented as number of patients (in percent), and p value calculated with Chi-square test and the Fisher exact test in case of small numbers

[d]POP-Q point C≥−3

Discussion

Comparison of LSC with bone anchor fixation and mesh limited to the apex to TVM revealed significantly higher overall POP-Q failure rate (symptomatic failure in any of the compartments) in the LSC group with no statistically significant differences regarding the vaginal vault. We anticipated a positive effect of fixation of the vaginal apex also on the anterior and posterior compartment due to restoration of the vaginal axis [19–21]. However, the results in the LSC cohort demonstrate that apical support alone does not adequately prevent prolapse of the anterior and posterior compartment and support the necessity of anterior and posterior fixation of the vaginal cuff at the time of LSC. This finding also has its repercussions on the power analysis which was based on overall failure rates in all compartments.

Different types of complications were seen in the two groups. Scores in the UDI domain genital prolapse improved significantly in both groups, but the postoperative genital prolapse score was lower (less complaints) in the TVM group.

The strengths of this study are the prospective design of the study and the use of standardized and validated instruments of measurement. Furthermore, since comparative data on these two main techniques for vaginal vault prolapse are limited, this is an actual and highly relevant topic in urogynecological practice [25]. The short follow-up of 6 months and the nonrandomized selection of intervention were important limitations of this study. Furthermore, an independent clinical investigator who was not involved in the management of the patients would ideally have performed the pre- and postoperative examinations.

Sometimes the vault may be prolapsed clinically to a significant extent and yet be measured as POP-Q stage I, demonstrating a limitation of the POP-Q scoring system with respect to the apical compartment [26]. We had two patients, included in the LSC cohort, with a vault prolapse and vaginal bulge symptoms (UDI score on domain genital prolapse≥16.6) despite an overall POP<stage II. In these two patients, the POPQ point C was≥−3 cm.

The high success rates of the LSC and TVM in the apical compartment were comparable to the rates reported in literature [3–9, 27]. However, the overall failure rate of 51 % in the LSC group was high compared with the 23 % failure rate after two years follow-up reported in a recent randomized controlled trial on LSC versus TVM for vaginal vault prolapse [12]. This may be explained by the fact that mesh was only applied to the apex without combining LSC with

Table 2 Peri- and postoperative data

Variable	LSC (n=45)	TVM (n=52)	p value
(Concomitant) surgery[a]	2 (4 %)	1 (2 %)	0.35
TVT-O	0	1 (2 %)	0.54
Laparoscopic adhesiolysis	1 (2 %)	0	0.46
Laparoscopic aspiration pseudocysts	1 (2 %)	0	0.46
Spinal analgesia[a]	0	33 (63 %)	<0.001
Operating time (min)[b]	120 (60–240)	70 (44–110)	<0.001
Blood loss (ml)[b]	50 (10–100)	100 (50–1,300)	<0.001
Duration urinary catheter (days)[b]	1 (1)	2 (1–10)	<0.001
Hospital stay (days)[b]	2 (0–5)	3 (0–8)	<0.001
Complications[a]			
Blood loss>500 ml	0 (0 %)	1 (2 %)	0.54
Bladder perforation	0 (0 %)	1 (2 %)	0.54
Repeat surgery for postoperative hemorrhage	0 (0 %)	1 (2 %)	0.54
Hematoma	0 (0 %)	2 (4 %)	0.28
Temporary urinary retention	0 (0 %)	10 (19 %)	0.001
Conversion laparotomy due to injury ileum	1 (2 %)	0 (0 %)	0.46
Temporary neurologic complaints caused by irritation left lumbar plexus	1 (2 %)	0 (0 %)	0.46
Outcome/complications at follow-up 6 months[a]			
Cumulative mesh exposure	1 (2 %)	4 (8 %)	0.19
Re-treatment for POP	2 (4 %)	0 (0 %)	0.21
Pain (lower abdomen/genital area)			
Baseline	9/43 (21 %)	11/44 (25 %)	0.65
At 6 months	1/40 (3 %)	1/45 (2 %)	0.50
De novo pain	0 (0 %)	0 (0 %)	0.99
Dyspareunia			
Baseline	3/18 (17 %)	4/17 (24 %)	0.29
At 6 months	3/21 (14 %)	3/18 (17 %)	0.33
De novo dyspareunia	2/18 (11 %)	1/17 (6 %)	0.40
Stress urinary incontinence			
Baseline	3/43 (7 %)	11/45 (24 %)	0.02
At 6 months	3/41 (7 %)	5/46 (11 %)	0.25
De novo stress urinary incontinence	2/41 (5 %)	2/41 (5 %)	0.38

TVT tension free vaginal tape—obturator system, *POP* pelvic organ prolapse, *LSC* laparoscopic sacral colpopexy, *TVM* total vaginal mesh

[a] Data presented as number of patients (in percent), and p value calculated with Chi-square test and the Fisher exact test in case of small numbers

[b] Data presented as median (range), and p value calculated with Mann–Whitney U test

anterior or posterior repairs (either laparoscopically applied mesh or with vaginal colporrhaphia) in the present study. In a cohort study on 22 LSC, an overall failure rate of 73 % after 2 years was found when a mesh was attached to the apex and the posterior wall only [8]. Anterior mesh application during LSC therefore also seems important. Adequate level I support has a critical role on the position of the anterior and posterior vagina [28, 29]. However, this adequate level I support has not prevented the occurrence of anterior and posterior wall prolapse in many cases in the LSC group. Combining the LSC with anterior and/or posterior repair, either performed laparoscopically or vaginally, might have resulted in better overall results in the LSC group. After evaluation of these results this has now become the standard procedure in LSC.

Our overall success rate of the TVM was high compared with the results of Maher et al. [12], but in that study the follow-up was 1.5 years longer and 12 out of the 55 patients with TVM were considered as failures due to lost to follow-up in that study. Our success rate of the TVM was low compared with a previously published cohorts of a total mesh [9, 10].

In contrast with the results of the study by Maher et al. [12], the symptom score of genital prolapse after 6 months was significantly lower (less complaints) in the TVM group, compared with the LSC group. Recurrent prolapse symptoms in the LSC group generally arose from the untreated anterior or posterior compartment. The application of mesh to the apex only in the LSC group might also explain this difference.

Table 3 POP-Q measurements at baseline and 6 months post surgery

POPQ point	Baseline		p value[a]	6 months		p value[a]	p value[b] within group
	LSC (n=45)	TVM (n=52)	LSC versus TVM	LSC (n=45)	TVM (n=52)	LSC versus TVM	LSC/TVM
Aa	−2 (−3 to 1)	3 (−3 to 3)	<0.001	−2 (−3 to 0)	−3 (−3 to 0)	<0.001	0.002/<0.001
Ba	−2 (−3 to 3)	3 (−2 to 9)	<0.001	−2 (−3 to 2)	−3 (−3 to 4)	<0.001	0.005/<0.001
C	0 (−3 to 4)	1 (−3 to 9)	0.41	−8 (−8 to −3)	−8 (−10 to 4)	0.074	<0.001/<0.001
GH	3 (2 to 5)	5 (2 to 7)	<0.001	3 (2 to 5)	3 (2 to 6)	0.21	1.00/<0.001
PB	3 (2 to 3)	3 (1 to 7)	0.13	3 (2 to 3)	3 (1 to 6)	<0.001	0.16/0.23
TVL	8 (7 to 9)	9 (5 to 10)	<0.001	8 (7 to 9)	9 (6 to 10)	<0.001	1.00/0.009
Ap	−2 (−3 to 2)	1 (−3 to 3)	<0.001	−2 (−3 to 0)	−3 (−3 to 0)	<0.001	<0.001/<0.001
Bp	−2 (−3 to 2)	2 (−3 to 9)	<0.001	−2 (−3 to 2)	−3 (−3 to 4)	<0.001	0.001/<0.001
POP-Q stage anterior	1 (0 to 3)	3 (1 to 4)	<0.001	1 (0 to 3)	0 (0 to 3)	<0.001	<0.001/<0.001
POP-Q stage apical	2 (0 to 3)	3 (0 to 4)	0.357	0 (0 to 1)	0 (0 to 3)	0.31	0.016/<0.001
POP-Q stage posterior	1 (0 to 3)	3 (0 to 4)	<0.001	1 (0 to 3)	0 (0 to 3)	<0.001	0.001/<0.001
Total POP-Q stage	2 (1 to 3)	3 (2 to 4)	<0.001	1 (0 to 3)	1 (0 to 3)	<0.001	<0.001/<0.001
Change C	–	–	–	7 (5 to 12)	7 (3–19)	0.97	–

POP pelvic organ prolapse, *POP-Q* pelvic organ prolapse quantification, *LSC* laparoscopic sacral colpopexy, *TVM* total vaginal mesh.

[a] Mann–Whitney U test

[b] Data presented as median (range)

[a] Wilcoxon signed-rank test

The types of complications were remarkably different between the two techniques. There was a high rate of temporary urinary retention in the TVM group. The complications with long lasting consequences were similar in both groups. Major complications such as bowel injury, de novo dyspareunia, de novo pain, and exposure did not differ between both groups in this study. In comparison with earlier studies on these two techniques, no major differences were found [6, 9, 10, 27]. In the RCT of Maher et al. [12], the reoperation rate in the

Table 4 Failure at 6 months for different definitions

Failure definition	LSC (N=45)	TVM (N=52)	p value[a]	OR (95 % CI)	RR (95 % CI)
(I) Apical compartment POP-Q stage ≥II with prolapse complaints or apical re-treatment	1 (2 %)	1 (2 %)	0.99	1.1 (0.07–18.7)	1.0 (0.9–1.1)
(II) POP-Q stage ≥II in one or more compartment	23[b] (51 %)	11 (21 %)	0.002	3.9 (1.6–9.4)	2.4 (1.3–4.4)
POP in every separate compartment					
Anterior	14[c] (31 %)	9 (17 %)	0.11	2.2 (0.8–5.6)	1.8 (1.0–2.2)
Posterior	10 (22 %)	4 (8 %)	0.04	2.2 (1.0–11.8)	2.9 (1.0–8.6)
Apical	1[d] (2 %)	2 (4 %)	0.39	0.6 (0.1–5.9)	0.5 (0.1–5.7)
(III) Overall POP-Q stage ≥II with prolapse complaints or re-treatment	7/42 (17 %)	1/52 (2 %)	0.02	10.2 (1.2–86.6)	1.2 (1.0–1.4)
(IV) POP at or beyond hymen with prolapse complaints or re-treatment	6/44 (14 %)	1/52 (2 %)	0.04	8.1 (0.9–69.7)	1.1 (1.0–1.3)
(V) Prolapse complaints or re-treatment	12/41 (29 %)	3/45 (7 %)	0.006	5.8 (1.5–22.4)	1.3 (1.1–1.6)

Data presented as numbers (in percent)

POP pelvic organ prolapse, *POP-Q* pelvic organ prolapse quantification, *LSC* laparoscopic sacral colpopexy, *TVM* total vaginal mesh, OR = odds ratio, *95% CI* 95 % confidence interval, *RR* relative risk

[a] Chi-square test and the Fisher exact test in case of small numbers

[b] Including one re-sacrocolpopexy and one anterior colporrhaphy within 6 months

[c] Including one anterior colporrhaphy within 6 months

[d] Including one sacrocolpopexy within 6 months

Table 5 Effect of surgery on symptoms and health-related quality of life scores

Domain	Baseline		6 months		p value within group[a]	p value between groups[b]
	LSC (n=43)	TVM (n=46)	LSC (n=40)	TVM (n=49)	(LSC/TVM)	LSC versus TVM baseline/6 m
UDI						
Genital prolapsed	67.9 (30.2)	63.0 (18.7)	11.3 (22.5)	2.0 (9.9)	<0.001/<0.001	0.49/0.01
OAB	34.6 (26.0)	32.2 (26.8)	17.6 (19.2)	15.4 (19.7)	<0.001/0.001	0.68/0.59
Incontinence	16.3 (20.7)	24.2 (26.8)	10.6 (17.4)	15.9 (21.8)	0.11/0.10	0.15/0.20
Obstructive micturition	34.5 (24.8)	28.1 (29.9)	15.4 (21.8)	12.2 (23.8)	<0.001/<0.001	0.28/0.51
Pain	25.4 (24.8)	27.7 (27.6)	12.5 (15.9)	10.1 (16.8)	0.001/<0.001	0.69/0.49
DDI						
Constipation	12.7 (19.8)	14 (18.7)	11.1 (20.4)	8.2 (15.1)	0.36/0.12	0.75/0.45
Obstructed defecation	13.4 (14.6)	12.0 (17.1)	7.5 (11.1)	9.1 (13.4)	0.003/0.10	0.69/0.56
Pain	6.2 (15.9)	9.6 (21.5)	6.7 (15.5)	7.1 (15.9)	0.99/0.56	0.40/0.89
Incontinence	4.4 (11.7)	9.8 (15.8)	5.0 (10.1)	4.3 (8.8)	0.99/0.03	0.07/0.72
IIQ						
Physical functioning	20.8 (26.9)	25.0 (28.2)	14.1 (24.0)	11.2 (21.1)	0.17/0.004	0.50/0.56
Mobility	26.4 (20.4)	32.0 (24.6)	24.5 (25.4)	15.7 (19.5)	0.57/0.003	0.25/0.08
Social functioning	12.4 (11.9)	15.9 (18.1)	7.6 (13.9)	6.7 (10.6)	0.10/0.01	0.35/0.74
Embarrassment	12.6 (20.7)	21.8 (26.1)	7.2 (13.9)	6.9 (12.3)	0.15/0.002	0.09/0.92
Emotional health	21.4 (21.4)	24.9 (25.6)	15.7 (21.1)	9.3 (13.3)	0.51/0.002	0.51/0.10

UDI, DDI, and IIQ data presented as mean (standard deviation). Scores range between 0 (least bother) to 100 (maximum bother)

UDI urogenital distress inventory, *DDI* defecatory distress inventory, *IIQ* incontinence impact questionnaire, *LSC* laparoscopic sacral colpopexy, *TVM* total vaginal mesh

[a] Paired t test

[b] Independent t test

LSC group was significantly lower, compared with the reoperation rate in the TVM group. This discrepancy with our results might be explained by the shorter follow-up as mentioned before.

Reports on major complications have recently been published on both techniques subject to this study [12, 30–34]. In the LSC group injury of the bowels, bowel herniation though a port site and lumber/sacral osteomyelitis with sepsis are possible life-threatening complications [12, 30–32]. In this study, one serosal lesion to the ileum injury occurred. This injury was recognized immediately and sutured after conversion to a laparotomy [24]. In the TVM group, acute massive hemorrhage, retroperitoneal hematoma, and infected pelvic hematoma have been reported, indicating major, possible life-threatening complications as well [12, 33]. A FDA Public Health Notification update informed the USA public that "surgical mesh for transvaginal repair of POP is an area of continuing serious concern" and "serious complications associated with surgical mesh for transvaginal repair of POP are not rare" [11]. A definition for a serious complications was not given. Severe/serious complications, such as de novo dyspareunia, de novo pain, and exposure did not differ between both groups in this study.

The LSC and the TVM both involve a significant learning curve [35]. Both techniques are associated with potential serious complications. The FDA promulgated a number of recommendations including proper training of the surgeon, certification, and counseling of the patient. Therefore centralization of these procedures in the hands of surgeons with proven experience seems mandatory.

Conclusions

Although either procedures (LSC or TVM) will be adequate in most patients with vault prolapse, specific indications for either technique may exist. For example, in elderly women with comorbidity, spinal analgesics and shorter duration of surgery connected with TVM may be advantageous. Furthermore, in patients with known pelvic/abdominal adhesions a TVM procedure could be preferable. In young, healthy, sexually active women, the more superficial vaginal insertion of mesh can be avoided when choosing LSC. In order to make a deliberate choice between these two types of surgery and to improve the guidance to our patients, further evaluation with long-term follow-up of both procedures is required, preferably by well-designed RCT's with a long-term follow-up of both procedures.

Declaration of Interest The authors report no conflicts of interest. The authors alone are responsible for the content and writing of the paper.

References

1. Dallenbach P, Kaelin-Gambirasio I, Dubuisson JB, Boulvain M (2007) Risk factors for pelvic organ prolapse repair after hysterectomy. Obstet Gynecol 110:625–632
2. Maher C, Feiner B, Baessler K, et al. (2010) Surgical management of pelvic organ prolapse in women. Cochrane Database Syst Rev 4:CD004014.
3. Agarwala N, Hasiak N, Shade M (2007) Laparoscopic sacral colpopexy with Gynemesh as graft material: experience and results. J Minim Invasive Gynecol 14:577–583
4. Ross JW, Preston M (2005) Laparoscopic sacrocolpopexy for severe vaginal vault prolapse: 5-year outcome. J Minim Invasive Gynecol 12:221–226
5. Cosson M, Rajabally R, Bogaert E et al (2002) Laparoscopic sacrocolpopexy, hysterectomy, and Burch colposuspension: feasibility and short-term complications of 77 procedures. JSLS 6:115–119
6. Higgs PJ, Chua HL, Smith AR (2005) Long term review of laparoscopic sacrocolpopexy. BJOG 112:1134–1138
7. Price N, Slack A, Jackson SR (2011) Laparoscopic sacrocolpopexy: an observational study of functional and anatomical outcomes. Int Urogynecol J 22:77–82
8. North C, Ali-Ross N, Smith A, Reid F (2009) A prospective study of laparoscopic sacrocolpopexy for the management of pelvic organ prolapse. BJOG 116:1251–1257
9. Milani AL, Withagen MI, Vierhout ME (2009) Trocar-guided total tension-free vaginal mesh repair of post-hysterectomy vaginal vault prolapse. Int Urogynecol J 20:1203–1211
10. McDermott CD, Terry CL, Woodman PJ, Hale DS (2011) Surgical outcomes following total Prolift: colpopexy versus hysteropexy. Aust N Z J Obstet Gynaecol 51:61–66
11. FDA U.S. Food and Drug Administration. Medical Devices. Available at http://www.fda.gov/medicaldevices/safety/alertsandnotices/publichealthnotifications/ucm061976.htm
12. Maher CF, Feiner B, DeCuyper EM, Nichlos CJ, Hickey KV, O'Rourke P (2011) Laparoscopic sacral colpopexy versus total vaginal mesh for vaginal vault prolapse: a randomized trial. Am J Obstet Gynecol 204(360):1–7
13. Bump RC, Mattiasson A, Bo K et al (1996) The standardization of terminology of female pelvic organ prolapse and pelvic floor dysfunction. Am J Obstet Gynecol 175:10–17
14. Van der Vaart CH, de Leeuw JR, Roovers JP, Heintz AP (2003) Measuring health-related quality of life in women with urogenital dysfunction: the urogenital distress inventory and incontinence impact questionnaire revisited. Neurourol Urodyn 22:97–104
15. Brummen HJ, Bruinse HW, Pol G, Heintz AP, Vaart CH (2006) Defecatory symptoms during and after the first pregnancy: prevalences and associated factors. Int Urogynecol J 17:224–230
16. van der Weiden RM, Withagen MI, Bergkamp AB, Mannaerts GH (2005) A new device for bone anchor fixation in laparoscopic sacrocolpopexy. The Franciscan laparoscopic bone anchor inserter. Surg Endosc 19:594–597
17. Visco AG, Weidner AC, Barber MD et al (2001) Vaginal mesh erosion after abdominal sacral colpopexy. Am J Obstet Gynecol 184:297–302
18. Antiphon P, Elard S, Benyoussef A, Fofana M, Yiou R, Gettman M et al (2004) Laparoscopic promontory sacral colpopexy: is the posterior recto-vaginal mesh mandatory. Eur Urol 45:655–661
19. Nichols DH, Milley PS, Randall CL (1970) Significance of restoration of normal vaginal depth and axis. Obstet Gynecol 36:251–256
20. Funt MI, Thompson JD, Birch H (1978) Normal vaginal axis. South Med J 71(1534–1535):1552
21. DeLancey JOL (2012) Surgery for cystocele III: do all cystoceles involve apical descent? Observations on cause and effect. Int Urogynecol J 23:665–667
22. Fatton B, Amblard J, Debodinance P, Cosson M, Jacquetin B (2007) Transvaginal repair of genital prolapse: preliminary results of a new tension-free vaginal mesh (Prolift technique)—a case series multicentric study. Int Urogynecol J 18:743–752
23. Withagen MI, Milani AL (2007) Which factors influenced the result of a tension free vaginal tape operation in a single teaching hospital? Acta Obstet Gynecol Scand 86:1136–1139
24. Withagen M, Vierhout M, Mannaerts G, van der Weiden R (2011) Laparoscopic sacrocolpopexy with bone anchor fixation: short-term anatomic and functional results. Int Urogynecol 23:481–486
25. Bot-Robin V, Lucot JP, Giraudet G, Rubod C, Cosson M (2012) Use of vaginal mesh for pelvic organ prolapse repair: a literature review. Gynecol Surg 9:3–15
26. Barber MD, Brubaker L, Nygaard I, Wheeler TL, Schaffer J, Chen Z, Spino C, For the Pelvic Floor Disorders Network (2009) Defining success after surgery for pelvic organ prolapse. Obstet Gynecol 114:600–609
27. Sanses TV, Shahryarinejad A, Molden S, Hoskey KA, Abbasy S, Patterson D, Saks EK, Weber Lebrun EE, Gamble TL, King VG, Nguyen AL, Abed H, Young SB, Fellows' Pelvic Research Network (2009) Anatomic outcomes of vaginal mesh procedure (Prolift) compared with uterosacral ligament suspension and abdominal sacrocolpopexy for pelvic organ prolapse: a Fellows' Pelvic Research Network study. Am J Obstet Gynecol 201(519):1–8
28. DeLancey JOL (1992) Anatomic aspects of vaginal eversion after hysterectomy. Am J Obstet Gynecol 166:1717–1724
29. Lowder JL, ParkAJ ER et al (2008) The role of apical vaginal support in the appearance of anterior and posterior vaginal prolapse. Obstet Gynecol 111:152–157
30. Thubert T, Pourcher G, Deffieux X (2011) Small bowel volvulus following peritoneal closure using absorbable knotless device during laparoscopic sacral colpopexy. Int Urogynecol J 22:761–763
31. Klauschie J, Suozzi B, O'Brien M, McBride A (2009) A comparison of laparoscopic and abdominal sacral colpopexy: objective outcome and perioperative differences. Int Urogynecol J 20:273–279
32. Nossier S, Kim Y, Lind L, Winkler H (2010) Sacral osteomyelitis after robotically assisted laparoscopic sacral colpopexy. Obstet Gynecol 116:513–515
33. Collins SA, Tulikangas PK, Lasala CA, Lind LR (2011) Complex sacral abscess 8 years after abdominal sacral colpopexy. Obstet Gynecol 118:451–454
34. Mokrzycki ML, Hampton BS (2007) Pelvic arterial embolization in the setting of acute hemorrhage as a result of the anterior Prolift procedure. Int Urogynecol J 18:813–815
35. Claerhout F, Roovers JP, Lewi P, Verguts J, De Ridder D, Deprest J (2009) Implementation of laparoscopic sacrocolpopexy—a single center's experience. Int Urogynecol J 20:1119–1125

Long-term follow-up after laparoscopic management of endometrial cancer

Benoit Rabischong · Demetrio Larraín · Guillaume Le Bouëdec · Michel Canis · Christophe Pomel · Kris Jardon · Fabrice Kwiatkowski · Jean-Louis Achard · Jacques Dauplat · Gerard Mage

Abstract The objective of this study was to evaluate long-term oncological outcomes of laparoscopic management of endometrial carcinoma (EC) in a large series of consecutive patients from two referral cancer centres. The study is a large retrospective study with 15-year follow-up. The clinical records of 207 consecutive women with clinical stage I EC managed by laparoscopy between 1990 and 2005 were reviewed. Laparoscopy included peritoneal washing, inspection of abdominal cavity, total laparoscopic hysterectomy + bilateral salpingo-oophorectomy and pelvic/para-aortic lymphadenectomy depending on the preoperative histology or frozen section results. Data collected included conversion rate, operative time, hospital stay, surgical complications, FIGO 1988 stage and 5-year survival. Laparoscopic procedures were converted to laparotomy in nine (4.3%) cases. Mean operative time was 173.2 min (70–300 min). Mean hospital stay was 5 days. The mean number of lymph nodes removed was 10 (2–25). Lymphadenectomy was considered not feasible in 20 cases (12.9%) due to technical difficulties. Intraoperative and postoperative complications were seen in 11 (5.6%) and 13 (6.6%) women, respectively. Histopathological results led to upstaging in 11.6% of cases. After a mean follow-up of 74.8 months (14–204 months), 5-year cause-specific and disease-free survival rates were 93.2% and 89.3%, respectively. Twenty-one (10.6%) patients developed recurrences. No port site metastases were identified. Laparoscopic management of EC is feasible, reproducible and does not worsen patient prognosis. It allows comprehensive surgical staging and the option of lymphadenectomy in a single surgical procedure without compromising the oncological radicality required. Our results show minimal morbidity and similar long-term outcomes than those obtained by laparotomy in the literature.

B. Rabischong · D. Larraín · M. Canis · K. Jardon · G. Mage
Department of Obstetrics Gynecology and Human Reproduction,
CHU Estaing,
1 Place Lucie Aubrac,
63003 Clermont-Ferrand, France

G. Le Bouëdec · C. Pomel · J.-L. Achard · J. Dauplat
Department of Gynecologic Oncology and Surgery,
Jean Perrin Cancer Center,
58 rue Montalembert,
63011 Clermont-Ferrand, France

F. Kwiatkowski
Department of Medical Research and Biostatistics,
Jean Perrin Cancer Center,
58 rue Montalembert,
63011 Clermont-Ferrand, France

B. Rabischong (✉)
1, Place Lucie Aubrac,
63003 Clermont-Ferrand CEDEX 1, France
e-mail: brabischong@chu-clermontferrand.fr

Keywords Endometrial cancer · Laparoscopy · Long-term follow-up · Survival

Background

Endometrial cancer (EC) is the most common gynaecological malignancy in developed countries, with more than 40,000 cases estimated to be diagnosed in 2009 in the USA [1] and 5,800 new cases diagnosed in 2005 in France [2].

Most women with EC develop postmenopausal bleeding, facilitating early diagnosis. Currently, more than 70% of cases are diagnosed whilst the tumour is confined to the uterus (clinical stage I) [3]. In such cases, surgery is the primary treatment.

According to the International Federation of Gynecology and Obstetrics (FIGO) [4], the staging surgery includes peritoneal washings, total hysterectomy and bilateral salpingo-oophorectomy. Although pelvic and para-aortic lymphadenectomy are recommended [5], they remain controversial.

In most centres worldwide, this surgical staging is more commonly performed via a midline vertical infraumbilical incision. Since the early 1990s, all the steps required for a comprehensive surgical staging are feasible by laparoscopy [6–10].

After these earliest reports [11–13], several retrospective studies [14–25] and recent trials [26–33] have demonstrated that laparoscopic staging of EC is feasible and safe, and results in shorter hospital stays and improved quality of life. Despite these established short-term advantages, there is no agreement about the survival benefit of laparoscopic staging procedures. The main reason for this is that survival data from well-designed prospective studies remain insufficient due to short-term follow-up [34]. Therefore, even if long-term outcomes after laparoscopic staging seem to be comparable to abdominal staging [18–22], they are not well documented yet.

The purpose of this study was to present our experience and both surgical and oncological outcomes for a large series of patients with early-stage EC managed completely via laparoscopy with a long-term follow-up.

Patients and methods

The medical records of 207 consecutive patients with early-stage (clinical stage I) EC who underwent laparoscopic staging at Clermont-Ferrand University Hospital and Jean Perrin Cancer Centre between February 1990 and December 2005 were retrospectively reviewed. Cases were identified from databases of both centres. Institutional Review Board exemption was granted by both centres because of the retrospective nature of this study.

Data collected included patient age, parity, menopausal status, body mass index (BMI), operating time, conversion to laparotomy, blood transfusion, intraoperative and post-operative complications, hospital stay, histological grade, number of lymph nodes yielded, surgical stage (FIGO 1988), adjuvant therapy, duration of follow-up and development of disease recurrence, site of recurrence or death.

It should be noted that although the FIGO staging was changed in 2009 [35], this change occurred after the creation of our database. Therefore, all our patients were staged and managed according to the old system. Moreover, most studies of laparoscopic management of EC, including the most recent trials [32–34], are based on the old system. Additionally, since no prognostic difference between the two systems for stage I EC has been noted [36], the old system is used in this report, unless otherwise stated.

Preoperative workup included pelvic examination, chest X-ray, standard preoperative blood analysis and abdomino-pelvic MRI in most of the cases.

We offered laparoscopy as first-line treatment to all patients, and during the study period, we performed primary laparotomy only in patients for whom laparoscopic approach was contraindicated.

Contraindications for laparoscopy included: severe cardiopulmonary disease precluding the Trendelenburg position, anaesthetic contraindication for pneumoperitoneum, limited vaginal access and/or a bulky uterus where vaginal removal might require morcellation, presence of gross adenopathies at MRI (more advanced disease is suspected) and severe obesity (BMI≥40) in the first 4 years of the study period. Previous laparotomy was not considered a contraindication for laparoscopy.

In all cases, laparoscopy started with a meticulous inspection of all pelvic and abdominal structures. In the event of evidence of peritoneal spread, we converted to laparotomy for completion of debulking and staging. The laparoscopic procedure included: peritoneal washing, total laparoscopic hysterectomy with bilateral salpingo-oophorectomy (TLH/BSO) and pelvic ± para-aortic lymphadenectomy according to the results of frozen section or preoperative histology. Operating times were recorded from the creation of the pneumoperitoneum to skin closure.

Pelvic lymphadenectomy was performed for all women with myometrial invasion, grade 3 tumours and those with high-risk histology (e.g. papillary serous or clear cell adenocarcinoma; Fig. 1).

Our technique of TLH/BSO was described previously [37]. To display vaginal fornices and uterine vessels, we routinely used a uterine manipulator (*Clermont-Ferrand*, Karl Storz, Tuttlingen, Germany) with a smooth tip (no screw thread) specially designed for oncological purposes. Although the coagulation of the tubes before uterine cannulation is not a systematic practice in our department, it was made in some cases according to surgeon preference.

Briefly, pelvic lymphadenectomy consisted of complete skeletonization of common, internal and external iliac vessels and harvesting of all fatty and lymphatic tissue above and below the obturator nerve. Nodes yielded were routinely retrieved in an endoscopic bag and sent to the pathologist for frozen section. Para-aortic lymphadenectomy extended to the renal vessels was performed only if the pelvic nodes were shown to be involved at frozen section (Fig. 1).

All surgeries were performed by 11 surgeons who were assisted by residents or fellows.

Adjuvant treatment was discussed together with radiotherapists, pathologists, and medical oncologists in a multidisciplinary meeting according to the protocol shown in Fig. 2. Adjuvant whole pelvic radiation ± brachytherapy

Fig. 1 Management protocol followed during the whole study period

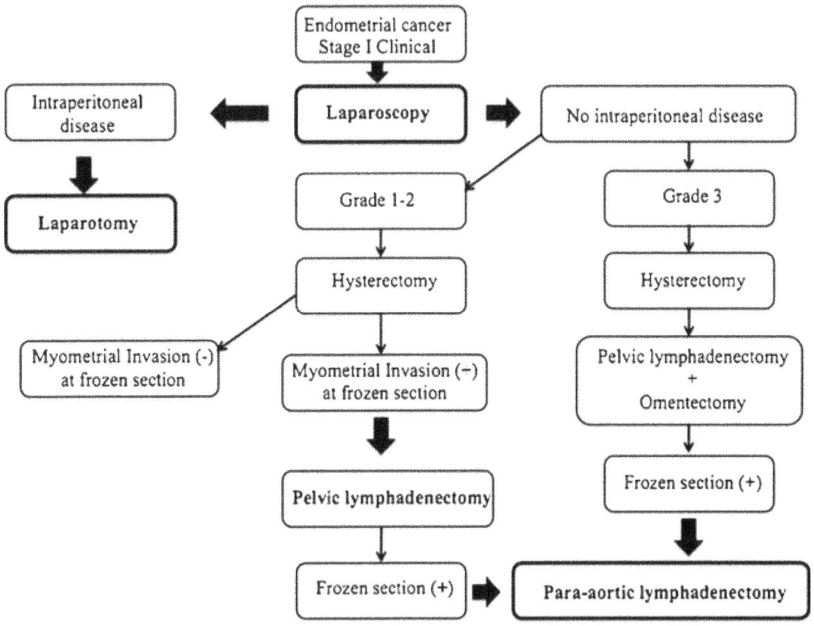

was recommended for all patients with grade 3 tumours and for those with surgical stage Ic or IIIa (positive cytology). Vaginal cuff brachytherapy was prescribed for patients with stage Ib grade 1/2. Patients with IIIa (adnexal involvement) and those with more advanced disease received extended field pelvic radiation and, in some cases, chemotherapy.

Follow-up visits were scheduled 1 month after surgery and then every 3 months for the first 2 years, and every 6 months thereafter. Recurrence-free and overall survival were estimated using Kaplan–Meier analysis, considering relapse or death as censoring events, respectively.

Data processing and statistical analysis were performed with SAS statistical software V8.02 (SAS Institute, Cary, NC, USA). Statistical significance was established at $p<0.05$.

Results and findings

Among 207 patients with clinical stage I EC managed by laparoscopy, 52 (25.1%) were obese (BMI≥30 kg/m^2), 36 (17.3%) were nulliparous, and 56 (27%) were ≥70 years old. Patient characteristics and clinical data are summarised in Table 1.

The laparoscopic procedure could successfully be completed in 198 (95.6%) patients, but it was converted to laparotomy in nine (4.3%) patients.

Reasons for conversion were the following: extrauterine/intraperitoneal disease (n=4), several pelvic and intraperitoneal adhesions precluding pelvic visualisation (n=2), severe subcutaneous emphysema and uncontrollable hypercapnia after hysterectomy (converted for lymphadenectomy, n=1),

Fig. 2 Postoperative management and different adjuvant therapies administered during the study period according to surgical stage and grade

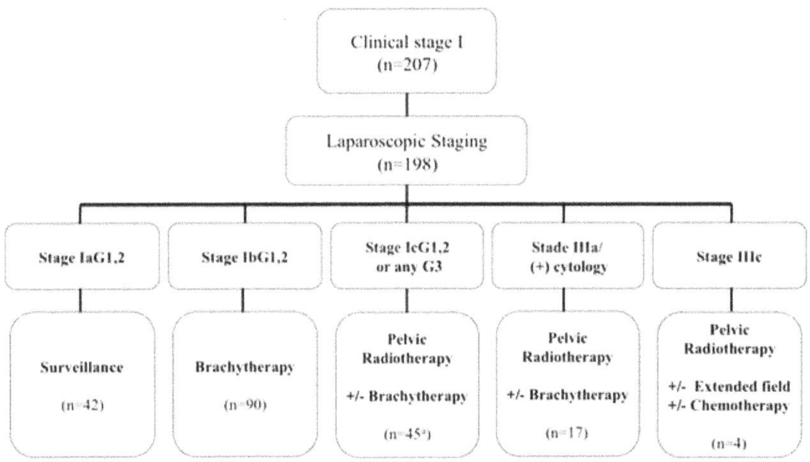

[a] Included 1 patient with stage IIaG1, and one with stage IIbG1

Table 1 Clinical characteristics (n=207)

Mean age (range)	63 years (36–88)
Age≥70 years	56 (27%)
Mean BMI (kg/m^2, range)	26.2 (16–56)
Obesity (BMI≥30)	52 (25.1%)
Nulliparity	36 (17.3%)
Postmenopausal status	184 (88.8%)

failure of pneumoperitoneum creation (BMI=32 kg/m^2, previous bowel resection, n=1) and difficult exposure due to morbid obesity (BMI=56 kg/m^2, n=1). These patients were excluded from the analysis.

Pelvic node dissection was performed according to our protocol in 87.1% of cases. The procedure was deemed not feasible in 20 (12.9%) cases because of morbid obesity (n=7), inadequate ventilation due to pneumoperitoneum and Trendelenburg position (n=7), several adhesions attributed to previous surgery (n=2), and gas embolism (n=1).

Three patients underwent para-aortic lymphadenectomy. For the first case, this was because of positive pelvic nodes at frozen section. The final histology reported three of ten metastatic para-aortic nodes. The second case was a patient with a clear cell tumour in which para-aortic lymphadenectomy was decided by the surgeon and eight negative para-aortic nodes were identified. The third case of lymph node dissection extended to the para-aortic chains was due to a false positive result of frozen section (endosalpingiosis).

Operative and postoperative complications occurred in 11 (5.6%) and 13 (6.6%) patients, respectively.

The mean operative time was 173.2 min (range 70–300 min) for TLH and pelvic lymphadenectomy, including the time waiting for frozen section evaluation. The mean length of hospital stay was 5 days (range 2–16 days). Surgical outcomes and complications are shown in Table 2.

Definitive surgical stage and grade are shown in Table 3. As a result of surgical staging, 23 patients (11.6%) were upstaged. Interestingly, there were two patients with stage IIIc tumours and positive pelvic lymph nodes for whom para-aortic lymphadenectomy was not performed because pelvic lymph nodes were negative at frozen section.

Reasons for upstaging were as follows: pelvic and/or para-aortic nodal metastases (n=3), positive cytology (n=13), adnexal metastases (n=3) or both (n=2). Two patients were upstaged due to cervical involvement. Adjuvant therapy was administered to 156 patients (Fig. 2). The mean follow-up was 74.8 months (range 14–204 months). At the last follow-up (March 2010), 21 (10.6%) women had recurrences, with a median recurrence interval of 35 months (range 6–143 months). No port site recurrences occurred in this series. Unexpectedly, one patient presented a delayed recurrence at 143 months after surgery. The sites of recurrence are summarised in Table 4. In order to be honest, we included among the recurrences two patients who probably had metastatic disease at the time of primary surgery. In these cases, preoperative evaluation could have led to understaging the disease (stage >I), given recurrence site and time since surgery (Table 4). Thirteen patients died from recurrent disease. Among patients with surgical stage I, one patient who had stage Ib clear cell carcinoma developed an early peritoneal recurrence 7 months after surgery. She died 24 months later from peritoneal carcinomatosis.

Overall and cause-specific survival rates were 88.9% and 93.2%, respectively (p=0.07, NS; Fig. 3a). The disease-free 5-year survival rate was 89.3% (Fig. 3b).

Discussion

Despite its retrospective design, this study remains an interesting data source. With its large series of consecutive patients with early-stage EC treated by laparoscopy over a long period of 15 years, this study in fact provides significant information about long-term survival and complications for these patients.

Surgical approach of endometrial cancer: the feasibility of laparoscopy

In agreement with several previous studies [14–33], our data support the statement that laparoscopic approach is feasible, safe and reproducible, offering patients all the advantages of a minimally invasive technique. Therefore, it seems that the only weakness in laparoscopic staging of EC is the increased operative time [22, 26, 30, 32]. We think that this is a reasonable concession given the lower morbidity, shorter hospital stay and improvement in quality of life [31–33]. These are major issues in EC patients who are frequently elderly, obese and with comorbid conditions. It should be noted that even if the mean hospital stay in our series was longer than previous reports [14–17], this can be explained by the fact that during the first 4 years of the study, patients stayed in the hospital for longer because we were more apprehensive about this "new" procedure. Nowadays, most patients are discharged on the second day after TLH, or even earlier in selected cases [38].

Vaginal hysterectomy has been reported as a safe, simpler and faster technique with low morbidity for the treatment of stage I EC in obese and elderly patients and those with significant coexisting medical conditions for whom total abdominal hysterectomy might be difficult or risky [39, 40]. However, the major objection to this approach is that it does not allow performing the complete

Table 2 Summary of surgical outcomes and complications

Mean operative time (TLH + pelvic lymphadenectomy)	173.2 min (70–300)	Intraoperative complications		11 (5.6%)
Conversion rate	9 (4.3%)	Haemorrhage	1	Controlled vaginally
Mean hospital stay (days)	5 (2–16)	Bladder injury	1	Treated laparoscopically during operation
Mean return bowel activity (days)	1.4 (1–3)	Subcutaneous emphysema	5	One case required late conversion to perform lymphadenectomy
Recurrence rate	21 (10.6%)	Gas embolism	1	Operative time 70 min. Favourable outcome
Para-aortic lymphadenectomy	3 (1.5%)	Blood transfusion	3	
Mean no. of pelvic nodes	10 (2–25)	Postoperative complications		13 (6.6%)
Lymphadenectomies indicated and not performed	20 (12.9%)	Hemoperitoneum	1	Required laparotomy and blood transfusion 48 h after surgery
Positive cytology	15 (7.6%)	Pulmonary embolism	1	Discharged in good conditions
Upstaged patients	23 (11.6%)	Vesicovaginal fistula	1	3 months after surgery. Managed laparoscopically
Cause-specific survival	93.2%	Intestinal sub-oclussion	1	Requiring readmission and medical treatment 3 weeks after surgery
Median recurrence-free interval	35 months	Phlebitis	2	
Mean follow-up	74.8 months	Port site hernia	1	
Overall survival	88.9%	Obturator neuropathy	3	Resolved spontaneously.
Disease-free survival	89.3%	Lymphedema/Lymphocyst	2	Resolved spontaneously.
Adjuvant therapy	156 (78.8%)	Vaginal cuff dehiscence	1	Previous radiotherapy. Cuff dehiscence 6 years after surgery. Re-closure without complications

surgical staging recommended by FIGO [4] to be carried out. Moreover, inspection of the abdominal cavity and peritoneal washings are not possible and, frequently, the ovaries cannot be removed [39].

In this study, more than 50% of the women were elderly or obese. We have shown that laparoscopy is an adequate approach for these patients since all FIGO guidelines with regard to surgical staging can be met by laparoscopy.

During the study period, our surgical technique underwent no major changes and the complication rate remained lower than reported in previous studies [41] despite the higher number of surgeons. This is very important since it

Table 3 Distribution of patients according to stage and histological grade

FIGO 1988 surgical stage	No. of patients (%)	Detail (%)	FIGO 2009 surgical stage
Ia	43 (21.7)		Stage Ia: 164 (82.8%)
Ib	96 (48.5)		Stage Ib: 36 (18.1%)
Ic	36 (18.2)		
IIa	1 (0.5)		Stage II: 1 (0.5%)
IIb	1 (0.5)		
IIIa	18 (9.1)	Positive cytology: 13 (6.6) Adnexal invasion: 3 (1.5) Both: 2 (1)	Stage IIIa: 5 (2.5%)
IIIc	3 (1.5)		Stage IIIc1: 2 (1%) Stage IIIc2: 1 (0.5%)
Grade			
1	154 (77.3)		
2	24 (12.1)		
3	21 (10.6)		

Table 4 Recurrence site and time to recurrence among 21 patients who relapsed

Case	1988 FIGO stage/grade	Recurrence site(s)	Time to recurrence (months)	Status
1	IbG3 (clear cell)	Peritoneal carcinomatosis	7	Deceased
2	IIIaG3, (+) cytology, (+) adnexa	Vagina	143	Alive
3	IIaG1	Vagina + central pelvis	58	Alive
4	IcG1	Aortic lymph nodes + liver + lungs	61	Alive
5	IIIaG1, (+) cytology	Central pelvis + bone	12	Deceased
6	IIIaG1, (+) cytology	Vagina + lungs	9	Deceased
7	IcG1	Liver + lungs	84	Alive
8	IbG1	Lungs	45	Deceased
9	IIIaG1, (+) cytology	Peritoneum	24	Deceased
10	IbG1	Central pelvis	42	Deceased
11	IaG1	Vagina	22	Alive
12	IbG2	Lungs	37	Deceased
13	IIIaG1, (+) cytology	Bone	15	Alive
14	IIIaG3, (+) cytology	Liver + lungs	13	Deceased
15[a]	IIIaG3 (clear cells), (+) adnexa	Aortic lymph nodes + liver	6	Deceased
16[a,b]	IIIcG1	Aortic lymph nodes	6	Alive
17	IaG1	Vagina + peritoneum	13	Deceased
18	IcG1	Central pelvis + aortic lymph nodes + lungs	29	Deceased
19	IbG3	Central pelvis	45	Alive
20	IcG3	Peritoneum	22	Deceased
21	IIIaG3, (+) cytology	Peritoneum + liver + lungs	16	Deceased

[a] Probably presence of metastatic disease at time of surgery. Clinically understaged

[b] Para-aortic lymphadenectomy not performed. False (−) frozen section of pelvic nodes

underlines the importance of using a standardised surgical technique in order to reduce complications and achieve procedure reproducibility [42].

Despite the claim that use of uterine cannulation is not necessary [30] and that it may led to dissemination of tumoral cells [43, 44], there is no evidence that uterine manipulation during laparoscopy increases the risk of cell spillage in the pelvic cavity [27, 28, 45]. To date, the prognostic importance of isolated positive cytology remains uncertain [46]. In fact, the new FIGO staging system deleted cytology as a variable dictating more advanced disease [35]. In this study, the rate of positive cytology and vaginal recurrence was comparable with those reported in previous studies in which patients were treated by laparotomy [47] or those in which TLH was performed without uterine cannulation [48]. Moreover, several studies comparing laparotomy with laparoscopy have shown that the rate of positive cytology was identical between the groups [41] even if the uterus was cannulated [24, 27]. Furthermore, in our experience, the uterine manipulator is essential

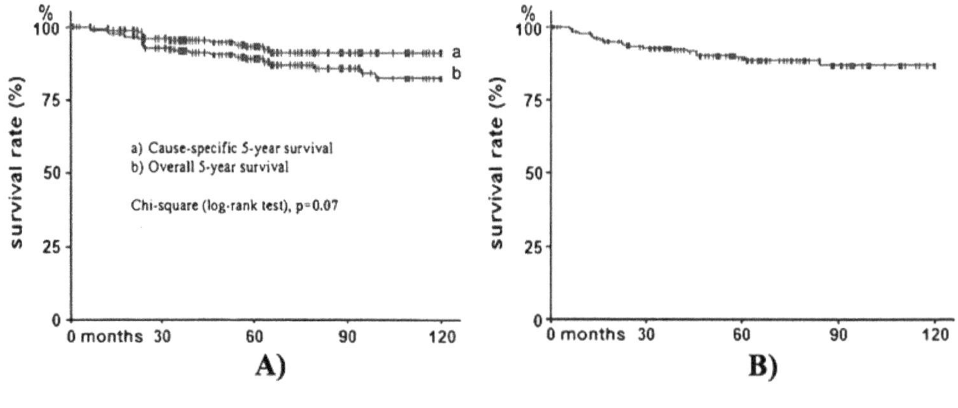

Fig. 3 a Overall and cause-specific 5-year survival rates projected by Kaplan–Meier curves (log-rank test, p=0.07, NS). **b** Disease-free 5-year survival curve

to improve exposure and prevent ureteral complications [37]. This is important since impaired exposure is a major reason for conversion [32], especially in obese women [49].

The rate of conversion to laparotomy was 4.3% in this series. It compares favourably with previous reports [24, 31, 32] and is consistent with the conversion rates reported for single-centre studies (<10%) [15, 20, 23] Unexpectedly, the recently published LAP-2 multicentric randomised controlled trial (RCT) [32] reported a conversion rate of 26%. This surprisingly high rate of conversion is probably more representative of the reality, without the bias of a specialised centre. However, it may be influenced by the higher prevalence of obesity among women in the USA compared with Europe [50] and the need for comprehensive surgical staging (including pelvic and para-aortic lymphadenectomy) to meet the study protocol [32].

These features make the LAP-2 protocol not fully applicable in many centres around the world where systematic pelvic and para-aortic lymphadenectomy is not the standard treatment for early-stage EC [22, 24, 27, 28, 41, 51].

Lymphadenectomy and endometrial cancer: the controversy

Despite the fact that lymphadenectomy is recommended as a standard component of surgical staging of EC [4, 5] and that there is agreement about its prognostic value, it remains a variable practice from institution to institution. Surveys of major gynaecological cancer centres demonstrate these differing approaches to management, with 54% of American centres [52] and 24% of centres in Western Europe [53] performing systematic lymphadenectomy for all women. Therefore, the reality is that about 50% of women still do not undergo lymphadenectomy at the time of their primary surgery [54].

The therapeutic benefit of lymphadenectomy is based on several retrospective studies that reported a significant survival advantage for patients undergoing lymph node dissection [54–58]. Conversely, and according to recent data, the surgical strategy for management of EC could undergo major changes. Two randomised trials have concluded that there is no benefit in performing systematic lymphadenectomy for clinical stage I EC in terms of overall, disease-specific and recurrence-free survival [59, 60]. In this context, older studies [61, 62] have demonstrated that in low-risk patients (endometrioid histology, grade 1 or 2, and without or with tumours invading <50% of the myometrium), the risk of nodal metastases is negligible. Furthermore, in the absence of positive pelvic lymph nodes or other risk factors associated with a poor prognosis, the probability of para-aortic lymph node metastases is extremely low [62, 63]. In this study, the number of patients with positive pelvic nodes was lower than in previous reports [23, 26, 59, 60, 64], but this could be explained by the fact that most of the patients in our series had low-risk tumours.

Recently, Mariani et al. [65] analysed the extension of lymphatic spread among 422 patients with clinical stage I EC. The authors reported that in patients with high-risk disease, the rate of lymphatic metastases above the inferior mesenteric artery was 16%, even with negative pelvic nodes. On the contrary, a recent paper including 1,942 patients showed that the risk of isolated para-aortic metastases was 1%, even with high-risk tumours, continuing the controversy concerning this issue [66]. In this study, most patients had low-risk tumours, and only three women underwent para-aortic lymphadenectomy. Therefore, the numbers are insufficient to draw any conclusion on the risk of isolated para-aortic metastases.

Based on the growing evidence suggesting that lymphadenectomies are not appropriate for low-risk patients [67] and the fact that the procedure is not totally free of complications [67, 68], the most rational approach is to adapt the indication of lymphadenectomy according to the patient's characteristics (age, performance status, comorbid conditions) and the histological characteristics of the tumour at preoperative biopsy or frozen section.

In our experience, as in others [69, 70], frozen section is a reliable method for triage of patients for lymphadenectomy, with a low rate of false-negative results.

Today, the therapeutic benefits of lymphadenectomy are still matter of debate, especially in early-stage disease [71]. In addition, there are still many questions to be answered about the role and extension of lymphadenectomy in EC. In this setting, the sentinel lymph node technique seems promising since it could clarify the current controversies regarding lymphatic dissemination of EC in the future [72, 73], although further studies are needed before it is put into clinical practice.

Although in our series only three of the patients with higher risk of recurrence underwent complete surgical staging including para-aortic lymphadenectomy, several randomised trials [74, 75] have demonstrated the safety of adjuvant radiotherapy in these patients despite the lack of comprehensive staging.

To date, with or without lymphadenectomy, the role of laparoscopy in the management of EC is established and the advantages of minimally invasive techniques are well known. Therefore, if lymphadenectomy proves to be necessary it should be attempted using a minimally invasive approach. This is very interesting since in our experience, and in agreement with several reports [32, 49], lymphadenectomy is the limiting step when performing laparoscopic staging due to impaired exposure.

This apparent "conflict" between a minimally invasive procedure and a comprehensive staging including complete lymphadenectomy could be resolved with the use of other techniques, such as the extraperitoneal laparoscopic approach [76] or robotic-assisted laparoscopy [77], in order to overcome the limitations of conventional laparoscopy.

Long-term results of laparoscopy in endometrial cancer patients

To be accepted as the gold standard, a surgical procedure must be feasible, effective, reproducible and safe. In addition, when treating cancer patients, it is mandatory to not compromise standard survival outcomes.

Several retrospective studies have shown no difference in survival and recurrence rates between laparotomy and laparoscopy; however, these studies are limited by their sample size and short-term follow-up [21–25]. To date, three RCTs have included survival data [26–28]. None of these studies have demonstrated any significant difference between laparoscopy or laparotomy with respect to recurrence, disease-free and overall survival. These trials lacked the power to prove this hypothesis, however, and only one of them has a mean follow-up >4 years [28].

Recently, Walker et al. [34] released initial survival data from the LAP-2 study conducted by the GOG at the 41st Annual Meeting of the Society of Gynecologic Oncologists. As expected, the authors showed that the 3-year overall survival was 89.8% in the laparoscopy group and 89.9% in the laparotomy group. They concluded that laparoscopy should be considered the standard for treatment for EC. We agree with these conclusions, but it is important to note that even if the sample size of the study was appropriate to address this issue, the follow-up is still too short. In this context, we think that there is still place for large retrospective series such as this one to support these conclusions. Although it is a retrospective study, its major strength is the long-term follow-up. Interestingly, in this and other studies with a longer follow-up, more than 30% of the recurrences reported occurred after 36 months [28].

In our study, the recurrence rate and disease-free 5-year survival were 10.6% and 89.3%, respectively, and are comparable with survival and recurrence data obtained by laparotomy [5]. Our results support the oncological safety of the laparoscopic approach. Therefore, to draw definitive conclusions from RCT, all that is needed is time. If the good results already published are confirmed in a few years, laparoscopy will become the gold standard technique for the management of early-stage EC.

Conclusion

Although long-term results of recent RCTs are still immature, available data demonstrate that the results of laparoscopy are equivalent or better than those achieved with laparotomy. From the data presented, we think that equivalent rates for both disease-free and overall survival can be expected. Therefore, after adequate training, laparoscopy should be preferred over laparotomy for the management of early-stage EC.

Declaration of interest The authors have no conflicts of interest to declare.

References

1. Jemal A, Siegel R, Ward E, Hao Y, Xu J, Thun MJ (2009) Cancer statistics, 2009. CA Cancer J Clin 59:225–249
2. Belot A, Grosclaude P, Bossard N, Jougla E, Benhamou E, Delafosse P et al (2008) Cancer incidence and mortality in France over the period 1980–2005. Rev Epidemiol Sante Publique 56:159–175
3. Creasman WT, Odicino F, Maisonneuve P, Quinn MA, Beller U, Benedet JL et al (2006) Carcinoma of the corpus uteri. FIGO 6th Annual Report on the Results of Treatment in Gynecological Cancer. Int J Gynaecol Obstet 95(Suppl 1):S105–S143
4. Sheperd JH (1989) Revised FIGO staging for gynaecological cancer. Br J Obstet Gynaecol 96:889–892
5. ACOG Practice Bulletin (2005) Clinical management guidelines for obstetrician-gynecologists. Management of endometrial cancer. Obstet Gynecol 106:413–424
6. Reich H, DeCaprio J, McGlynn F (1989) Laparoscopic hysterectomy. J Gynecol Surg 5:213–215
7. Canis M, Mage G, Chapron C, Wattiez A, Pouly JL, Bruhat MA (1993) Laparoscopic hysterectomy. A preliminary study. Surg Endosc 7:42–45
8. Wattiez A, Raymond F, Canis M, Chapron C, Pouly JL, Mage G et al (1993) External iliac lymphadenectomy by celioscopy: surgical technique. Ann Chir 47:523–528
9. Childers JM, Hatch KD, Tran AN, Surwit EA (1993) Laparoscopic para-aortic lymphadenectomy in gynecologic malignancies. Obstet Gynecol 82:741–747
10. Querleu D (1993) Laparoscopic paraaortic node sampling in gynecologic oncology: a preliminary experience. Gynecol Oncol 49:24–29
11. Childers JM, Surwit EA (1992) Combined laparoscopic and vaginal surgery for the management of two cases of stage I endometrial cancer. Gynecol Oncol 45:46–51
12. Childers JM, Brezechffa PR, Hatch KD, Surwitt EA (1993) Laparoscopically assisted surgical staging (LASS) of endometrial cancer. Gynecol Oncol 51:33–38
13. Mage G, Bournazeau JA, Canis M, Glowaczower E, Masson FN, Raiga J et al (1995) Treatment of endometrial clinical stage I endometrial adenocarcinoma by laparoscopic surgery. Seventeen cases. J Gynecol Obstet Biol Reprod (Paris) 24:485–490
14. Hidlebaugh DA, Orr RK (1997) Staging endometrial carcinoma. Clinical and financial comparison of laparoscopic and traditional approaches. J Reprod Med 42:482–488
15. Gemignani ML, Curtin JP, Zelmanovich J, Patel DA, Venkatraman E, Barakat RR (1999) Laparoscopic assisted vaginal hysterectomy for endometrial cancer: clinical outcomes and hospital charges. Gynecol Oncol 73:5–11
16. Holub Z, Jabor A, Bartos P, Eim J, Urbánek S, Pivovarniková R (2002) Laparoscopic surgery for endometrial cancer: long term results of a multicentric study. Eur J Gynaecol Oncol 23:305–310

17. Occelli B, Samouelian V, Narducci F, Leblanc E, Querleu D (2003) The choice of approach in the surgical management of endometrial carcinoma: a retrospective serie of 155 cases. Bull Cancer 90:347–355
18. Magrina JF, Mutone NF, Weaber AL, Magtibay PM, Fowler RS, Cornella JL (1999) Laparoscopic hysterectomy with bilateral salpingo-oophorectomy for endometrial cancer: morbidity and survival. Am J Obstet Gynecol 181:376–381
19. Eltabbakh GH (2002) Analysis of survival after laparoscopy in women with endometrial carcinoma. Cancer 95:1894–1901
20. Kuoppala T, Tomas E, Heinonen PK (2004) Clinical outcomes and complications of laparoscopic surgery compared with tradicional surgery in women with endometrial cancer. Arch Gynecol Obstet 270:25–30
21. Magrina JF, Weaber AL (2004) Laparoscopic treatment of endometrial cancer: five-year recurrence and survival rates. Eur J Gynaecol Oncol 25:439–441
22. Zapico A, Fuentes P, Grassa A, Arnanz F, Otazua J, Cortés-Prieto J (2005) Laparoscopic-assisted vaginal hysterectomy versus abdominal hysterectomy in stage I and II endometrial cancer. Operating data, follow up and survival. Gynecol Oncol 98:222–227
23. Cho YH, Kim DY, Kim YM, Kim YT, Nam JH (2007) Laparoscopic management of early uterine cancer: 10-year experience in Asan Medical Center. Gynecol Oncol 106:585–590
24. Nezhat F, Yadav J, Rahaman J, Gretz H, Cohen C (2008) Analysis of survival after laparoscopic management of endometrial cancer. J Minim Invasive Gynecol 15:181–187
25. Obermair A, Manolitsas TP, Leung Y, Hammond IG, McCartney AJ (2004) Total laparoscopic hysterectomy for endometrial cancer: patterns of recurrence and survival. Gynecol Oncol 92:789–793
26. Malzoni M, Tinelli R, Cosentino F, Perone C, Rasile M, Iuzzolino D et al (2009) Total laparoscopic hysterectomy versus abdominal hysterectomy with lymphadenectomy for early-stage endometrial cancer: a prospective randomized study. Gynecol Oncol 112:126–133
27. Tozzi R, Malur S, Koehler C, Schneider A (2005) Laparoscopy versus laparotomy in endometrial cancer: first analysis of survival of a randomized prospective study. J Minim Invasive Gynecol 12:130–136
28. Zullo F, Palomba S, Falbo A, Russo T, Mocciaro R, Tartaglia E et al (2009) Laparoscopic surgery vs laparotomy for early stage endometrial cancer: long-term data of a randomized controlled trial. Am J Obstet Gynecol 200(296):e1–e9
29. Zorlu CG, Simsek T, Ari ES (2005) Laparoscopy or laparotomy for the management of endometrial cancer. JSLS 9:442–446
30. Fram KM (2002) Laparoscopically assisted vaginal hysterectomy versus abdominal hysterectomy in stage I endometrial cancer. Int J Gynecol Cancer 12:57–61
31. Zullo F, Palomba S, Russo T, Falbo A, Costantino M, Tolino A et al (2005) A prospective randomized comparison between laparoscopic and laparotomic approach in women with early stage endometrial cancer: a focus on the quality of life. Am J Obstet Gynecol 193:1344–1352
32. Walker JL, Piedmonte MR, Spirtos NM, Eisenkop SM, Schlaerth JB, Mannel RS et al (2009) Laparoscopy compared with laparotomy for comprehensive surgical staging of uterine cancer: Gynecologic Oncology Group Study LAP2. J Clin Oncol 27:5331–5336
33. Kornblith AB, Huang HQ, Walker JL, Spirtos NM, Rotmensch J, Cella D (2009) Quality of life of patients with endometrial cancer undergoing laparoscopic International Federation of Gynecology and Obstetrics staging compared with laparotomy: a Gynecologic Oncology Group Study. J Clin Oncol 27:5337–5342
34. Walker JL, Piedmonte MR, Spirtos NM, Eisenkop SM, Spiegel G, Mannel RS et al (2010) Recurrence and survival after randomization to laparoscopy versus laparotomy for comprehensive surgical staging of uterine cancer: Gynecologic Oncology Group Study LAP2. 2010 SGO 41st Annual Meeting, Abstract LBA1
35. Creasman W (2009) Revised FIGO staging for carcinoma of the endometrium. Int J Gynaecol Obstet 105:109
36. Lewin S, Herzog T, Barrena Medel N, Deutsch I, Sun X, Burke W et al (2010) Comparative performance of the new versus old FIGO staging system for endometrial cancer. Gynecol Oncol 116(Suppl 1):6–7, Abstract 10
37. Wattiez A, Soriano D, Cohen SB, Nervo P, Canis M, Botchorishvili R et al (2002) The learning curve of total laparoscopic hysterectomy: comparative analysis of 1647 cases. J Am Assoc Gynecol Laparosc 9:339–345
38. de Lapasse C, Rabischong B, Bolandard F, Canis M, Botchorishvili R, Jardon K et al (2008) Total laparoscopic hysterectomy and early discharge: satisfaction and feasibility study. J Minim Invasive Gynecol 15:20–25
39. Chan JK, Lin YG, Monk BJ, Tewari K, Bloss JD, Berman ML (2001) Vaginal hysterectomy as primary treatment of endometrial cancer in medically compromised women. Obstet Gynecol 97:707–711
40. Massi G, Savino L, Susini T (1996) Vaginal hysterectomy versus abdominal hysterectomy for the treatment of stage I endometrial adenocarcinoma. Am J Obstet Gynecol 174:1320–1326
41. Hahn HS, Kim HJ, Yoon SG, Kim WC, Choi HJ, Kim HS et al (2010) Laparoscopy-assisted vaginal versus abdominal hysterectomy in endometrial cancer. Int J Gynecol Cancer 20:102–109
42. Altgassen C, Possover M, Krause N, Plaul K, Michels W, Schneider A (2000) Establishing a new technique of laparoscopic pelvic and para-aortic lymphadenectomy. Obstet Gynecol 95:348–352
43. Lim S, Kim HS, Lee KB, Yoo CW, Park SY, Seo SS (2008) Does the use of an uterine manipulator with an intrauterine balloon in total laparoscopic hysterectomy facilitate tumor cell spillage into the peritoneal cavity in patients with endometrial cancer? Int J Gynecol Cancer 18:1145–1149
44. Sonoda Y, Zerbe M, Smith A, Lin O, Barakat RR, Hoskins WJ (2001) High incidence of positive peritoneal cytology in low-risk endometrial cancer treated by laparoscopically assisted vaginal hysterectomy. Gynecol Oncol 80:378–382
45. Eltabbakh GH, Mount SL (2006) Laparoscopic surgery does not increase the positive peritoneal cytology among women with endometrial carcinoma. Gynecol Oncol 100:361–364
46. Wethington SL, Barrena Medel NI, Wright JD, Herzog JT (2009) Prognostic significance and treatment implications of positive peritoneal cytology in endometrial adenocarcinoma: unraveling a mystery. Gynecol Oncol 115:18–25
47. Turner DA, Gershenson DM, Atkinson N, Sneige N, Wharton AT (1989) The prognostic significance of peritoneal cytology for stage I endometrial cancer. Obstet Gynecol 74:775–780
48. Wong CK, Wong YH, Lo LS, Tai CM, Ng TK (2005) Laparoscopy compared with laparotomy for the surgical staging of endometrial carcinoma. J Obstet Gynaecol Res 31:286–290
49. Scribner DR Jr, Walker JL, Johnson GA, McMeelin DS, Gold MA, Mannel RS (2002) Laparoscopic pelvic and paraaortic lymph node dissection in the obese. Gynecol Oncol 84:426–430
50. Pischon T, Nöthlings U, Boeing H (2008) Obesity and cancer. Proc Nutr Soc 67:128–145
51. Ghezzi F, Cromi A, Uccella S, Siesto G, Giudici S, Serati M et al (2010) Laparoscopic versus open surgery for endometrial cancer: a minimum 3-year follow-up study. Ann Surg Oncol 17:271–278
52. Maggino T, Romagnolo C, Landoni F, Sartori E, Zola P, Gardducci A (1998) An analysis of approaches to the management of endometrial cancer in North America: a CTF study. Gynecol Oncol 68:274–279
53. Maggino T, Romagnolo C, Zola P, Sartori E, Landoni F, Gardducci A (1995) An analysis of approaches to the treatment

of endometrial cancer in western Europe: a CTF study. Eur J Cancer 31A:1993–1997
54. Smith DC, Macdonald OK, Lee CM, Gaffney DK (2008) Survival impact of lymph node dissection in endometrial carcinoma: a surveillance, epidemiology, and end results analysis. Int J Gynecol Cancer 18:255–261
55. Kilgore LC, Partridge EE, Alvarez RD, Austin JM, Shingleton HM, Noojin F 3rd et al (1995) Adenocarcinoma of the endometrium: survival comparisons of patients with and without pelvic node sampling. Gynecol Oncol 56:29–33
56. Mohan DS, Samuels MA, Selim MA, Shalodi AD, Ellis RJ, Samuels JR et al (1998) Long-term outcomes of therapeutic pelvic lymphadenectomy for stage I endometrial adenocarcinoma. Gynecol Oncol 70:165–171
57. Chan JK, Cheung MK, Huh WK, Osann K, Husain A, Teng NN et al (2006) Therapeutic role of lymph node resection in endometrioid corpus cancer: a study of 12,333 patients. Cancer 107:1823–1830
58. Todo Y, Kato H, Kaneuchi M, Watari H, Takeda M, Sakuragi N (2010) Survival effect of para-aortic lymphadenectomy in endometrial cancer (SEPAL Study): a retrospective cohort analysis. Lancet 375:1165–1172
59. ASTEC Study Group, Kitchener H, Swart AM, Qian Q, Amos C, Parmar MK (2009) Efficacy of systematic pelvic lymphadenectomy in endometrial cancer (MRC ASTEC trial): a randomised study. Lancet 373:125–136
60. Benedetti Panici P, Basile S, Maneschi F, Alberto Lissoni A, Signorelli M, Scambia G et al (2008) Systematic pelvic lymphadenectomy vs no lymphadenectomy in early-stage endometrial carcinoma: randomized clinical trial. J Natl Cancer Inst 100:1707–1716
61. Creasman WT, Morrow CP, Bundy BN, Homesley HD, Graham JE, Heller PG (1987) Surgical pathologic spread patterns of endometrial cancer: a Gynecologic Oncology Group study. Cancer 60:2035–2041
62. Boronow RC, Morrow CP, Creasman WT, Disaia PJ, Silverberg SG, Miller A (1984) Surgical staging in endometrial cancer: clinical–pathologic findings of a prospective study. Obstet Gynecol 63:825–832
63. Morrow CP, Bundy BN, Kurman RJ, Creasman WT, Heller P, Homesley HD (1991) Relationship between surgical pathological risk factors and outcome in clinical stage I and II carcinoma of the endometrium: a Gynecologic Oncology Group study. Gynecol Oncol 40:55–65
64. Chi DS, Barakat RR, Palayekar MJ, Levine DA, Sonoda Y, Alektiar K et al (2008) The incidence of pelvic lymph node metastasis by FIGO staging for patients with adequately surgically staged endometrial adenocarcinoma of endometrioid histology. Int J Gynecol Cancer 18:269–273
65. Mariani A, Dowdy SC, Cliby WA, Gostout BS, Jones MB, Wilson TO et al (2008) Prospective assessment of lymphatic dissemination in endometrial cancer: a paradigm shift in surgical staging. Gynecol Oncol 109:11–18
66. Abu-Rustum NR, Gomez JD, Alektiar KM, Soslow RA, Hensley ML, Leitao MM Jr et al (2009) The incidence of isolated paraaortic nodal metastasis in surgically staged endometrial cancer patients with negative pelvic lymph nodes. Gynecol Oncol 115:236–238
67. May K, Bryant A, Dickinson HO, Kehoe S, Morrison J (2010) Lymphadenectomy for the management of endometrial cancer. Cochrane Database Syst Rev 1:CD7585
68. Cragun JM, Havrilesky LJ, Calingaert B, Synan I, Secord AA, Soper JT et al (2005) Retrospective analysis of selective lymphadenectomy in apparent early-stage endometrial cancer. J Clin Oncol 23:3668–3675
69. Quinlivan JA, Petersen RW, Nicklin JL (2001) Accuracy of frozen section for the operative management of endometrial cancer. BJOG 108:798–803
70. Egle D, Grissemann B, Zeimet AG, Müller-Holzner E, Marth C (2008) Validation of intraoperative risk assessment on frozen section for surgical management of endometrial carcinoma. Gynecol Oncol 110:286–292
71. Seamon LG, Fowler JM, Cohn DE (2010) Lymphadenectomy for endometrial cancer: the controversy. Gynecol Oncol 117:6–8
72. Barranger E, Delpech Y, Coutant C, Dubernard G, Uzan S, Darai E (2009) Laparoscopic sentinel node mapping using combined detection for endometrial cancer: a study of 33 cases—is it a promising technique? Am J Surg 197:1–7
73. Abu-Rustum NR, Khoury-Collado F, Pandit-Taskar N, Soslow RA, Dao F, Sonoda Y et al (2009) Sentinel lymph node mapping for grade 1 endometrial cancer: is it the answer to the surgical staging dilemma? Gynecol Oncol 113:163–169
74. Creutzberg CL, van Putten WL, Koper PC, Lybeert ML, Jobsen JJ, Wárlám-Rodenhuis CC et al (2000) Surgery and postoperative radiotherapy versus surgery alone for patients with stage-1 endometrial carcinoma: multicentre randomised trial. PORTEC Study Group. Post Operative Radiation Therapy in Endometrial Carcinoma. Lancet 355:1404–1411
75. Nout RA, Smit VP, Putter H, Jürgenliemk-Schulz IM, Jobsen JJ, Lutgens LC et al (2010) Vaginal brachytherapy versus pelvic external bean radiotherapy for patients with endometrial cancer of high-intermediate risk (PORTEC-2): an open-label non-inferiority, randomised trial. Lancet 375:816–823
76. Dowdy SC, Aletti G, Cliby WA, Podratz KC, Mariani A (2008) Extra-peritoneal laparoscopic para-aortic lymphadenectomy—a prospective cohort study of 293 patients with endometrial cancer. Gynecol Oncol 111:418–424
77. Gehrig PA, Cantrell LA, Shafer A, Abaid LN, Mendivil A, Boggess JF (2008) What is the optimal minimally invasive surgical procedure for endometrial cancer staging in the obese and morbidly obese woman? Gynecol Oncol 111:41–45

17

Laparoscopic removal of large submucous myomas

Rakesh Sinha · Meenakshi Sundaram · Chaitali Mahajan · Shweta Raje · Pratima Kadam · Gayatri Rao · Rinkita Sinha

Abstract The aim of this study was to analyze the feasibility and technique of removing large submucous myomas laparoscopically. This technique decreases the complications of removing the submucous myoma hysteroscopically. The design was based on a retrospective review (Canadian Task Force Classification II-1) in a dedicated high volume gynecological laparoscopy centre. The subjects were twenty-two women who underwent laparoscopic removal of submucous myomas at our center. Laparoscopic removal of submucous myoma was done in all patients in whom the size of the myoma was more than 5 cm. The results revealed the following: (1) median clinical size of the uterus was 12 weeks (6, 18); (2) median size of the myoma was 7 cm (5, 10); (3) median weight of the specimen was 200 g (60, 460); (4) median total duration of surgery was 75 min (40, 120); (5) median total blood loss was 50 ml (10, 500); and the total morcellation time was 15 min (5, 45). Laparoscopic myomectomy for large submucous myomas is a technically feasible procedure. It can be performed by experienced surgeons irrespective of the size or depth of the myoma. It prevents the complications of hysteroscopic removal of the myoma.

Keywords Myomas · Myomectomy · Submucous myomas · Laparoscopic myomectomy · Hysteroscopic myomectomy

R. Sinha · M. Sundaram · C. Mahajan · S. Raje · P. Kadam · G. Rao · R. Sinha
Bombay Endoscopy Academy and Centre for Minimally Invasive Surgery (BEAMS Hospital),
Mumbai, India

M. Sundaram (✉)
674, 16th Cross Road, Behind Khar Gymkhana,
Khar Pali, Khar (W),
Mumbai 400 052, India
e-mail: drmeena25@yahoo.com

Introduction

Uterine leiomyomas are one of the most common benign smooth muscle tumors in women, with a prevalence of 20–40% in women over the age of 35 years [1]. Submucous myomas are those that most frequently cause menorrhagia and infertility [2]. Hysteroscopic myomectomy is considered the first-line conservative surgical therapy for the management of symptomatic submucous fibroids [3]. Most studies have suggested beneficial effects in treating both menstrual abnormalities and infertility with this procedure. The few studies that have reported on long-term outcomes for fibroid-related menstrual abnormalities indicate that hysteroscopic myomectomy is associated with a 10–35% risk of surgical re-intervention, including repeat myomectomy, open myomectomy or hysterectomy [3]. Uterine bleeding, perforation and fluid overload are major complications which can occur during hysteroscopic myomectomy if not performed by an experienced surgeon. Prolonged surgery can cause fluid overload leading to electrolyte imbalances and its subsequent complications [4]. This can occur especially during hysteroscopic resection of large submucous myomas. To avoid the complications of hysteroscopy, laparoscopic removal of large submucous myomas can be done. In our centre, if the size of the submucous myoma is more than 5 cm on ultrasonography, we prefer to remove them by laparoscopic myomectomy.

Materials and methods

Twenty-two women who had submucous myomas more than 5 cm underwent laparoscopic myomectomy. The mean age was 34 years. Eleven patients were nulliparous, six women had previous normal delivery and the other five had previous caesarean section. The indication for myomectomy was menorrhagia in all women, two complained of fibroid uterus and one had lump in the abdomen. The clinical size of the uterus varied from 6 weeks to a maximum of 18 weeks. The average maximum diameter of the myoma measured by ultrasonography was 7.5 cm. All patients underwent pelvic ultrasound examination and basic blood investigations. Patients were kept on a liquid diet 2 days before the procedure and a laxative was given 12 h before the surgery to empty the bowel. Antibiotic prophylaxis was given to all patients included in the study. Subcutaneous low-dose heparin and a sequential compression device were also given to all patients for prophylaxis against possible thromboembolic episodes.

Operative procedure

The surgeries are performed under general anesthesia with the patient in modified lithotomy position. A diagnostic hysteroscopy is done in all cases. The submucous myomas are visualised (Figs. 1, 2 and 3). The size and extent of the myoma inside the cavity were assessed. The angle of the myoma with respect to the uterine cavity is assessed. If the myoma has more than 50% intramural extension and the size of the myoma is more than 5 cm, then we proceed to do a laparoscopic myomectomy.

Veress needle is inserted at the Palmer's point. The Palmer's point [5] (a point 3 cm below the left costal margin in the midclavicular line) is a safe zone in all patients other than those with splenomegaly.

After insufflation with carbon dioxide, a 5-mm trocar is inserted blindly in the left upper quadrant above the level of the umbilicus almost close to the Palmer's point. A 10-mm optical port is inserted supraumbilically. This port is inserted under vision through the left lateral port. We used three 5-mm accessory ports; the port placed initially in the left lateral upper quadrant is used as the first accessory port. The second port is placed under vision in the right lateral upper quadrant and the third port is placed in the left lateral lower quadrant.

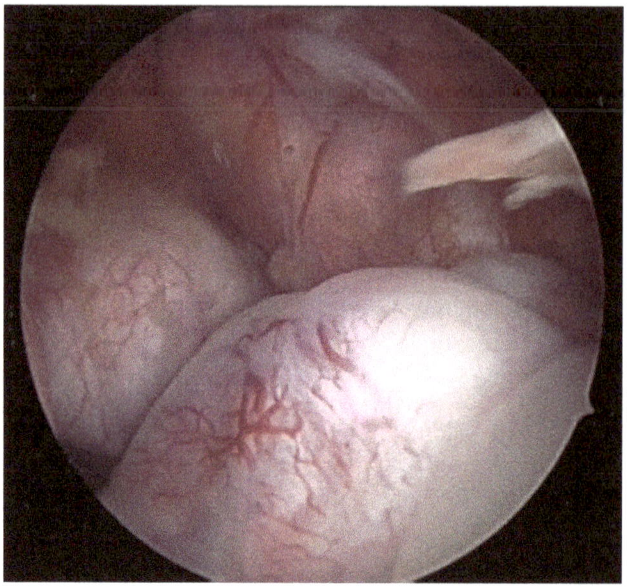

Fig. 2 Multiple submucous myomas on hysteroscopy

At laparoscopy, the uterus is usually uniformly enlarged or shows evidence of fibroid projecting from one of the walls. The adnexa are visualised. A horizontal incision is made on the fundus of the uterus or on the most prominent part of the fibroid (Fig. 4). As the incision is widened and deepened, the submucous fibroid can be visualised. The 5-mm myoma spiral is used to enucleate the myoma. By

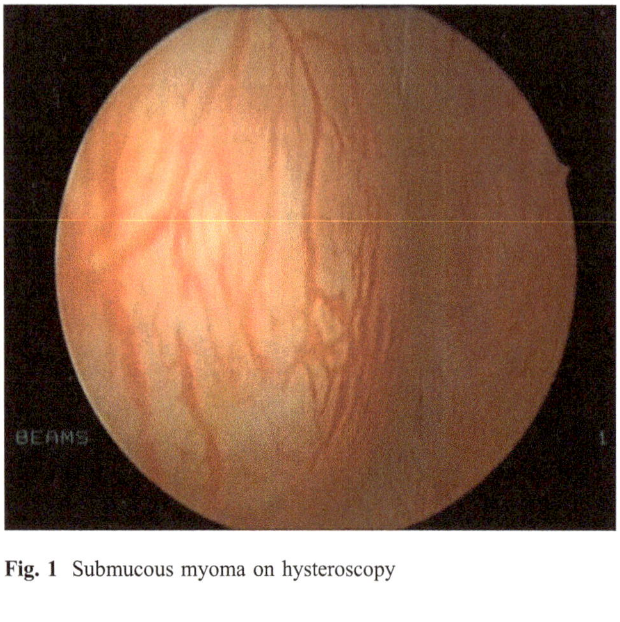

Fig. 1 Submucous myoma on hysteroscopy

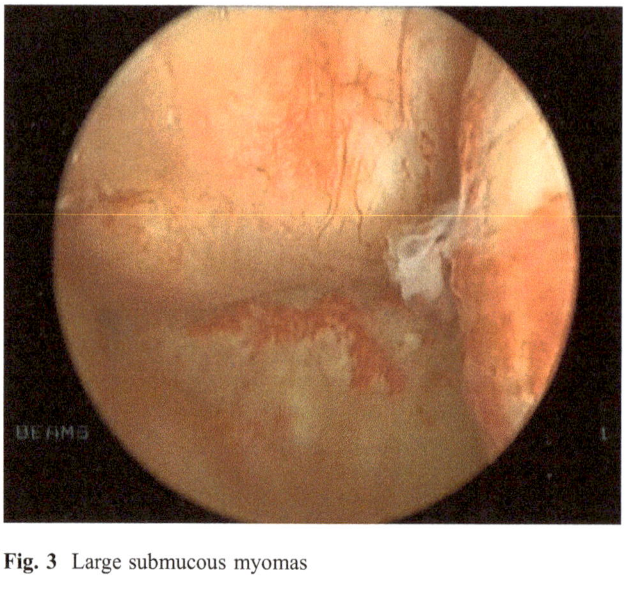

Fig. 3 Large submucous myomas

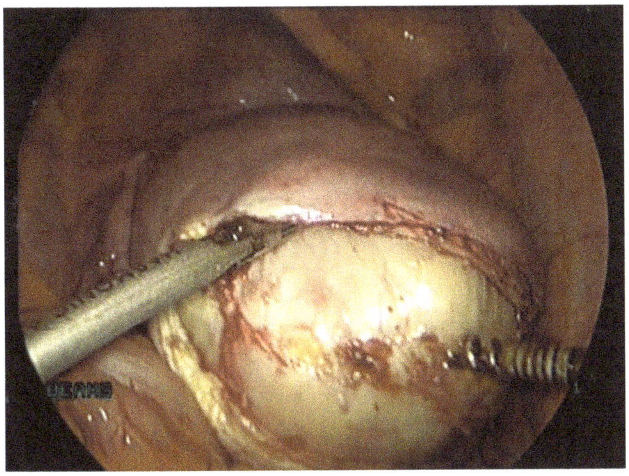

Fig. 4 Horizontal incision on the myoma laparoscopically

gentle traction and countertraction, the myoma is enucleated completely (Fig. 5). Precaution should be taken while enucleating the myoma to prevent damage to the underlying endometrium (Fig. 6). The endometrium is separated from the myoma carefully and reposited in the cavity. Even if the endometrial cavity is opened incidentally (Fig. 7), it is reposited and the myoma bed is sutured. We do not suture the endometrial lining.

The myometrial bed is sutured in two layers: first, mattress to obliterate the dead space and second, figure of eight interrupted sutures (Fig. 8). Adhesion barrier is placed on the suture line. In some patients where the myoma is very large, we also ligate the uterine vessels bilaterally before myomectomy. In such cases, the uterovesical fold of peritoneum is opened initially and the bladder is pushed down. The uterine vessels are identified bilaterally and ligated with no: 1-0 delayed absorbable sutures. Once the uterines are ligated, the myoma gets devascularised and the blood loss during the procedure is considerably reduced [6]. The enucleated

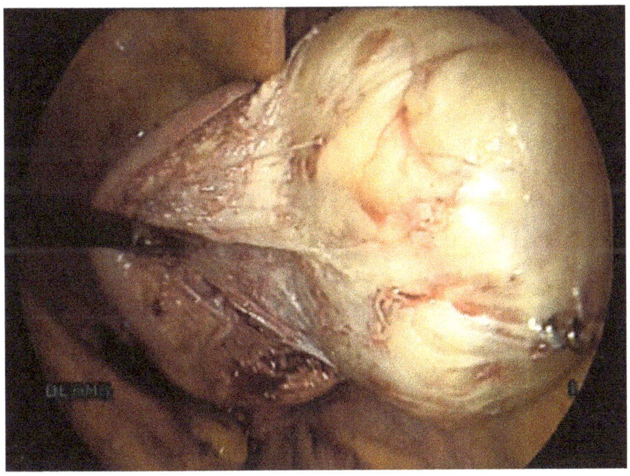

Fig. 5 Enucleation of myoma

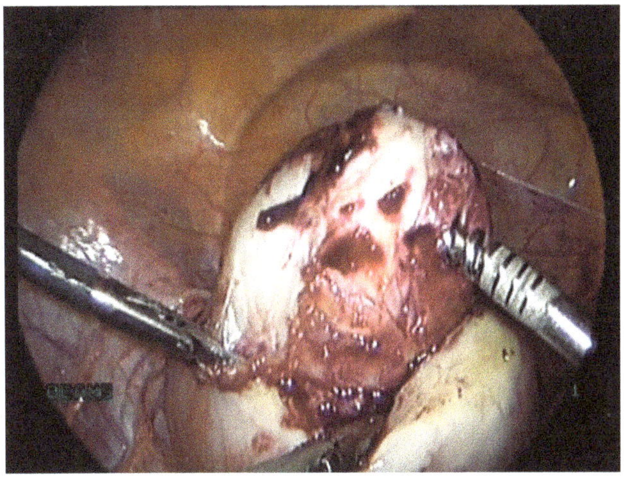

Fig. 6 Enucleation of the submucous myoma preserving the endometrium

myoma is then retrieved by an electromechanical morcellator through a 12-mm port (Figs. 9 and 10).

The total blood loss is calculated. The time taken for surgery from the insertion of Veress to the last skin suture is noted. Skin is sutured with 3-0 delayed absorbable subcuticular sutures. The specimen is sent for histopathological examination. The urinary catheter is removed after 12 h. Patients are started on liquid diet 6 h after the surgery.

Data analysis

Analysis was done using SPSS for Windows, Version 14.0 (SPSS Inc., Chicago, IL). Results are expressed as median (minimum, maximum). All procedures were performed laparoscopically. The following data were obtained: (1) median clinical size of the uterus was 12 weeks (6, 18); (2) the median size of the myoma was 7 cm (5, 10); (3) the

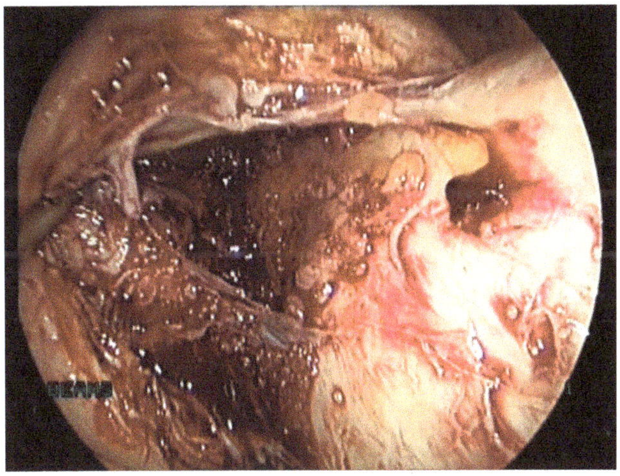

Fig. 7 Opened endometrial cavity during myoma enucleation

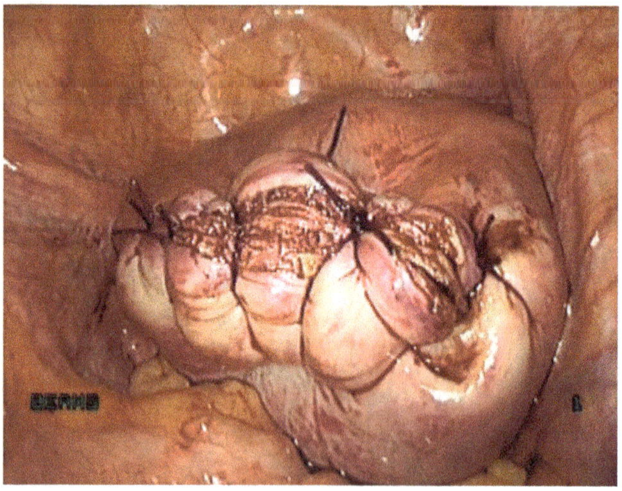

Fig. 8 Sutured myoma bed

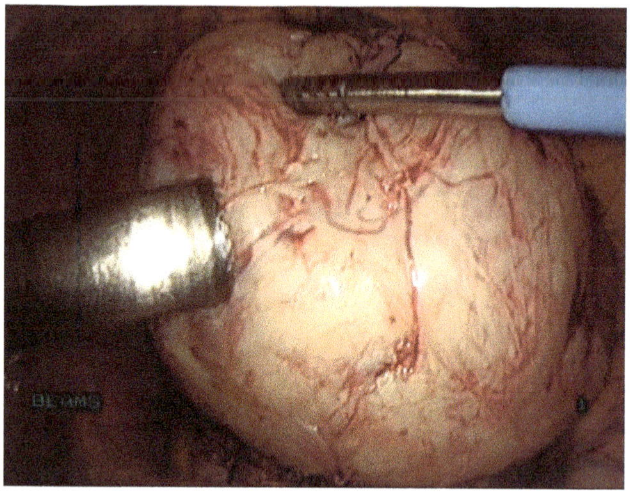

Fig. 10 Myoma retrieved by morcellation

median weight of the specimen was 200 g (60, 460); (4) the median total duration of surgery was 75 min (40, 120); (5) the median total blood loss was 50 ml (10, 500); and (6) the total morcellation time was 15 min (5, 45). Histopathological examination showed leiomyoma in all patients.

The data reveal that there is no complication associated with laparoscopic resection in any of the patients .Even large submucous myomas can be removed with minimal blood loss.

Discussion

Hysteroscopic myomectomy is a therapeutic option for the treatment of submucous fibroids. However, transcervical resection of fibroids with deep intramural extension is performed only in selected patients [7]. A major concern is that complete hysteroscopic resection might result in uterine perforation or fluid overload [4]. As hysteroscopic myomectomy is at times a highly complex procedure, its real feasibility must be evaluated correctly preoperatively in order to minimize the morbidity and mortality that can occur during the procedure.

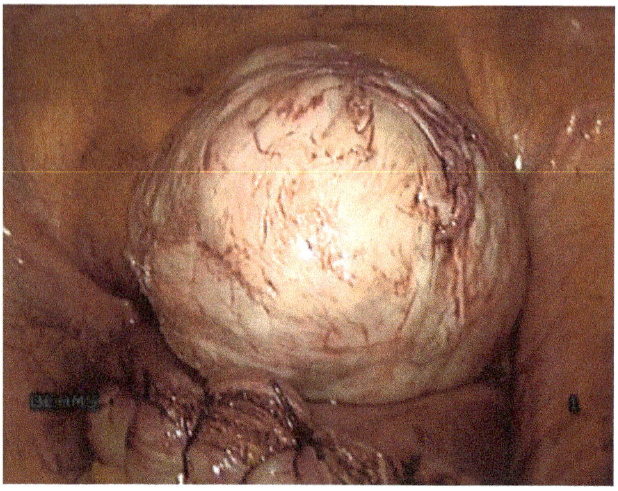

Fig. 9 Submucous myoma removed laparoscopically

Conventionally, hysteroscopic myomectomy is not advisable if the myoma is larger than 5 or 6 cm, if more than 50% of the endometrial surface is affected by myoma size or number, or if the size of the uterine cavity has been limited to that of 16 weeks of gestation [8]. Some authors have described two stage hysteroscopic myomectomy for removal of large submucous fibroids [9]. Myomas with the greatest diameter within the uterine wall have been associated with increased operating time and potential side effects, such as heavy hemorrhage, difficulty to control uterine perforation and water intoxication, and often require a second-stage operation to remove the myoma when the remaining portion of the submucous fibroid has been pushed into the uterine cavity by continuous myometrial contraction [10].

In order to avert the complications of hysteroscopic myomectomy and avoid an incomplete excision, we perform laparoscopic myomectomy for patients with large submucous fibroids more than 5 cm. Laparoscopic approach to remove these fibroids prevented the complications of hysteroscopy, and intraoperative blood loss during laparoscopic removal was minimised by uterine artery ligation.

A study by Wang et al. [11] concluded that, in the presence of a submucous fibroid larger than 4 cm and with an intramural extension greater than 50%, laparoscopic rather than hysteroscopic myomectomy can be performed for the sake of safety and, if needed, for the concomitant removal of fibroids of a nonsubmucous type. However, this particular approach should be performed only by surgeons skilled in laparoscopic suturing.

The concerns of laparoscopic removal of submucous fibroids are mainly: opening the endometrial cavity, healing of suture line, and possibility of subsequent pregnancy and risk of uterine rupture during pregnancy. The events leading to dehiscence are thought to include suboptimal suturing of the uterine incision and/or impaired wound healing from extensive use of coagulation or any tissue-destroying modality [12]. Studies have shown that if the uterine myometrium is well approximated with sutures, there is no increased risk of uterine rupture even if the endometrial cavity was opened.

Seracchioli et al. [13] described laparoscopic myomectomy for deeply penetrating fibroids as a safer option. They described that the risk factors for uterine rupture in subsequent pregnancy include failure to adequately approximate the myometrium, using the wrong suture, electrically caused necrosis and surgeon's inexperience. They avoided the extensive use of thermal energy for haemostasis because it might lead to poor vascularisation and tissue necrosis with an increased risk of uterine rupture and fistula formation.

Conclusion

We believe that for the experienced laparoscopic surgeon skilled in endoscopic suturing, achieving good uterine closure is possible even in difficult conditions. Hence, laparoscopic myomectomy is a better treatment option for patients with submucous fibroids more than 5 cm in size and if the intrauterine extension is more than 50%. The major advantage is that the procedure prevents the risk of hysteroscopy complications.

Declaration of interest The authors report no conflicts of interest. The authors alone are responsible for the content and writing of the paper.

References

1. Solomon LA, MD VL, Schimp DO (2005) Clinical update of smooth muscle tumors of the uterus. J Minim Invasive Gynecol 12:401–408
2. Narayan R, Goswamy RK (1994) Treatment of submucous fibroids and outcome of assisted conception. J Am Assoc Gynecol Laparosc 1(4 Pt 1):307–311
3. Indman PD (2006) Hysteroscopic treatment of submucous myomas. Clin Obstet Gynecol 49(4):811–820
4. Sinha M, Hegde A, Sinha R (2007) Parotid area sign: a clinical test for the diagnosis of fluid overload in hysteroscopic surgery. J Minim Invasive Gynecol 14:161–168
5. Sinha R, Hegde A (2005) Safe entry techniques during laparoscopy. J Minim Invasive Gynecol 12:463–465
6. Sinha R, Sundaram M, Nikam YA et al (2008) Total laparoscopic hysterectomy with earlier uterine artery ligation. J Minim Invasive Gynecology 15(3):355–359
7. Wamsteker K, Emanuel MH, de Kruif JH (1993) Transcervical hysteroscopic resection of submucous fibroids for abnormal uterine bleeding: results regarding the degree of intramural extension. Obstet Gynecol 82:736–740
8. Neuwirth RS (1995) Hysteroscopic submucous myomectomy. Obstet Gynecol Clin North Am 22:541–558
9. Donnez J, Polet R, Smets M, Bassil S, Nisolle M (1995) Hysteroscopic myomectomy. Curr Opin Obstet Gynecol 7:311–316
10. Crosignani PG, Vercellini P, Meschia M, Oldani S, Bramante T (1996) GnRH agonists before surgery for uterine leiomyomas. a review. J Reprod Med 41:415–421
11. Wang CJ, Soong YK, Lee CL (2007) Laparoscopic myomectomy for large intramural and submucous fibroids. Int J Gynecol Obstet 97:206–207
12. Gary N, Frishman MD, Marcus W, Jurema MD (2005) Myomas and myomectomy. J Minim Invasive Gynecol 12:443–456
13. Seracchioli R, Colombo FM, Bagnoli A et al (2003) Laparoscopic myomectomy for fibroids penetrating the uterine cavity: is it a safe procedure? Br J Obstet Gynaecol 110:236–240

Evaluation of immediate laparoscopic surgery for gynecologic disorders

Haruhiko Kanasaki • Aki Oride • Kentaro Nakayama • Kohji Miyazaki

Abstract The purpose of this study was to obtain information to aid in deciding the timing of immediate laparoscopic surgery for gynecological disorders. We evaluated immediate laparoscopic surgery (within 12 h after admission) performed at our institution between January 2005 and March 2010. Of the total 287 laparoscopic surgeries performed for patients with gynecological disorders during this period, 70 (24.4%) were immediate laparoscopic surgeries, 33 (47.1%) of which were for ectopic pregnancy, and 24 (34.3%) for ovarian tumor. Among the 24 surgeries for ovarian tumor, there were almost equal proportions of surgeries for mature cystic teratoma (ten cases, 41.7%) and endometrioma (nine cases, 37.5%). As to the breakdown of immediate surgery by pathology, immediate surgeries were performed in 20.8% of mature cystic teratoma cases and in 12.9% of endometrioma cases during this study period. In the 24 immediate surgeries for ovarian tumor, 10 cases (41.7%) had neither torsion nor rupture, 7 cases (29.2%) had torsion with mature cystic teratoma, serous cystadenoma or follicular cyst, and 7 cases (29.2%) had rupture of the tumor, all of which were endometrioma. Preoperatively, there were no significant differences between torsion and non-torsion cases in serum white blood cell (WBC) count or C-reactive protein (CRP) levels in peripheral blood. However, serum WBC and CRP levels tended to be elevated in cases of rupture with endometrioma. Especially in patients with ovarian tumor, presumed pathology is important in deciding the timing of immediate laparoscopic surgery.

H. Kanasaki (✉) · A. Oride · K. Nakayama · K. Miyazaki
Department of Obstetrics and Gynecology,
Shimane University School of Medicine,
89-1 Enya Cho,
Izumo 693–8501 Shimane Prefecture, Japan
e-mail: kanasaki@med.shimane-u.ac.jp

Keywords Endometrioma · Immediate surgery · Laparoscopy · Ovarian tumor · Ovarian torsion

Background

Laparoscopic surgery has increasingly been applied in recent years to treat a number of gynecological disorders. Compared with laparotomy, laparoscopy has several benefits such as better cosmetic results, a more rapid recovery, shorter hospital stay, less blood loss, and reduced postoperative pain [1, 2]. Thus, physicians either prefer or are required to perform unscheduled laparoscopic surgery (within 12 h after admission) for emergency cases. In such cases for women, ectopic pregnancy and ovarian torsion are the two most common disorders [3, 4]. Due to possible maternal morbidity and occasionally mortality, the timely and appropriate treatment of ectopic pregnancy is important. For ovarian torsion too, diagnosis and treatment in a timely and appropriate manner is important because delay may have grave consequences, such as functional loss of the ovary.

Immediate surgery should be performed to prevent disease progression and to remove symptoms such as abdominal pain. However, as laparoscopic surgery requires sufficient numbers of experienced staff (including physicians, anesthesiologists, nurses and clinical engineers) compared with laparotomy, in rural areas where the total number of doctors has been reducing, immediate laparoscopic surgery, especially at night, imposes a burden on gynecologists and anesthesiologists. Since 2005, laparoscopic surgery has been performed by fixed operators at our institution, Shimane University Hospital. From January 2005 to March 2010, 287 patients underwent laparoscopic surgery for gynecological disorders at the hospital. Among the total laparoscopic surgeries performed, immediate surgeries were retrospectively evaluated to obtain information to help decide the timing of the immediate laparoscopic surgeries.

Methods

A retrospective medical record review was conducted at Shimane University Hospital in Shimane prefecture, Japan. The medical records of all women who underwent laparoscopy for gynecologic disorders at some time between January 1, 2005 and March 31, 2010 (n=287) were reviewed. Only women who underwent laparoscopy within 12 h after admission were assigned to the immediate surgery group (n=70, 24.4%). Medical history was taken by a physician, and all patients gave informed consent for the surgery. A single investigator reviewed each record and abstracted the data.

Due to the limited number of operators for laparoscopy, both laparoscopy and laparotomy have been applied in emergency cases at our hospital. Furthermore, laparotomy is performed if patients do not insist on laparoscopy. The first author (H.K.) participated in all of the immediate laparoscopies reviewed in the present study. Pathologic specimens were also studied by one senior pathologist. In cases where pregnancy-related symptoms were doubtful, urinary hCG levels were checked. Before surgery, all patients underwent physical examination, pelvic examination, and trans-abdominal or trans-vaginal ultrasonography. Blood counts and a blood coagulation test as well as biochemical examination were also evaluated for peripheral blood.

In laparoscopy surgery, after general anesthesia, a 10-mm trocar was inserted just below the umbilicus and insufflated with carbon dioxide at a pressure of 10 mmHg. On direct view, two trocars (12 or 5 mm) were placed through lower abdominal incisions. For management of benign ovarian cyst, after an incision was made on the antimesenteric surface of the cyst, two atraumatic grasping forceps were used to pull the cyst wall and the normal ovarian parenchyma in opposite directions so that the cyst wall could be stripped from the bed of normal ovarian tissue. If the ovary and adnexal lesion were completely distorsioned and showed necrotic change in color, oophorectomy, and adnexectomy using the Ligasure™ vessel sealing system (Coviden, Boulder, CO) was conducted.

Difference in the levels of serum white blood cell (WBC) count and C-reactive protein (CRP) were determined using an unpaired t test. $P<0.05$ was considered statistically significant (student's t test).

Findings

From a total of 287 laparoscopic surgeries performed to treat gynecological disorders at our hospital from January 2005 to March 2010, immediate laparoscopic surgery (within 12 h after admission) was carried out in 70 cases (24.4%). Immediate surgery was chosen principally to eliminate pain or avoid risks associated with delayed surgery.

Of the 70 immediate surgeries performed, 33 (47.1%) were for ectopic pregnancy, 24 (34.3%) for ovarian tumor, 9 (12.9%) for ovarian hemorrhage, 3 (4.3%) for ovarian hyperstimulation syndrome, and in 1 case (1.4%) the patient wanted to undergo laparoscopic tubal ligation within 12 h after vaginal delivery. Among the 33 cases of ectopic pregnancy, rupture of the fallopian tube was noted in 10 cases (41.7%). Laparotomy was routinely performed in patients in shock, but immediate laparoscopy was not performed in cases of ectopic pregnancy with shock. Postoperative pathological findings of the 24 cases of ovarian tumor are shown in Fig. 1. Among these cases, ten (41.7%) had mature cystic teratoma, nine (37.5%) endometrioma, and two (8.3%) serous cystadenoma. Laparoscopic surgery was performed for a total of 172 cases of ovarian tumor in the study period, 70 (40.7%) of which were for endometrioma and 48 (27.9%) for mature cystic teratoma.

Despite there being a larger total number of surgeries for endometrioma than for mature cystic teratoma, there were still a considerable number of immediate surgeries for mature cystic teratoma. The breakdown of immediate surgery by ovarian pathology during the study period is shown in Table 1. Among the 48 cases of mature cystic teratoma, immediate surgery was performed in 10 cases (20.8%), whereas among the 70 cases of endometrioma,

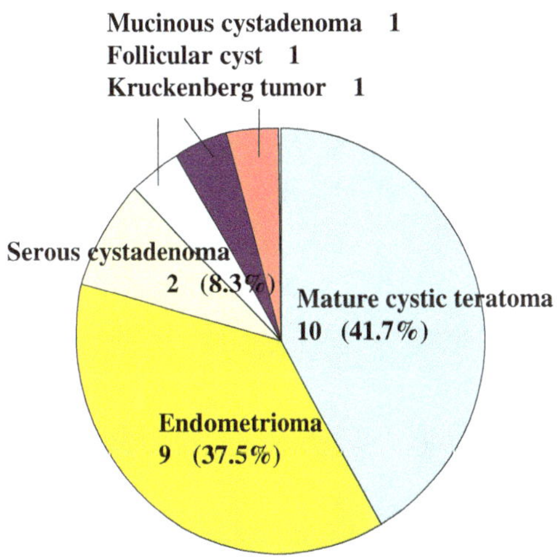

Fig. 1 Pathological findings of the ovary in immediate laparoscopy cases

Table 1 Pathological findings of cases with ovarian tumor and rate of immediate surgery

	Total laparoscopy (n=172)	Immediate laparoscopy (n=24)	%
Mature cystic teratoma	48	10	20.8
Endometrioma	70	9	12.9
Serous cystadenoma	38	2	5.3
Mucinous cystadenoma	9	1	11.1
Others	7	2	28.6

immediate surgery was performed in 9 cases (12.9%). Immediate surgery for mature cystic teratoma was more likely to be performed due to sudden onset of symptoms.

For patients with ovarian tumor, immediate laparoscopic surgery was performed in order to avoid irreversible adnexal damage due to ovarian torsion or eliminate abdominal pain caused by tumor rupture. As for the operative findings for the 24 cases of ovarian tumor, in 10 cases (41.7%), neither torsion nor rupture was observed, and removal of the tumor improved the symptoms. Ovarian torsion was observed in seven cases (29.2%), namely four with mature cystic teratoma, two with serous cystadenoma, and one with follicular cyst. Among these seven cases of ovarian torsion, ovarectomy was performed in two cases. In one case, unilateral adnexa were completely twisted with necrotic changes of the ovary and, in another case, although there were no such necrotic changes, bilateral oophorectomy was performed because the patient was 55 years old. In the remaining five cases, detorsion and cystectomy of the ovarian tumor were performed because the adnexal damage was not irreversible. Furthermore, torsion of endometrioma was not observed. Rupture of ovarian tumor, however, was found in seven cases (29.2%) of endometrioma.

For ovarian tumors, accurate preoperative diagnosis is important in deciding the timing of surgery. To predict irreversible damage due to adnexal torsion, serum WBC and CRP levels in peripheral blood are generally used as markers for necrotic change. To examine the usefulness of these markers in the accurate diagnosis of ovarian torsion, preoperative differences in serum WBC and CRP levels were compared between a torsion group (n=7), in which at least one complete adnexal twist was observed, and a control group (n=8). Here, it is important to note again that torsion of endometrioma was not observed in this study so cases of endometrioma were excluded from the control group. For both serum WBC count and CRP levels, there was no significant difference between the two groups (Fig. 2).

Seven of the nine patients with endometrioma had rupture of endometrioma. Preoperative WBC and CRP levels in these cases are shown in Table 2. Since non-ruptured endometrioma was found only in two cases, we could not statistically compare the laboratory data between a control group and a ruptured group. Generally, serum WBC and CRP levels tended to be elevated in ruptured cases. In some cases, both WBC and CRP were elevated, and in other cases, only one of them was elevated.

Discussion

Immediate laparoscopic surgeries performed for gynecologic disorders at our institution were reviewed in the present study. The first author (H.K.) introduced laparoscopic surgery in the institution from January 2005, and since then, almost 300 surgeries have been performed by the same staff.

Recently, laparoscopic surgery has become the first choice for treating ectopic pregnancy and benign ovarian tumors due to its several benefits such as faster recovery, enhanced visualization, shorter hospital stays [1, 2], and

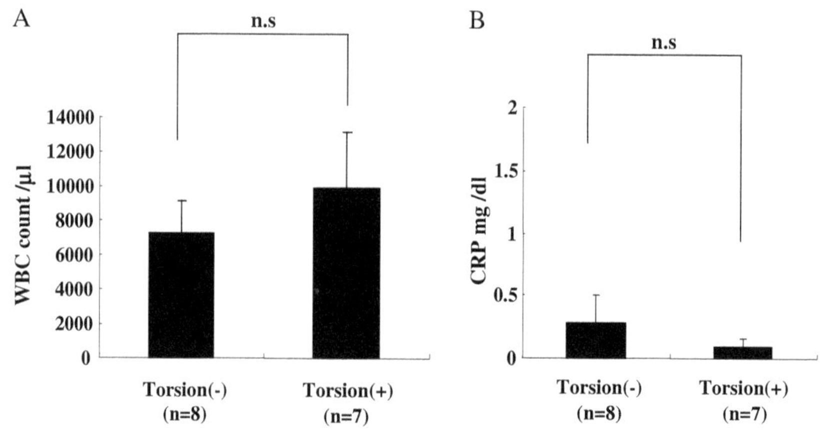

Fig. 2 Preoperative serum WBC (**a**) and CRP levels (**b**) in patients with ovarian torsion

Table 2 Preoperative serum WBC and CRP levels in the patients with endometrioma

	Patient age (years)	WBC (ml)	CRP (mg/dl)
Ruptured cases (n=7)	40	5970	4.0
	22	11230	0.2
	24	17420	–
	28	11610	10.31
	27	6620	9.06
	27	24700	0.9
	32	8420	3.72
Unruptured cases (n=2)	22	6100	0.2
	27	6850	0.07

less potential for adhesion formation [5]. In addition, single incision laparoscopic surgery and natural orifice translumenal endoscopic surgery have attracted widespread attention for the cosmetic benefits they afford [6, 7]. Given these benefits and the popularization of laparoscopic surgery, we gynecologists need to decide whether to perform a laparoscopy or laparotomy when faced with patients who present with acute abdomen or patients who require unscheduled laparoscopic surgery.

It is generally agreed that laparoscopy requires special techniques and operators need special, time-consuming training. Therefore, not all gynecologists can perform laparoscopic surgery for patients who require emergency treatment. In addition, a number of devices such as monitors, forceps, and camera monitors should be prepared, and understanding and cooperation between anesthesiologists and other surgical staff are necessary, especially when working overtime. This review of our cases of unscheduled (immediate) laparoscopic surgery was designed to create a guide to help physicians decide the timing of immediate laparoscopy.

Among the immediate laparoscopies evaluated, almost half of them were performed for patients with ectopic pregnancy. Although higher persistent trophoblast rates with laparoscopic surgery have been reported by other studies [5, 8], laparoscopic surgery is generally favored because of its benefits such as less blood loss and lower costs. Banz et al. concluded that laparoscopic salpingostomy, which was performed for 84.9% of a total of 473 women with ectopic pregnancy during their 9-year study period, was a safe and effective treatment [3]. In the present study period (January 2005 to March 2010), a similarly high proportion of ectopic pregnancies (94.3%; 33 of 35) were treated successfully with immediate laparoscopy at our institution.

Of the immediate laparoscopies performed overall, 34.3% were for the treatment of ovarian tumor. Through a review of the pathological findings, we noted that immediate laparoscopy was more likely to be carried out in cases of mature cystic teratoma in the ovary than in cases of endometrioma (20.8% and 12.9%, respectively) (Table 1). All patients who underwent immediate surgery presented with signs and symptoms such as pain, vomiting, nausea, and tenderness, from which we suspected torsion or rupture of an ovarian tumor. However, for the 24 cases of immediate laparoscopy for ovarian tumor, 10 (41.7%) had neither torsion nor rupture. In other words, we could have avoided ten immediate surgeries and probably scheduled them with adequate preparation.

Obvious torsion was observed in 7 of the 24 cases of ovarian tumor in the present study. Torsion was noted in mature cystic teratoma, serous cystadenoma, and follicular cyst. There were no cases of torsion of endometrioma. Accurate diagnosis of ovarian torsion is difficult, and previous studies have demonstrated a low rate of accurate preoperative prediction [4, 9]. Signs of necrotic change indicated by elevated WBC and CRP levels are uncommon for ovarian torsion [10]. There were no significant differences in the serum levels of WBC and CRP between torsion cases and non-torsion cases in the present study (Fig. 2). As serum markers are not reliable enough to diagnose ovarian torsion accurately, sonographic findings of ovarian tumor (e.g., appearance of cystic, solid or complex mass, adnexal location that is cranial to the uterine fundus, thickening of adnexal wall, unilateral ovarian enlargement with multiple peripherally located follicles, and cystic hemorrhage) would be more useful as a predictor and to decide upon immediate surgery for ovarian torsion [11]. Doppler studies are also a promising tool for the diagnosis of ovarian torsion [12].

Rupture of ovarian tumor was found in seven cases, all of which were endometrioma. Prediction of ovarian tumor rupture is not an easy matter unless the tumor diameter has diminished or it is detected in the fluid of the pelvic cavity by diagnostic imaging. Although we did not statistically analyze serum WBC and CRP levels in the patients with ruptured endometrioma due to the low number of cases, the levels tended to be elevated. Endometrioma is relatively diagnosed by transvaginal ultrasound scan with its characteristic feature of homogeneous low level echoes in a cystic mass [13]. Thus, we need to suspect tumor rupture in cases of pelvic pain and endometrioma when serum WBC and CRP levels are elevated. Ovarian endometrioma is often accompanied by endometriosis in the pelvic cavity which forms adhesions. Pelvic adhesion may restrict mobility of the uterine adnexal region which can result in rupture but not torsion.

Conclusion

In this study, we reviewed immediate laparoscopic surgeries performed to treat gynecologic disorders at our institution.

Immediate surgery was principally performed in cases of ectopic pregnancy, which accounted for almost half of the cases (46.5%). Immediate laparoscopies for ovarian tumor were the next most frequent immediate surgeries performed. In the cases of ovarian tumor where immediate laparoscopy was selected based on clinical symptoms, no evidence of ovarian torsion or rupture was observed in 41.1%. Ovarian torsion was observed only in cases that had mature cystic teratoma, serous cystadenoma or follicular cyst. Furthermore, there were no cases of torsion of endometrioma, but there were cases of rupture, all with endometrioma. Serum WBC and CRP levels are not reliable indicators for the diagnosis of ovarian torsion, but they tend to be elevated in rupture of endometrioma. Laparoscopy is generally recognized to have several benefits such as faster recovery, shorter hospital stays, and less potential for adhesion formation. In addition, postoperative pain is light compared to that following laparotomy. Accordingly, laparoscopy is one of the techniques we gynecologists should learn and be sufficiently practiced in. The trends for immediate laparoscopic surgery that we found in our review can help physicians decide whether laparoscopy should be performed immediately, even during the night, or whether it is possible to watch and wait and schedule laparoscopy with adequate preparation.

Declaration of interest The authors report no conflicts of interest. The authors alone are responsible for the content and writing of the paper.

References

1. Mais V, Ajossa S, Piras B, Marongiu D, Guerriero S, Melis GB (1995) Treatment of nonendometriotic benign adnexal cysts: a randomized comparison of laparoscopy and laparotomy. Obstet Gynecol 86:770–774
2. Yuen PM, Yu KM, Yip SK, Lau WC, Rogers MS, Chang A (1997) A randomized prospective study of laparoscopy and laparotomy in the management of benign ovarian masses. Am J Obstet Gynecol 177:109–114
3. Banz C, Chalvatzas N, Kelling K, Beyer D, Hornemann A, Diedrich K, Kavallaris A (2010) Laparoscopic management of ectopic pregnancy during a 9-year period. Fertil Steril 94:2780–2782
4. Bar-On S, Mashiach R, Stockheim D, Soriano D, Goldenberg M, Schiff E, Seidman DS (2010) Emergency laparoscopy for suspected ovarian torsion: are we too hasty to operate? Fertil Steril 93:2012–2015
5. Lundorff P, Hahlin M, Kallfelt B, Thorburn J, Lindblom B (1991) Adhesion formation after laparoscopic surgery in tubal pregnancy: a randomized trial versus laparotomy. Fertil Steril 55:911–915
6. Tacchino R, Greco F, Matera D (2009) Single-incision laparoscopic cholecystectomy: surgery without a visible scar. Surg Endosc 23:896–899
7. Giday SA, Dray X, Magno P, Buscaglia JM, Shin EJ, Surti VC, Assumpcao L, Marohn MR, Ruben D, Zhigalin A, Pipitone LJ, Kantsevoy SV (2010) Infection during natural orifice transluminal endoscopic surgery: a randomized, controlled study in a live porcine model. Gastrointest Endosc 71:812–816
8. Murphy AA, Nager CW, Wujek JJ, Kettel LM, Torp VA, Chin HG (1992) Operative laparoscopy versus laparotomy for the management of ectopic pregnancy: a prospective trial. Fertil Steril 57:1180–1185
9. Daponte A, Pournaras S, Hadjichristodoulou C, Lialios G, Kallitsaris A, Maniatis AN, Messinis IE (2006) Novel serum inflammatory markers in patients with adnexal mass who had surgery for ovarian torsion. Fertil Steril 85:1469–1472
10. Origoni M, Cavoretto P, Conti E, Ferrari A (2009) Isolated tubal torsion in pregnancy. Eur J Obstet Gynecol Reprod Biol 146:116–120
11. Shadinger LL, Andreotti RF, Kurian RL (2008) Preoperative sonographic and clinical characteristics as predictors of ovarian torsion. J Ultrasound Med 27:7–13
12. Albayram F, Hamper UM (2001) Ovarian and adnexal torsion: spectrum of sonographic findings with pathologic correlation. J Ultrasound Med 20:1083–1089
13. Shwayder JM (2008) Pelvic pain, adnexal masses, and ultrasound. Semin Reprod Med 26:252–265

19

Abdominal cerclage after failed transvaginal cervical cerclage

Anwar Moria · Nouf Aljaji · Louise Miner · Togas Tulandi

Abstract This study aimed to evaluate the efficacy of abdominal cerclage by laparotomy and by laparoscopy among women who had failed transvaginal cerclage. We evaluated all women with cervical insufficiency that underwent abdominal cerclage between the years 2000 and 2010. Of a total of 20 patients, 12 patients underwent abdominal cerclage by laparoscopy and 8 others by laparotomy. The procedure was done in the pregnant state in four patients in the laparoscopy group and in all patients in the laparotomy group. There was no significant difference in the operative time between the laparoscopy and the laparotomy group. The median duration of hospitalization in the laparoscopy group was 6 h and in the laparotomy group was 96 h. Of 18 pregnancies, 16 resulted in a live birth (88.9%). Abdominal cerclage in women who have failed a transvaginal cervical cerclage is associated with a high live birth rate.

Keywords Cervical incompetence · Cervical insufficiency · Cervical cerclage · Abdominal cerclage · Cervicoisthmic cerclage

Background

Cervical cerclage has been used to prevent preterm birth in high-risk women with cervical insufficiency, with a short and/or dilated cervix, and in those with a high risk of preterm delivery. It is usually applied through the vagina after confirmation of fetal viability. Abdominal cervical cerclage was first described in 1965 [1]. This approach is different from the traditional vaginal McDonald [2] or Shirodkar [3] cerclage. The cerclage is placed at the cervicoisthmic junction through an abdominal approach after reflecting the bladder away. The advantages of abdominal cerclage include more proximal placement of the suture providing a better support for the pregnancy, decreased risk of suture migration, absence of a foreign body in the vagina that could promote infection, and the ability to leave the suture in situ for future pregnancies. In a review, Zaveri et al. concluded that women with a failed transvaginal cervical cerclage in a previous pregnancy had a lower risk of perinatal death or delivery of less than 24 weeks if an abdominal cerclage was placed instead of repeat transvaginal cerclage [4]. The purpose of our study was to evaluate the efficacy of abdominal cerclage by laparotomy and by laparoscopy among women with cervical insufficiency who had failed transvaginal cervical cerclage.

Materials and methods

We evaluated the charts of all women who underwent abdominal cervical cerclage from the year 2000 to 2010 at the Sir Mortimer B. Davis, Jewish General Hospital. The indication of abdominal cerclage was at least one failed transvaginal cervical cerclage. Information was retrieved from the hospital's medical file and crosschecked with the clinic charts. Cases of emergency transvaginal cervical cerclage were excluded. The research ethics office of the hospital approved the study.

A. Moria · N. Aljaji · L. Miner · T. Tulandi
Department of Obstetrics and Gynecology, McGill University, Montreal, QC, Canada

T. Tulandi (✉)
687 Pine Ave. West,
Montreal, Quebec H3A 1A1, Canada
e-mail: togas.tulandi@mcgill.ca

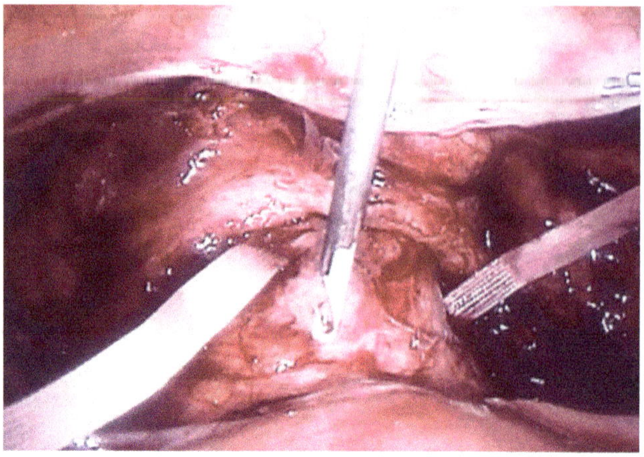

Fig. 1 The Mersilene tape has been placed surrounding the cervix. Note the opening at the tip of the suturing device

Between the years 2000 and 2004, abdominal cerclage was conducted by laparotomy around 12 weeks of gestation after confirmation of fetal heart activity and was performed by the patient's treating obstetrician. As of 2005, all abdominal cerclage was performed by the senior author (TT) through laparoscopy. In both techniques, we started by dissecting the bladder peritoneum off the cervix and we used 5-mm Mersilene tape (Ethicon Inc., Peterborough, Ontario, Canada) for the cerclage. In the laparotomy technique, the suture was inserted through the avascular area of the paracervical tissue medial to the uterine vessels and at the level of the uterine isthmus.

The laparoscopic abdominal cerclage was performed as we previously described [5]. In short, we used a disposable EndoClose suturing device (Tyco Health Care, Gasport, UK) piercing the body of the cervix medial to the uterine vessels without dissecting the ureter and the vessels. The tapered end of the tape was inserted into the distal opening of the device and retracted anteriorly. The procedure was repeated on the opposite site and the knot was tied anteriorly (Figs. 1 and 2). We evaluated operative time, intra- and postoperative complications, the duration of hospitalization, and outcome of pregnancies.

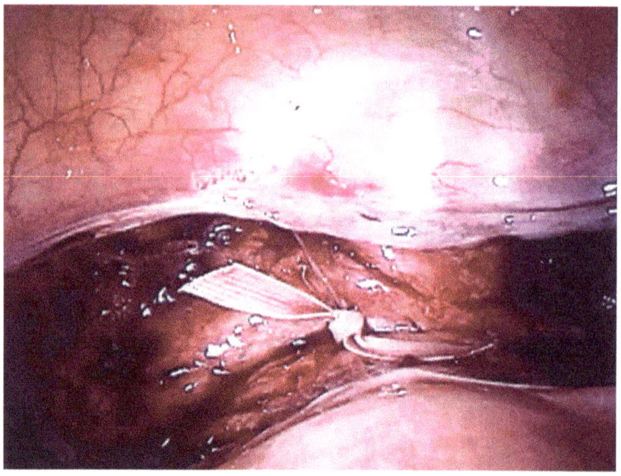

Fig. 2 Completion of the abdominal cerclage with the knot on the anterior wall of the cervix

Table 1 Profiles of 20 women who had failed transvaginal cerclage and subsequently underwent abdominal cervical cerclage

	Laparoscopy	Laparotomy
Number	12	8
Age (years)	34.4±1.3	34.2±0.8
BMI	24.9±1.6	23.3±2.4
Operative time (min)	64.2±6.1	66.1±10.0

BMI body mass index

Statistical analysis

We used Shapiro–Wilk test to evaluate the distribution of the data. Comparisons were analyzed using Student's *t* test or Mann–Whitney *U* test when appropriate. A *P* value of less than 0.05 was considered significant.

Findings

Of a total of 20 patients, 12 patients underwent abdominal cerclage by laparoscopy and 8 others by laparotomy. The procedure was done in the pregnant state in four patients in the laparoscopy group and in all patients in the laparotomy group. The age and body mass index of both groups of patients were comparable (Table 1). We did not encounter any excessive bleeding during surgery in both groups of patients. There was no significant difference in the operative time between the laparoscopy and the laparotomy group. The median duration of hospitalization in the laparoscopy group was 6 h and in the laparotomy

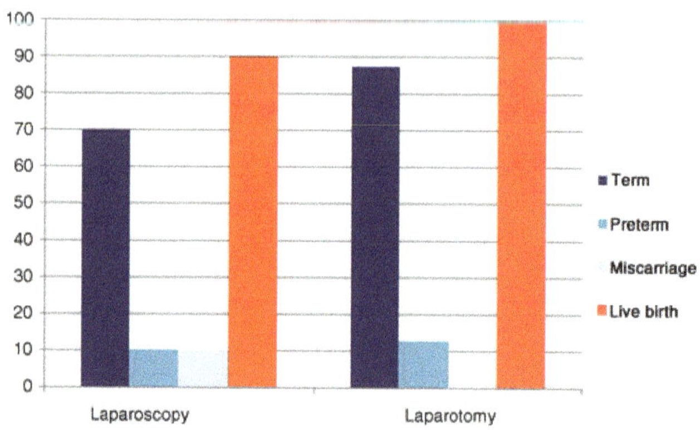

Fig. 3 Pregnancy outcome in 18 pregnancies among women who had failed transvaginal cerclage and subsequently underwent abdominal cervical cerclage

group was 96 h (interquartile range 80–108) ($P<0.0001$; 95% CI, 66–114).

At the time of this writing, two patients in the laparoscopic group who recently underwent the procedure had not conceived and another was lost from follow-up leaving nine evaluable cases for obstetrical outcome. Seven patients had successful term pregnancy; one patient experienced a miscarriage at 14 weeks of gestation. She underwent curettage with the abdominal cerclage in situ, and in the subsequent pregnancy she delivered at 34 gestational weeks. Another patient had severe oligohydramnios at 19 gestational weeks and underwent laparoscopic removal of the cerclage. Of a total of eight patients in the laparotomy group, seven patients had a successful term pregnancy and another had premature delivery at 29 weeks of gestation. Overall, 16 of 18 pregnancies resulted in a live birth (88.9%, Fig. 3).

There was no postoperative complication in the laparoscopy group. In the laparotomy group, one patient had wound infection and another had urinary tract infection in the immediate postoperative period.

Discussion

In our study, abdominal cervical cerclage resulted in 88.9% live birth rate. This is in agreement with a previous study in 2009 [6], where the fetal salvage rate was 89%. They used criteria for a presumptive diagnosis of cervical insufficiency including failed transvaginal cerclage in 58% of cases. Conversion to laparotomy was needed in 10% of cases due to bleeding from the uterine vessels and impaired visibility [6].

In contrast, all of our patients had a history of failed transvaginal cerclage. Further, our laparoscopic technique was slightly different. Instead of using Prolene suture, we used 5-mm Mersilene tape [5]. We also utilized an EndoClose suturing device that was inserted medial to the uterine vessels piercing the cervical body. Unlike the conventional abdominal cerclage, dissection of the vessels and ureter was not needed simplifying the procedure. Indeed, none of the laparoscopic procedures were converted to laparotomy, and bleeding was minimal.

Although there is a clear obstetrical advantage of abdominal cerclage over transvaginal cervical cerclage in high-risk populations, abdominal cerclage has not been popular. This is due to the need for two surgical procedures; the first is to perform the cerclage and the second is for cesarean delivery. In addition, there has been a concern that if a miscarriage or fetal demise was to occur, a hysterotomy would have to be performed. However, today, abdominal cerclage can be performed by laparoscopy. In the case of a miscarriage, curettage can still be done with the cerclage in place. In the case of second trimester loss, the cerclage can be removed by laparoscopy precluding the need for hysterotomy [7].

Previous reports and ours demonstrated that one could perform abdominal cerclage before pregnancy. Indeed, surgery in the non-pregnant state is associated with decreased operative bleeding and no risk of miscarriage or rupture membrane. Moreover, it requires only one surgery in the pregnant state which is the cesarean delivery. Groom et al. in 2003 reported 19 women with preconceptional abdominal cerclage insertion and a fetal survival rate of 100% in women who were able to get pregnant [8]. This is compared favorably with our results in the women who underwent abdominal cerclage in the pregnant state where all of our cases subsequently had a live birth.

The advantages of laparoscopic surgery are well established including minimal blood loss and short hospital stay. All of our laparoscopic cases were discharged around 6 h after the procedure. As expected, the hospital stay was longer in the laparotomy group. Despite the simplicity of laparoscopic technique, we found no difference in the operative time. This could be related to the challenge in threading the tapered Mersilene suture into the opening of the suturing device. We recently found that the use of Carter-Thomason CloseSure system facilitates the procedure. The device can be used to pierce the body of the cervix; its tip can be opened like forceps and could grasp the suture easily.

One of the weaknesses of our study is the small sample size. This could be due to our strict indication of the procedure.

Conclusion

We conclude that abdominal cerclage in women who have failed a transvaginal cervical cerclage is associated with a high live birth rate and it could be performed by laparoscopy.

Conflicts of interest The authors report no conflicts of interest. The authors alone are responsible for the content and writing of the paper.

References

1. Benson RC, Durfee RB (1965) Transabdominal cervico uterine cerclage during pregnancy for the treatment of cervical incompetency. Obstet Gynecol 25:145–155
2. McDonald I (1957) Suture of the cervix for inevitable miscarriage. J Obstet Gynaecol Br Imp 64:346–353
3. Shirodkar V (1955) A new method of operative treatment of habitual abortions in the second trimester of pregnancy. Antiseptic 52:299–300

4. Zaveri V, Aghajafari F, Amankwah K, Hannah M (2002) Abdominal versus vaginal cerclage after a failed transvaginal cerclage: a systematic review. Am J Obstet Gynecol 187:868–872
5. Al-Fadhli R, Tulandi T (2004) Laparoscopic abdominal cerclage. Obstet Gynecol Clin 31:497–504
6. Whittle WL, Singh SS, Allen L, Glaude L, Thomas J, Windrim R, Leyland N (2009) Laparoscopic cervico-isthmic cerclage: surgical technique and obstetric outcomes. Am J Obstet Gynecol 201:364.e1–364.e7
7. Agdi M, Tulandi T (2008) Placement and removal of abdominal cerclage by laparoscopy. Reprod Biomed Online 16:308–310
8. Groom KM, Bryony AJ, Edmonds DK, Benett PR (2004) Preconception transabdominal cervicoisthmic cerclage. Am J Obstet Gynecol 191:230–234

20

Increasing experience in laparoscopic staging of early ovarian cancer

Henk W. R. Schreuder · Thyrza O. S. Pattij · Ronald P. Zweemer · Marchien W. van Baal · René H. M. Verheijen

Abstract We assessed the effect of increasing experience of a single surgeon (learning curve) in the laparoscopic staging procedure for women with early ovarian cancer and compared the results with the literature. We retrospectively analysed a total of 25 women with apparent early-stage ovarian cancer who underwent a laparoscopic staging procedure by the same surgeon. Three time periods, based on date of surgery, were compared with respect to operating time, amount of lymph nodes harvested and surgical outcome. There was no significant difference in operation time, estimated blood loss and hospital stay between the three periods. There was, however, a significant increase in the median number of pelvic and para-aortal lymph nodes harvested (group1=6.5, group 2=8.0 and group 3=21.0; $P<0.005$). For the total period, median operation time was 235 min and median estimated blood loss was 100 ml. The median length of hospital stay was 4.0 days. Two intra-operative and two postoperative complications occurred. The upstaging rate was 32%. The mean interval between initial surgery and laparoscopic staging was 51.2 days. Mean duration of follow-up was 43 months, range (1–116 months). Five (20%) patients had recurrences, and two (8%) patients died of the disease. In conclusion, there is a significant learning curve for the laparoscopic full staging procedure in ovarian cancer. In our study this is mainly reflected in the amount of lymph nodes harvested and not in the total operating time.

H. W. R. Schreuder (✉) · T. O. S. Pattij · R. P. Zweemer · R. H. M. Verheijen
Division of Woman and Baby, Department of Surgical and Oncological Gynecology, University Medical Centre Utrecht, P.O. Box 85500, Room F05-126,
3508 GA Utrecht, The Netherlands
e-mail: h.w.r.schreuder@umcutrecht.nl

M. W. van Baal
Department of Obstetrics and Gynaecology, Flevo Hospital, Almere, The Netherlands

Keywords Early ovarian cancer · Laparoscopy · Staging · Learning curve

Background

The risk of an unexpected ovarian malignancy is estimated to be 1% or less in premenopausal women and 3.0% in postmenopausal women [1]. The majority of these adnexal cysts and masses are managed by general gynaecologists, which may lead to inadequate staging of ovarian cancer during the primary operation [2, 3]. As a consequence these patients have two options: (1) second surgery to be optimally staged since optimal staging is an independent prognostic parameter for survival or (2) chemotherapy, since non-optimal staged patients benefit from adjuvant chemotherapy [4]. In patients there are subgroups who have little or nothing to gain from adjuvant chemotherapy and it appears to be safe to withhold adjuvant chemotherapy from patients with early-stage disease who are optimally staged [5].

The traditional procedure for staging ovarian cancer is through laparotomy with a midline incision, exposing the whole peritoneal cavity [6]. Since 1994 several mainly small studies have been published by a limited group of centres on the results of a laparoscopic approach to the staging of early ovarian cancer [7–22]. Laparoscopic staging proves to be accurate and feasible in ovarian cancer patients and has the advantages of minimal invasive surgery. These advantages include less blood loss [8, 17, 18, 21], optical magnification of laparoscopic inspection [12, 14, 17], shorter hospital stay [8, 10–12, 16–18, 21], shorter time interval to adjuvant chemotherapy [10, 17] and faster return of bowel movements [17, 18]. Laparoscopic staging provides similar complication rates as open surgery [8, 16]. Despite studies proving the feasibility, accuracy and safety of laparoscopic staging in early ovarian cancer, laparotomy is still advocated by the majority of centres. One of the reasons for a slow implementation of minimal invasive techniques in complex oncological surgery may be a long learning curve. The learning curve of the laparoscopic staging procedure in ovarian cancer has never been addressed. However Eltabbakh et al. demonstrated clearly a learning curve in the laparoscopic staging procedure for endometrial cancer [23]. Our study primarily focuses on the learning curve of a single surgeon in the laparoscopic staging procedure in women with early ovarian cancer and the surgical outcome of these patients.

Patients and methods

A retrospective chart review was undertaken and identified 25 cases of laparoscopic staging of apparent early-stage ovarian cancer, all operated by the same surgeon (RV) in the period from June 2001 to October 2009. To obtain clinical and pathologic information, we reviewed the patient's medical records. The following information was obtained: age, BMI, surgical procedure, pre- and postoperative FIGO stage, histopathology, days between first operation and staging laparoscopy, operation time, estimated blood loss, number of pelvic and para-aortic nodes, complications, hospital stay, nature of subsequent treatment, delay in chemotherapy, length of follow-up, recurrence and mortality. Postoperative complications were defined as occurring within 30 days after the procedure. Most ovarian carcinomas were diagnosed at final histopathology, after a first operation where a malignancy was not anticipated. After the final pathologic diagnosis, patients were scheduled for a laparoscopic staging procedure. Preoperative investigations after the diagnosis of malignancies included: CA 125 measurement, ultrasound and CT scan. All but two patients were clinically expected to have stage I disease, the other two patients were expected to have stage II disease. All histological types of ovarian cancers were included. Patient characteristics are shown in Table 1.

Table 1 Patient characteristics

Characteristics	Number
Patients	25
Mean age in years (range)	49.7 (18–79)
BMI in kg/m^2 (range)	24.6 (17.4–36.5)
Histological types	
Adenocarcinoma	16
Clear cell	4
Borderline	4
Other	1
FIGO stage (before staging)	
IA	12
IB	1
IC	9
IIC	2
Unknown	1
Tumour grade	
Grade 1	10
Grade 2	7
Grade 3	5
Unknown	3
Procedures at initial surgery	
Cystectomy	3
Adnectomy	11
Bilateral adnectomy	5
Hysterectomy + adnectomy	1
Hysterectomy + bilateral adnectomy	4
No initial surgery	1
Ovarian preservation procedure at secondary surgery	4
Mean age in years (range)	32.3 (18–41)
Histologic type	
Borderline	2
Adenocarcinoma	2

Laparoscopic staging procedure

All patients were operated by the same surgeon, using the same technique. Four trocar ports were used. The first 11-mm trocar was inserted into the umbilical area, one 10-mm trocar above the symphysis, one 10-mm at the left upper quadrant and a 5-mm trocar at the right upper quadrant of the lower abdomen. A thorough exploration of all pelvic and abdominal organs and peritoneal surface was conducted. Cytological washings of the peritoneal cavity were taken, and any suspicious lesion was biopsied next to random biopsies from the diaphragm, left and right paracolic gutter, peritoneal reflection of the bladder and pouch of Douglas. Residual adnexal tissue and/or the residual infundibulo-pelvic ligament on the side of the originally involved ovary was removed. Comprehensive surgical staging further involved transperitoneal lymph node sampling from the pelvic and para-aortic regions up to the left renal vein, followed by an infra- or supracolic omentectomy (using a vessel-sealing technique). A hysterectomy was not routinely performed. The uninvolved ovary, when unsuspicious on visual inspection, was left in situ in fertility-sparing procedures, in which case a wedge biopsy was taken.

Learning curve

To assess the effect of increasing experience, of the surgeon in the laparoscopic staging procedure, the patients were arranged in chronological order based on the date of their staging surgery. The patients were divided in equal groups according to three periods. Group I (n=9) had surgery in 2001–2003, group II (n=8) had surgery in 2004–2006 and group III (n=8) had surgery in 2007–2009. The groups were compared for surgical outcomes: operating time, estimated blood loss, number of lymph nodes harvested, complications and hospital stay.

Literature search

A PubMed search was performed to retrieve all articles concerning laparoscopic staging procedures in women with ovarian cancer between 1980 and January 2010. Search terms used included: 'ovarian cancer', 'early ovarian cancer', 'early-stage ovarian cancer', 'ovarian carcinoma', 'ovarian neoplasm's', 'adnexal tumor', 'fallopian tube neoplasm's', 'fallopian tube cancer', 'laparoscopy', 'laparoscopic surgery', 'staging', 'staging surgery' and 'laparoscopic staging'. The relevant studies we found were compared to our series on the basis of above parameters.

Statistical analysis

To analyse non-continuous variables we used the Kruskal–Wallis test. P values <0.05 were considered significant. Statistic analysis was performed using the statistical software package SPSS 15.0 (SPSS Inc, Chicago, IL).

Findings

A total of 25 patients underwent laparoscopic staging for presumed early-stage ovarian cancer. Most patients (n=24) had a secondary staging (restaging) procedure after referral, one patient was primarily staged. Patient's characteristics are outlined in Table 1. The surgical outcome is outlined in Table 2. The median operation time was 235 min (range 100–285, mean 224). Intraoperative complications were two arterial bleedings. One patient lost 1,000 ml of blood, the other patient 1,500 ml and required a blood transfusion during surgery. No conversion to laparotomy was needed. Postoperative complications were two port site haematomas in different patients, which resolved spontaneously. In 19 patients pelvic lymph nodes were collected (median 8.0, mean 12.2) and in 24 patients' para-aortic lymph nodes were collected (median 6.0, mean 5.8). The median number of total lymph nodes harvested was 8.0 (range 3–31, mean 12.2).

Table 2 Surgical outcome

Variable	
Operation time (min)	235 (100–285)
Estimated blood loss (ml)	100 (10–1,500)
Total LNN[a]	
Pelvic lymph nodes (n=19)	8.0 (3–31)
Para-aortic lymph nodes (n=24)	6.0 (2–12)
Overall (n=24)	8.0 (3–31)
Time between operations (days)	54±21
Upstaging (n)	8 (32%)
Intraoperative complications (n)	2 (8%)
Postoperative complications (n)	2 (8%)
Postoperative hospital stay (days)	4.0 (2–6)
Time to adjuvant chemotherapy (days)	21 (±10.3)
Follow-up (months)	43 (±31.5)

Data are expressed as median (range), mean±standard deviation or number (in percentage)

[a] In those patients where a pelvic and/or para-aortic lymphadenectomy was performed

The operating time and total number of lymph nodes collected are shown in a scatter plot chronologically arranged by date of surgery (Fig. 1). The operating times are widely spread, but the total number of lymph nodes harvested show an increase during time. Based on final pathological assessment, eight patients were upstaged. From presumed stage IA, two patients were upstaged to stage IC, one to stage IIB, one to stage IIC, one to stage IIIA, two patients were upstaged from presumed stage IC to stage IIIC and one patient was upstaged from IIC to stage IIIC. Eleven patients did not need adjuvant chemotherapy; all other patients received adjuvant chemotherapy. These patients all had stage IC or higher or a grade 3 tumour. Mean duration of follow-up was 43 months. Five patients had a recurrence. One mucinous borderline tumour (2001 FIGO stage IC, no lymph node dissection) and four carcinomas recurred. In two patients recurrence appeared as carcinomatous pleuritis or peritonitis. Both these patients were completely staged and had a clear cell carcinoma (2003 FIGO IIC and 2006 FIGO stage IC); they died from the disease. The other patients are all alive without disease.

To demonstrate a possible learning curve over time, the patients were divided into three groups and compared with respect to operating time, estimated blood loss, hospital stay and number of pelvic and para-aortic lymph nodes. Median operating time, estimated blood loss and hospital stay did not show a significant difference between the three groups. But there was a significant increase in the total number of lymph nodes collected (P=0.003, Table 3). Table 4 shows an overview of the original literature

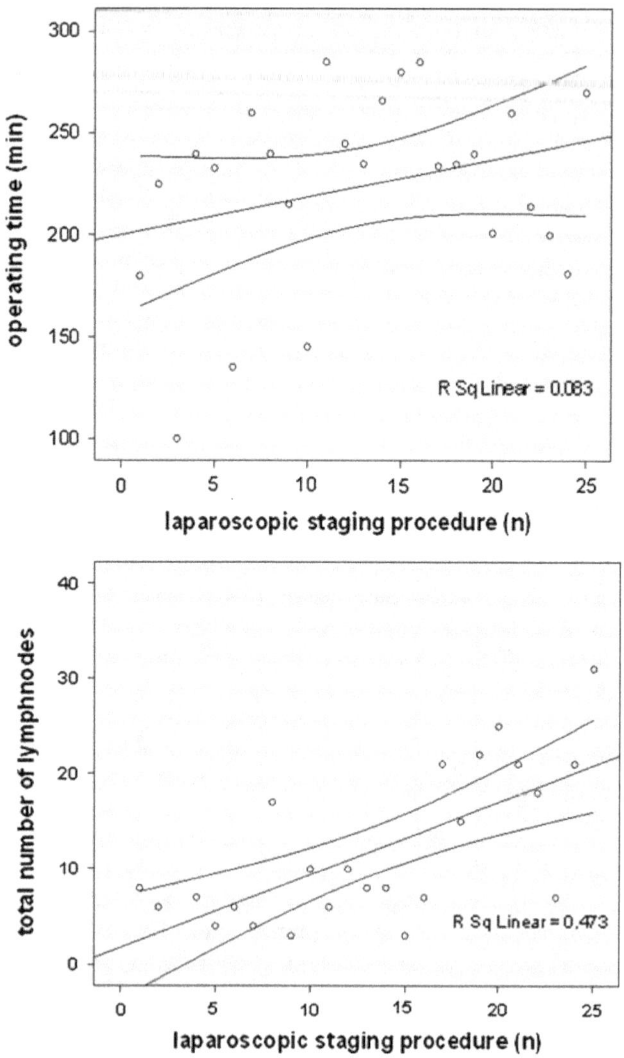

Fig. 1 Operating time and number of lymph nodes. Surgical procedures in chronological order: operating time (n=25) and total number of lymph nodes [pelvic + para-aortal (n=24) (scatter plot)]

regarding the laparoscopic staging procedure in early ovarian cancer. We added the present study in this table.

Discussion

We expected that with increase of the surgeon's experience in performing laparoscopic staging procedures, the effect would be a shorter operating time and a higher number of pelvic and para-aortal lymph nodes harvested. However we did not find a decrease in operating time as a function of the surgeon's experience in laparoscopic staging. This might be due to the relatively limited number of cases. We did find a significant increase in the amount of lymph nodes harvested. The variation in operating time may be due to differences in the extent of surgery performed during laparoscopic staging. In the relatively small group we were unable to correct for these differences. Depending on what is done at initial surgery, the staging procedure for early ovarian cancer should be completed at the second operation (restaging). In our series all patients had an omentectomy, which was usually performed infracolicly. In nine patients a unilateral and in three patients, a bilateral salpingo-oophorectomy was performed, four patients had an ovarian excision (to preserve fertility) and in nine patients, a bilateral salpingo-oophorectomy had already been performed during the initial surgery. In six patients (four carcinomas and two borderline tumours, all before 2004), there was no pelvic lymphadenectomy performed. In the earlier years, less emphasis was laid on the role of pelvic lymphadenectomy and during the years, the guidelines changed. In one patient, with a borderline tumour, a para-aortic lymphadenectomy was not performed. In one patient a hysterectomy was performed, and two patients had an appendectomy because of a mucinous tumour. A laparoscopic procedure including a hysterectomy takes longer. Childers et al. found a mean operating time of 149 min in patients who did not undergo a hysterectomy during their laparoscopic staging, and a mean operating time of 196 min in patients who did undergo a hysterectomy [9]. We do not routinely perform a full hysterectomy in a laparoscopic staging procedure. In view of the lack of evidence that the uterus may be involved when the tumour (seemingly) does not extend beyond the ovaries, it is not justifiable to routinely include such, potentially harmful, operation [24, 25]. However in a case of endometroid ovarian carcinoma, we perform an endometrial curettage. We did not find recurrences in a retained uterus, confirming that it is safe to leave the hysterectomy. Regarding fertility-sparing surgery in early ovarian cancer, several authors reported that it seems to be safe to leave the uterus and the remaining ovary [15]. Despite the fact that we couldn't find a decrease in operating time, it is likely that the increase of lymph nodes harvested demonstrates a learning curve in the laparoscopic management of women with early-stage ovarian carcinoma. This aspect of the learning curve was also found by Eltabbakh et al. In this study, a laparoscopic assisted vaginal hysterectomy with bilateral salpingo-oophorectomy and pelvic lymph node sampling was performed in patients staged for endometrial cancer. Next to a significantly reduced operating time, the authors describe a significant increase in the amount of pelvic lymph nodes harvested with gaining experience [23].

Although there are studies proving laparoscopic staging to be accurate and feasible [8, 10–12, 14, 16–18, 21], many gynaecologic oncologists are still reluctant to adopt laparoscopic staging of ovarian cancer. Apart from inexperience with minimal invasive surgery, reluctance seems mainly based on doubts about the adequacy of the procedure. In particular to the number of lymph nodes obtained, possible risk of port site metastases, lack of tactile

Table 3 Surgical outcome in time periods

	Group I (first period), n=9	Group II (second period), n=8	Group III (third period), n=8	P value
Operative time (min)	225.0 (100–260)	245.0 (145–285)	207.5 (181–270)	0.095
EBL (ml)	50.0 (10–1,000)	50.0 (20–200)	100.0 (20–1,500)	0.682
Total number lymph nodes[a]	6.5 (3–17)	8.0 (3–21)	21.0 (7–31)	0.003
Pelvic[a]	7.5 (1–12)	3.0 (1–13)	13.0 (4–19)	0.023
Para-aortic[a]	5.5 (2–7)	4.0 (2–8)	9.0 (3–12)	0.017
Hospital stay (days)	3.0 (2–5)	4.0 (3–6)	3.5 (3–6)	0.069

Data expressed as medians with range

[a] In those patients where a pelvic and/or para-aortic lymphadenectomy was performed

sensation and risk of intraoperative mass rupture have been questioned [8, 11, 12, 16–18, 22].

Several studies found similar numbers of lymph nodes obtained during laparoscopic and laparotomic staging [11, 21]. The overall number of lymph nodes obtained in our study is lower than in other studies. This could be due to the fact that we describe the learning curve from the first case. In other studies the surgeons are already experienced in the laparoscopic staging procedure and completed their learning curve before the series they describe. This is substantiated by the fact that the mean number of lymph nodes in the last eight patients (group 3) is indeed comparable with other authors. Besides we do not routinely perform a full lymph node dissection, but rather a sampling. In retrospect, the number of lymph nodes harvested in the first periods was too low. Future surgeons can avoid this by learning the procedure from a gynaecologic surgeon who already performed many lymph node dissections. Another concern is the risk of port site metastases due to direct wound contamination or implantation by instruments [17]. Nagarsheth et al. demonstrated that the risk of port site metastases (ranging from 0% to 2.3%) is comparable to the incidence of implantation metastases observed after conventional laparotomy [18, 26]. The risk seems to be higher in patients with recurrent ovarian cancer or primary peritoneal malignancies in the presence of ascites [16, 26]. In our study no port site metastases were seen.

Intraoperative mass rupture in the primary laparoscopic staging procedure of early-stage ovarian cancer is also been thought to be a risk [27]. However in secondary staging procedures, there is no risk of intraoperative mass rupture, since the tumour has already been removed in the first procedure. Intraoperative mass rupture leads to subsequent contamination of the peritoneal cavity with tumour cells and upstages the unexpected ovarian cancer from stage IA to stage IC. Upstaging of the tumour can create the need for adjuvant chemotherapy in patients with potentially curable disease [18]. A multivariate analysis showed that capsular rupture caused by the surgeon did not significantly affect the prognosis in stage I and II ovarian cancer [28]. In contrast to many others, Vergote et al. reported in a larger multivariate analysis that tumour rupture during surgery has a negative effect on prognosis [29]. However, whether or not tumour rupture has a prognostic effect, it should not be considered specific to the laparoscopic procedure. The incidence of iatrogenic rupture of ovarian cancer cysts is similar in the laparoscopy and laparotomy groups [17, 19].

The rate of upstaging (having a higher stage after secondary staging procedure then presumed after the initial operation) found in this study is 32%, percentages found in other studies range between 0% (only nine patients described) [20] and 41.7% [12]. The high percentage of 41.7% found by Jung et al. is not entirely comparable to percentages found in other studies because they included a relatively high percentage of primary staging procedures. Our upstaging percentage is similar to upstaging rates in laparotomic staging ranging from 21.2% [17] to 47% [21].

The mean operation time in our series is comparable to the operating times reported by other authors, ranging from 149 to 377 min [9, 11]. The operating times found in studies with a laparotomy control group range from 218 to 290 min [18, 21]. The operation time for the laparoscopic procedures is generally longer than for a laparotomy. This should however be weighted against the patients' benefit from a less traumatic technique, quicker recovery, shorter hospitalisation and the opportunity to start chemotherapy earlier [10].

In the literature, postoperative stay for laparoscopic staging ranges from 2 to 10.6 days [12, 30]. We found a median of 4.0 days (range 2–6 days). Jung et al. found a mean postoperative stay of 10.6 days, which is substantially longer than in the most other studies. The postoperative stay in the laparotomic control groups ranges 5.8–14.5 days [8, 17].

In our series, four complications occurred. The complication rate for the laparoscopic staging procedure in early-stage ovarian cancer found in the literature ranges from 4.2% [12] to 37.5% [7]. The complication rate in laparoscopy is similar to or even less compared with laparotomy [8, 11].

Conclusion

This study is primarily focused on the effect of increasing experience of a single surgeon ('learning curve') in the

Table 4 Overview of literature for the laparoscopic staging procedure in early-stage ovarian cancer

Laparoscopy	Number	Restaging/primary staging	OR time (min)	Delay (weeks)	Hospital stay (days)	PLN (*n*)	PALN (*n*)	EBL (ml)	Upstaging (*n*, %)	Compl (*n*, %)	Follow-up (months)	R (*n*)	M (*n*)
Present series	25	24/1	224 (100–285)	7.3 (3.1–13.3)	4.0 (2–6)	13.8 (3–31)	5.8 (2–12)	193 (10–1,500)	8 (32%)	4 (16%)	43 (1–116)	5	2
Nezhat et al. [16]	36	9/25	229 (59–386)	NA	2.37 (1–5)	14.84 (0–45)	12.23 (0–53)	195 (25–500)	7 (19.4%)	4 (11.1%)	56	3	0
Muzii et al. [15]	27	27/0	180 (130–300)	6.8 (2–9)	3 (2–7)	NA	NA	200 (100–700)	7 (26%)	1 (3.7%)	20 (7–38)	1	0
Jung et al. [12]	24	5/19	253.7±65.7	NA	10.6±4.0	22.5±8.9	11.0±5.8	567.0±170.9	10 (41.7%)	1 (4.2%)	10 (2–39)	1	1
Park et al. [17]	19	7/12	221±83	19 (7–34)	8.9±6.1	27.2±9.7	6.6±6.2	240±228	4 (21.1%)	2 (10.5%)	17 (2–40)	0	0
Park et al. [18]	17	6 / 11	303.8±84.9	35.8	9.4±4.1	13.7±5.6	8.9±7.1	231.2±117.9	1 (5.9%)	2 (11.8%)	19 (5–56)	2	1
Colomer et al. [10]	20	7/13	223 (180–320)	4.7 (2–11.4)	3.2 (1–7)	18 (14–21)	11.3 (7–23)	NA	4 (20%)	2 (10%)	24.7 (1–61)	1	0
Ghezzi et al. [11]	15	5/10	377±47	8 (5–14)	3 (2–12)	25.2±9.3	6.5±3.9	250 (50–1,000)	4 (26.7%)	2 (6.7%)	16 (4–33)	0	0
Chi et al. [8]	20	13/7	321±64	NA	3.1±0.7	L, 5.8±2.9 R, 6.5±3.9	L, 2.9±1.7 R, 3.8±1.8	235±138	NA	0	NA	NA	NA
Spirtos et al. [21]	58	58/0	187.9±59.8	NA	3.35±5.10	L, 9.0±6.0 R, 9.6±5.2	L, 5.3±3.3 R, 5.0±3.4	171.9±128	8 (13.8%)	11 (19%)	NA	NA	0
Leblanc et al. [14]	53	42/11	238 (120–370)	8.3±4.8	3.1 (1–5)	14 (4–27)	20 (7–40)	NA	8 (19%)	4 (7.5%)	54 (8–116)	5	2
Krivak et al. [30]	19	0/19	201 (90–350)	NA	2 (1–8)	NA	NA	271 (50–1,500)	7 (36%)	4 (16%)	32	NA	NA
Tozzi et al. [22]	24	11/13	176 (102–306)	12 (4–21)	7 (5–12)	19.8 (14–29)	19.6 (5–35)	NA	NA	1 (4.1%)	46 (2–72)	2	0
Leblanc et al. [13]	28	25/3	230±67.5	8.3 (2–26)	3.3 (1–6)	13.7 (4–27)	19.7 (5–40)	NA	6 (21%)	1 (3.7%)	38 (2–89)	1	1
Amara et al. [7]	4	3/1	290 (190–335)	NA	1.75 (1–2)	NA	NA	NA	NA	0	NA	NA	NA
Pomel et al. [19]	10	10/0	313	NA	4.75 (2–8)	7.1 (3–13)	8.8 (6–12)	NA	NA	2 (20%)	NA	NA	NA
Childers et al. [9]	14	5/9	149 (120–240)	NA	1.6 (0–3)	NA	NA	NA	8 (57%)	2 (14.3%)	NA	NA	NA
Querleu and Leblanc [20]	9	9/0	227 (130–360)	NA	2.8 (1–5)	NA	8.6 (5–17)	<300	0%	0	NA	NA	NA
Laparotomy													
Park et al. [17]	33	NA	275±63	13 (9–16)	14.5±5.6	33.9 ±14.5	8.8±8.1	568±451	7 (21.2%)	9 (27.3%)	23 (1–44)	0	0
Park et al. [18]	19	NA	290±121	32	14.1±4.2	19.3±10.1	6.4±3.9	505.3±279.8	6 (31.6%)	7 (36.8%)	14 (5–61)	0	0
Ghezzi et al. [11]	19	NA	272±81	NA	7 (4–14)	25.1±5.8	7±4.5	400 (150–1,000)	6 (31.6%)	8 (42.1%)	60 (32–108)	4	0
Chi et al. [8]	30	NA	276±68	NA	5.8±2.6	L, 7.1±4.3 R, 7.6±3.8	L, 4.8±4.2 R, 4.4±2.8	367±208	NA	2 (7%)	NA	NA	NA
Spirtos et al. [21]	17	NA	218±73	NA	7.31±9.3	L, 8.2±5.0 R, 9.14±9.9	L, 4.6±2.6 R, 4.4±2.7	352.8±415.0	8 (47%)	NA	NA	NA	0

Delay between initial OR and staging, *PLN* pelvic lymph nodes, *PALN* para-aortic lymph nodes, *EBL* estimated blood loss, *Compl* complications, *R* Recurrence, *M* Mortality (depending on what authors describe *NA* not available, – range, ± standard deviation)

laparoscopic staging of women with early ovarian cancer. We demonstrated a significant learning curve for the laparoscopic full staging procedure in early ovarian cancer. In our study the effect of the increased experience of the surgeon is mainly reflected in the increased number of lymph nodes harvested and not by the total operating time. Minimal invasive surgery requires a high level of skill and delicate dissection, and many gynaecologic oncologists have not yet been trained in this procedure. The laparoscopic staging procedure is a complex procedure and should best be learned under direct supervision of a skilled gynaecologic laparoscopic surgeon. If more gynaecologic oncologists would develop their experience with laparoscopic staging, this could have a great impact on applying laparoscopic surgery on a wider scale among women with early-stage ovarian cancer.

Declaration of interest The authors report no conflicts of interest. The authors alone are responsible for the content and writing of the paper.

Reference

1. Muzii L, Angioli R, Zullo M, Panici PB (2005) The unexpected ovarian malignancy found during operative laparoscopy: incidence, management, and implications for prognosis. J Minim Invasive Gynecol 12(1):81–89
2. Engelen MJ, van der Zee AG, de Vries EG, Willemse PH (2006) Debulking surgery for ovarian epithelial cancer performed by a gynaecological oncologist improved survival compared with less specialised surgeons. Cancer Treat Rev 32 (4):320–323
3. Mayer AR, Chambers SK, Graves E, Holm C, Tseng PC, Nelson BE, Schwartz PE (1992) Ovarian cancer staging: does it require a gynecologic oncologist? Gynecol Oncol 47(2):223–227
4. Trimbos JB, Vergote I, Bolis G, Vermorken JB, Mangioni C, Madronal C, Franchi M, Tateo S, Zanetta G, Scarfone G, Giurgea L, Timmers P, Coens C, Pecorelli S (2003) Impact of adjuvant chemotherapy and surgical staging in early-stage ovarian carcinoma: European Organisation for Research and Treatment of Cancer-Adjuvant ChemoTherapy in Ovarian Neoplasm trial. J Natl Cancer Inst 95(2):113–125
5. Winter-Roach BA, Kitchener HC, Dickinson HO (2009) Adjuvant (post-surgery) chemotherapy for early stage epithelial ovarian cancer. Cochrane Database Syst Rev 3:CD004706
6. Benedet JL, Bender H, Jones H III, Ngan HY, Pecorelli S (2000) FIGO staging classifications and clinical practice guidelines in the management of gynecologic cancers. FIGO Committee on Gynecologic Oncology. Int J Gynaecol Obstet 70(2):209–262
7. Amara DP, Nezhat C, Teng NN, Nezhat F, Nezhat C, Rosati M (1996) Operative laparoscopy in the management of ovarian cancer. Surg Laparosc Endosc 6(1):38–45
8. Chi DS, Bu-Rustum NR, Sonoda Y, Ivy J, Rhee E, Moore K, Levine DA, Barakat RR (2005) The safety and efficacy of laparoscopic surgical staging of apparent stage I ovarian and fallopian tube cancers. Am J Obstet Gynecol 192(5):1614–1619
9. Childers JM, Lang J, Surwit EA, Hatch KD (1995) Laparoscopic surgical staging of ovarian cancer. Gynecol Oncol 59(1):25–33
10. Colomer AT, Jimenez AM, Bover Barcelo MI (2008) Laparoscopic treatment and staging of early ovarian cancer. J Minim Invasive Gynecol 15(4):414–419
11. Ghezzi F, Cromi A, Uccella S, Bergamini V, Tomera S, Franchi M, Bolis P (2007) Laparoscopy versus laparotomy for the surgical management of apparent early stage ovarian cancer. Gynecol Oncol 105(2):409–413
12. Jung US, Lee JH, Kyung MS, Choi JS (2009) Feasibility and efficacy of laparoscopic management of ovarian cancer. J Obstet Gynaecol Res 35(1):113–118
13. Leblanc E, Querleu D, Narducci F, Chauvet MP, Chevalier A, Lesoin A, Vennin P, Taieb S (2000) Surgical staging of early invasive epithelial ovarian tumors. Semin Surg Oncol 19(1):36–41
14. Leblanc E, Querleu D, Narducci F, Occelli B, Papageorgiou T, Sonoda Y (2004) Laparoscopic restaging of early stage invasive adnexal tumors: a 10-year experience. Gynecol Oncol 94(3):624–629
15. Muzii L, Palaia I, Sansone M, Calcagno M, Plotti F, Angioli R, Panici PB (2009) Laparoscopic fertility-sparing staging in unexpected early stage ovarian malignancies. Fertil Steril 91 (6):2632–2637
16. Nezhat FR, Ezzati M, Chuang L, Shamshirsaz AA, Rahaman J, Gretz H (2009) Laparoscopic management of early ovarian and fallopian tube cancers: surgical and survival outcome. Am J Obstet Gynecol 200(1):83–86
17. Park JY, Kim DY, Suh DS, Kim JH, Kim YM, Kim YT, Nam JH (2008) Comparison of laparoscopy and laparotomy in surgical staging of early-stage ovarian and fallopian tubal cancer. Ann Surg Oncol 15(7):2012–2019
18. Park JY, Bae J, Lim MC, Lim SY, Seo SS, Kang S, Park SY (2008) Laparoscopic and laparotomic staging in stage I epithelial ovarian cancer: a comparison of feasibility and safety. Int J Gynecol Cancer 18(6):1202–1209
19. Pomel C, Provencher D, Dauplat J, Gauthier P, Le BG, Drouin P, Udet-Lapointe P, Dubuc-Lissoir J (1995) Laparoscopic staging of early ovarian cancer. Gynecol Oncol 58(3):301–306
20. Querleu D, Leblanc E (1994) Laparoscopic infrarenal paraaortic lymph node dissection for restaging of carcinoma of the ovary or fallopian tube. Cancer 73(5):1467–1471
21. Spirtos NM, Eisekop SM, Boike G, Schlaerth JB, Cappellari JO (2005) Laparoscopic staging in patients with incompletely staged cancers of the uterus, ovary, fallopian tube, and primary peritoneum: a Gynecologic Oncology Group (GOG) study. Am J Obstet Gynecol 193(5):1645–1649
22. Tozzi R, Kohler C, Ferrara A, Schneider A (2004) Laparoscopic treatment of early ovarian cancer: surgical and survival outcomes. Gynecol Oncol 93(1):199–203
23. Eltabbakh GH (2000) Effect of surgeon's experience on the surgical outcome of laparoscopic surgery for women with endometrial cancer. Gynecol Oncol 78(1):58–61
24. Schlaerth AC, Chi DS, Poynor EA, Barakat RR, Brown CL (2009) Long-term survival after fertility-sparing surgery for epithelial ovarian cancer. Int J Gynecol Cancer 19(7):1199–1204
25. Zanetta G, Chiari S, Rota S, Bratina G, Maneo A, Torri V, Mangioni C (1997) Conservative surgery for stage I ovarian carcinoma in women of childbearing age. Br J Obstet Gynaecol 104(9):1030–1035

26. Nagarsheth NP, Rahaman J, Cohen CJ, Gretz H, Nezhat F (2004) The incidence of port-site metastases in gynecologic cancers. JSLS 8(2):133–139
27. Tozzi R, Schneider A (2005) Laparoscopic treatment of early ovarian cancer. Curr Opin Obstet Gynecol 17(4):354–358
28. Kodama S, Tanaka K, Tokunaga A, Sudo N, Takahashi T, Matsui K (1997) Multivariate analysis of prognostic factors in patients with ovarian cancer stage I and II. Int J Gynaecol Obstet 56(2):147–153
29. Vergote I, De BJ, Fyles A, Bertelsen K, Einhorn N, Sevelda P, Gore ME, Kaern J, Verrelst H, Sjovall K, Timmerman D, Vandewalle J, Van GM, Trope CG (2001) Prognostic importance of degree of differentiation and cyst rupture in stage I invasive epithelial ovarian carcinoma. Lancet 357(9251):176–182
30. Krivak TC, Elkas JC, Rose GS, Sundborg M, Winter WE, Carlson J, MacKoul PJ (2005) The utility of hand-assisted laparoscopy in ovarian cancer. Gynecol Oncol 96(1):72–76

21

Techniques to reduce shoulder pain after laparoscopic surgery for benign gynaecological disease

Buket Taş · Anders Meller Donatsky · Ismail Gögenur

Abstract Due to the well-known advantages of minimal invasive surgery, the majority of procedures for benign gynaecological diseases are performed by laparoscopy. Although laparoscopic surgery results in improved patient satisfaction, a considerable portion of patients have complaints of post-operative shoulder pain. This review presents an overview of the currently evaluated techniques to reduce shoulder pain after laparoscopic surgery for benign gynaecological disease. According to the Preferred Reporting Items for Systematic Reviews and Meta-Analysis guidelines, a systematic review was conducted using Medline, Embase and Cochrane databases. Randomised clinical trials reporting techniques to reduce shoulder pain after laparoscopic gynaecologic procedures for benign diseases were included. Eighty-eight articles were screened for inclusion. A total of 15 articles were included in the final review. The following studies described the techniques used to reduce shoulder pain: six studies evaluated the effect of local anaesthetics, three studies evaluated the effect of pulmonary recruitment manoeuvre and three studies evaluated the effect of intraperitoneal drainage. The remaining three studies evaluated the effect of saline installation, minilaparoscopy and gasless laparoscopy by using the Laprolift®. Overall, the pulmonary recruitment manoeuvre and intraperitoneal drainage were found to reduce the incidence and severity of shoulder pain (SP). Based on the current evidence, safety and possibility to implement the technique in daily practice, pulmonary recruitment manoeuvre can be recommended to reduce both the incidence and severity of SP.

Keywords Laparoscopy · Gynaecology · Shoulder pain · Gynaecologic surgery

Introduction

Laparoscopic surgery in patients with benign gynaecological diseases has several advantages compared to open surgery such as faster recovery, reduced hospital stay, lower morbidity and better cosmetic results [1–4]. Although laparoscopic surgery results in improved patient satisfaction, a considerable portion of patients have complaints of post-operative shoulder pain (SP). Post-operative SP is hypothesised to be a result of pneumoperitoneum achieved by carbon dioxide insufflation which induces peritoneal stretching, irritation of the diaphragm and phrenic nerve resulting in referred pain to the shoulder [5]. The precise aetiology is not fully known.

The incidence of SP in the first post-operative day is 35 to 61 % [6–8]. The severity ranges from mild to severe, and some patients even have SP for more than 72 h after surgery [9]. While the exact pathogenesis of post-operative SP is not fully understood, different techniques to reduce the incidence and severity of SP after benign gynaecological laparoscopy have been evaluated in the literature.

The aim of this study was to critically appraise the effectiveness of different techniques in reducing post-operative SP after laparoscopic surgery in terms of the incidence and/or severity of SP. If enough high-quality studies were retrieved and if a clinically relevant and statistically significant difference was demonstrated, we aimed to give a recommendation for daily practice.

B. Taş
Erasmus Medical Centre Rotterdam, 's- Gravedijkwal 230,
3015 CE Rotterdam, The Netherlands

A. M. Donatsky · I. Gögenur
Department of Surgery, University Hospital of Copenhagen,
Herlev, Herlev Ringvej 75,
2730 Herlev, Denmark

B. Taş (✉)
Verboomstraat 30,
3082 JN Rotterdam, The Netherlands
e-mail: bukettas@hotmail.com

Methods

Search strategy

On the basis of the Preferred Reporting Items for Systematic Reviews and Meta-Analysis, a systematic review was conducted. The literature search was conducted by a clinical librarian in the Medline, Embase and Cochrane databases. All randomised controlled trials (RCTs) published in the English language were selected for screening based on the following search terms: "shoulder pain" and "gynecologic" and "laparoscopy". No restriction in the year of publication was applied. The exact search terms are demonstrated in the appendix wherein a combination of MeSH terms and free text words was applied.

Study selection

Two independent reviewers selected all relevant articles. First, the authors eliminated independently and simultaneously all duplicates and articles that were not relevant by looking at the titles and/or abstracts. Subsequently, the relevant articles were selected on the basis of reading the full text manuscripts. The eligibility criteria for inclusion were based on study design and outcome measurements. The outcome measurements include incidence of shoulder pain, severity of shoulder pain on any scale and the need for post-operative analgesics. For study design, only RCTs reporting techniques to reduce SP after benign laparoscopic gynaecologic procedures under general anaesthesia were included. For outcome measurements, only studies reporting the incidence and/or the severity of "shoulder pain" or "shoulder tip pain" were included. The severity of shoulder pain could be assessed on any scale.

The two reviewers identified the articles that met the eligibility criteria. The final inclusion of articles was based on reading the full article. If disagreement regarding inclusion occurred, an agreement was reached by discussion. Finally, to identify other relevant RCTs, a manual search was made in the reference lists of the reviewed papers.

Data extraction

The following data were extracted from the included RCTs: year of publication, total number of participants and respective allocation, laparoscopic procedure, intervention type, administration method and location for intraperitoneal solutions, significant and non-significant results on incidence and/or severity of SP measured on any scales at rest/cough/mobilisation and post-operative analgesic consumption. The data extracted are presented in tables for each intervention type.

Results

The search strategy identified 88 articles which were screened for inclusion. Fifteen RCTs were included in the final review. Reasons for exclusion are presented in the flow chart (Fig. 1). Of the included RCTs, six studies evaluated the effect of intraperitoneal local anaesthetics [10–15], three studies evaluated the effect of pulmonary recruitment manoeuvre (PRM) [5, 8, 16] and three studies evaluated the effect of drainage [17–19]. The remaining three studies have been grouped together as "other techniques" and evaluated the effect of intraperitoneal saline installation [20], minilaparoscopy [21] and gasless laparoscopy by using Laprolift® [22]. One of the studies primarily evaluating PRM also had an intervention arm evaluating intraperitoneal saline vs. nothing [15]. The results from this arm have been included in "other techniques".

Due to the heterogeneity of the included studies, it was not possible to convert the outcome measurements into dichotomous data or continuous data in order to demonstrate an overall effect. Therefore, no estimates of treatment effects or meta-analyses are presented in this systematic review. Instead, we preferred to indicate if a significant effect was demonstrated ($p<0.05$). As it would have no direct consequences on the results presented here, we decided making an evaluation of risk of bias for the included studies.

Intraperitoneal local anaesthetics

Six RCTs evaluated the effect of intraperitoneal local anaesthetics [10–15]. The results are presented in Table 1. The administration method, location and type of intraperitoneal local anaesthetics varied between studies (Table 1). The severity of SP was assessed by using the visual analogue scale (VAS) in all studies [10–15]. One study assessed SP at rest using VAS and SP during coughing on a four-point scale [14]. Three studies reported VAS at rest and during coughing/mobilisation [11, 13, 14]. One study assessed VAS at rest [15]. The final two studies did not report the method of the VAS assessment [10, 12]. In one study, the control group received no intraperitoneal solution [13]. In the remaining five studies, the control group received saline solution [10–12, 14, 15]. None of the studies found a significant reduction in the incidence of SP [11–15]. Only two out of six studies found a significant reduction in SP severity [10, 14]. One of these only found a significant reduction of SP severity during coughing in the first post-operative hour [14]. All studies reported post-operative analgesic consumption. A significant decrease in analgesic requirement was found in three out of six studies [10, 11, 14].

Pulmonary recruitment manoeuvre

Three RCTs evaluated the effect of PRM [5, 8, 16]. The results are presented in Table 2. All studies reported both the

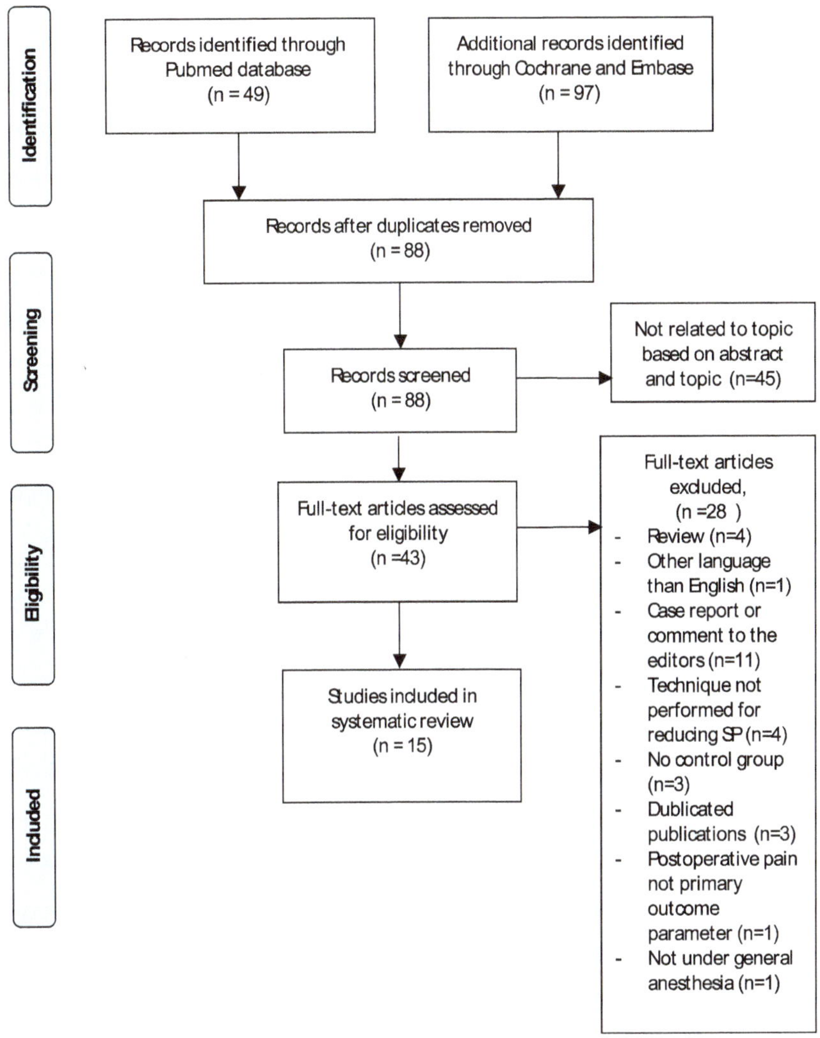

Fig. 1 Flow diagram demonstrating the selection process of included studies

incidence and severity of SP [5, 8, 16]. In all studies, post-operative SP was assessed using VAS and PRM resulted in a significant reduction in the incidence of SP [5, 8, 16]. Two studies also found a significant reduction in the severity of SP [8, 16]. Two studies measured the VAS scores at rest [8, 16], and the last study did not report whether they measured the VAS at rest or during cough/mobilisation [5]. The significant effect of PRM on SP severity was found 4–24 h after surgery and 12 h after discharge [16] and at 24 h post-operatively [8]..

Two out of three studies reported post-operative analgesic consumption [8, 16]. In one of these studies, a significant reduction in post-operative analgesic requirements was found [16].

Drainage

Three RCTs evaluated the effect of drainage [5, 8, 16]. The results are presented in Table 3. Two studies assessed the severity of SP by using VAS [17, 18], and one assessed the severity by a follow-up questionnaire [19]. One study measured the severity of SP both at rest and during coughing [19]. The last two studies did not report whether the measurement was done at rest and/or during coughing/mobilisation [17, 18]. One study reported both the incidence and severity of SP [18] and found a significant reduction in both (severity at 24 h and 48 h post-operatively) [18]. The last two studies reported only the severity of SP and found a significant reduction compared with the control group (12–72 h post-operatively [17] and at 4 and 48 h post-operatively [19]). Two studies reported post-operative analgesic consumption, and both found a significant reduction in the post-operative analgesic requirements [18, 19].

Other techniques

The remaining three RCTs investigated the effect of gasless laparoscopy using Laprolift® [22], minilaparoscopy [21] and intraperitoneal saline [8]. The results are presented in Table 4. None of the studies reported on SP incidence. All studies reported the severity of SP using VAS. The only intervention that reduced the severity of SP was intraperitoneal saline

Table 1 The effect of intraperitoneal local anaesthetics (LA) on the incidence and severity of shoulder pain (SP)

Reference	Publication year	Number	Procedure	Intervention	Control	Administration	Site	Incidence SP	Severity SP	Post-operative analgesics
Benhamou et al. [10]	1994	50, 25/25	Sterilisation	Lidocaine	Saline	Infusion	Right subdiaphragmatic area	N/A	↓	↓
Callesen et al. [11]	1999	80, 40/41	Sterilisation	Ropivacaine	Saline	Infusion	Pelvic cavity	–	–	↓
Johnson et al. [12]	1994	77, 39/38	Sterilisation, laparoscopy	Bupivacaine	Saline	Flushed	Abdominal cavity	N/A	–	–
Kaufman et al. [13]	2008	40, 20/20	Salpingo-oophorectomy, ovarian cystectomy	Ropivacaine	Nothing	Nebulization	Abdominal cavity	–	–	–
Ozer et al. [14]	2005	51, 26/25	Not specified	Bupivacaine	Saline	Subphrenic catheter	Right subdiaphragmatic area	–	↓	↓
Chou et al. [15]	2005	79, 26/27	Not specified	Bupivacaine	Saline	Infusion	Pelvis cavity, subdiaphragmatic area	–	–	–

N/A not available, ↓ significant decrease, – not significant

administration [17]. One of the studies evaluating PRM also evaluated intraperitoneal saline in a separate arm and found a significant reduction in both the incidence and severity of SP [8]. This reduction was also found when intraperitoneal saline was compared to PRM [8].

Discussion

In this systematic review, PRM showed overall promising results in reducing both the incidence and severity of SP after laparoscopic surgery for benign gynaecological disease. Despite this, only one study found reduced post-operative analgesic requirement. Another promising technique was drainage, although this alternative raises concerns regarding complications. The use of intraperitoneal local anaesthetics had limited effect on the incidence and severity of SP. Intraperitoneal saline on the other hand had an effect, but the evidence is limited to two studies.

Several causes of SP after laparoscopic surgery have been reported in the literature, but the leading hypothesis is based on carbon dioxide (CO_2) in the abdominal cavity. It is thought that pneumoperitoneum causes diaphragmatic irritation by overstretching the diaphragmatic muscle fibres resulting in a pain sensation mediated by the phrenic nerve [23]. Jackson et al. investigated the association between the dimension of the gas bubbles in the peritoneal cavity and the severity of pain and found a correlation between the residual gas volume and post-laparoscopic pain [23]. To support the theory of overstretched diaphragmatic muscle fibres, it has also been shown that low insufflation rate reduces post-operative SP [24]. Rapid distension is associated with tearing of blood vessels, traumatic traction of the nerves and release of inflammatory mediators [6] leading to post-operative pain.

Intraperitoneal administration of local anaesthetics has been evaluated for several different laparoscopic procedures [25–29]. It is based on the theory that the instillation of local anaesthetics in the peritoneal cavity blocks the visceral afferent signalling, thereby resulting in reduced nociception [30]. The literature presented in this review does not support the use of local anaesthetics for SP reduction in benign gynaecological laparoscopy. None of the studies could demonstrate a reduction in incidence, and only two out of six studies reported a significant reduction in the severity of SP [10, 14]. Despite this, three out of six studies found a significant reduction of post-operative analgesic consumption [10, 11, 14]. The present evidence does not support a widespread use of intraperitoneal local anaesthetics in benign gynaecological laparoscopy for reduction of SP. Besides a local effect in the peritoneal cavity, the analgesic effect of intraperitoneal local anaesthetics could also be mediated through systemic absorption. There are measurable plasma levels of local anaesthetics shortly after

Table 2 The effect of pulmonary recruitment manoeuvre (PRM) on the incidence and severity of shoulder pain (SP)

Reference	Publication year	Number	Procedure	Intervention	Incidence of SP	Severity of SP	Post-operative analgesics
Phelps et al. [5]	2008	100, 46/54	Elective outpatient gynaecologic surgery	PRM vs. nothing	↓	–	N/A
Sharami et al. [16]	2010	131, 67/64	Minor laparoscopic gynaecologic surgery	PRM vs. nothing	↓	↓	↓
Tsai et al. [8]	2011	104, 53/51	Laparoscopic surgery for benign gynaecologic lesions	PRM vs. nothing	↓	↓	–
Tsai et al. [8]	2011	107, 53/54	Laparoscopic surgery for benign gynaecologic lesions	PRM vs. INSI	↑	↑	–

N/A not available, ↓ significant decrease, ↑ significant increase, – not significant

intraperitoneal administration due to absorption over the peritoneal surface. A potential risk with administration of intraperitoneal local anaesthetics is that the dosage is difficult to control. Although plasma levels of local anaesthetics have been reported to be close to and above safe threshold, no clinical toxicity or adverse effects have thus far been reported [31]. It cannot be ruled out that local anaesthetics can be used to reduce SP after laparoscopic surgery for benign gynaecological disease, but further studies are warranted before a general recommendation can be made.

The most promising data were found in the studies evaluating the effect of PRM. PRM was associated with an overall reduction in both the incidence and the severity of SP [5, 8, 16]. PRM works by removing residual CO_2 from the peritoneal cavity by manually delivering pulmonary inflations with a pressure of between 40 and 60 cmH_20. The positive pressure causes the lungs to expand and the diaphragm to descend, resulting in the evacuation of residual CO_2 from the peritoneal cavity [5, 8, 16]. There is heterogeneity concerning the maximal pressure used during inflation. One study applied a pressure of 60 cmH_20 [5]. Although there are concerns that this ventilation pressure can result in pneumothorax, the authors did not report any cardiovascular or pulmonary complications. Another study applied the PRM technique with a reduced pressure (40 cmH_2O) and also found a significant reduction in the incidence and severity of SP without cardiovascular or pulmonary complications [16]. Thus, it seems that a significant reduction in SP can be achieved with lower pressures, thus minimising the potential risk of complications. One of the studies which applied the PRM technique also compared PRM to intraperitoneal saline. This study arm reported a reduction in both the incidence and severity of SP when saline was compared to PRM. The authors hypothesised that this reduction is due to a longer lasting effect of intraperitoneal saline compared to PRM. A possible explanation of this longer lasting effect is that intraperitoneal saline acts as a buffer system. The CO_2 in the abdominal cavity resolves in the water and becomes carbonic acid. From here, the carbonic acid is transformed to bicarbonate through the red blood cell in the intravascular space. In the lungs, the bicarbonate is again transformed to CO_2 which is exhaled by the patient [8].

Intraperitoneal drainage was also associated with a reduction in both the incidence and severity of SP [17–19]. The application of a drain to reduce SP is based on the assumption that it allows residual CO_2 to be removed from the abdominal cavity. Open and closed suction drainage was associated with a reduction in the severity [17, 18] and incidence of SP [18, 19]. In two of the three RCTs, there was also a reduction in the post-operative analgesic requirements [18, 19]. However, it can be discussed if it is a cost-effective and safe procedure [19]. Although there were no complications reported in any of the studies [17–19], the use of drains can potentially lead to complications such as wound infections, increased abdominal wall pain, decreased pulmonary function, restricted mobilisation and prolonged hospital stay [32]. With the application of PRM, which is also based on removing residual CO_2

Table 3 The effect of drainage on the incidence and severity of shoulder pain (SP)

Reference	Publication year	Number	Procedure	Intervention	Incidence of SP	Severity of SP	Post-operative analgesics
Swift et al. [17]	2002	67, 30/37	Laparoscopic gynaecologic surgery for benign disease	Open drain 4 h post-operatively	N/A	↓	N/A
Abbott et al. [19]	2001	161, 82/79	Diagnostic/minor gynaecologic laparoscopy	Open drain 4 h post-operatively	N/A	↓	↓
Shen et al. [18]	2003	164, 80/84	Laparoscopic assisted vaginal hysterectomy	Closed suction drainage	↓	↓	↓

N/A not available, ↓ significant decrease

Table 4 The effect other interventions on the incidence and severity of shoulder pain (SP)

Reference	Publication year	Number	Procedure	Intervention	Incidence of SP	Severity of SP	Post-operative analgesics
Guido et al. [22]	1998	54, 30/24	Laparoscopic tubal ligation	Gasless laparoscopy with Laprolift®	N/A	–	N/A
Ghezzi et al. [21]	2011	76, 38/38	Hysterectomy	Minilaparoscopic vs. conventional hysterectomy	N/A	–	–
Tsai et al. [8]	2011	106, 54/51	Laparoscopic surgery for benign gynaecologic lesions	Saline instillation	↓	↓	–
Suginami et al. [20]	2009	40, 21/19	Laparoscopic gynaecologic surgery	Saline instillation	N/A	↓	–

N/A not available, ↓ significant decrease, – not significant

from the abdominal cavity, none of these complications exist. In addition, the PRM technique can be performed in a much shorter time duration compared to drainage and allows for faster mobilisation. Thus, it seems that for removing residual CO_2, the PRM technique is favourable compared to drainage with respect to ease of implementation and potential post-operative complications.

Another technique that is also based on removing residual CO_2 from the abdominal cavity is intraperitoneal saline instillation. Intraperitoneal saline instillation is believed to reduce SP by two different mechanisms of action. First, it increases the intraperitoneal pressure which displaces the residual carbon dioxide from the peritoneal cavity. Secondly, it acts as a physiological buffer whereby the residual carbon dioxide is dissolved [8, 20]. Both RCTs evaluating this technique found a significant reduction in the severity of SP, and Tsai et al. also found a significant reduction in the incidence of SP. In this study, they even found that saline instillation was more effective than the PRM technique [8]. In this systematic review, all studies, except one evaluating local anaesthetics, used a placebo group with intraperitoneal saline. The fact that saline does seem to reduce SP could account for the discouraging results found in the studies comparing local anaesthetics vs. saline. In our opinion, future studies evaluating local anaesthetics should primarily compare it to a control group using no instillation. The pain-reducing effect of saline may be due to the buffer system described above as well as to the displacement of trapped CO_2 from the peritoneal cavity at the end of surgery.

Gasless laparoscopy performed with Laprolift® is an alternative surgical technique to conventional laparoscopy with pneumoperitoneum. The technique eliminates the effect of residual CO_2 in the peritoneal cavity completely. Despite this, no reduction in SP severity could be found in this study [22]. The occurrence of SP without pneumoperitoneum indicates that the pathogenesis of SP is complex and multifactorial. This technique is particularly indicated in elderly patients with pulmonary/cardiac comorbidities, where increased abdominal pressure and the use of CO_2 can have potential side effects.

The last study aimed to reduce post-operative pain by minimising the surgical trauma. This study compared the effect of minilaparoscopy vs. conventional laparoscopic hysterectomy and did not report a significant difference in the severity of SP. Keeping in mind the hypnotised pathogeneses for SP, this technique should have a little impact on SP as the only difference between the two techniques is the port sizes (port size of 3 vs. 5 mm) [21].

There are several limitations to this systematic review. Due to the heterogeneity of the included studies, it is difficult to compare them and impossible to perform a meta-analyses. Another limitation is the quality. Outcome parameters were often not clearly defined. Evaluation of sample size and power calculation was not performed in all the included studies. Most RCTs included in this review did not describe in detail how they assessed pain (during rest/coughing/mobilisation) neither did they describe the timing of VAS measurements. Description of the inclusion and exclusion criteria were not well defined or not reported at all. Another point of limitation is that some studies did not report the indication for laparoscopic surgery. Finally, this systematic review used language restriction. Only studies written in English were included. This may introduce language bias and lead to erroneous conclusions.

Several different techniques to reduce SP have been evaluated in the literature. A definite conclusion is difficult based on the retrieved evidence presented. This was due to the heterogeneity of the included studies, the study size and the quality of included studies. Overall the pulmonary recruitment manoeuvre and drainage show promising results in reducing both the incidence and severity of SP. In an era of fast-track surgery with early mobilisation, the routine use of drainage is not recommended and only increases the risk of post-operative complications. Another promising method is intraperitoneal saline, although the evidence is too weak to make any definite conclusions. The results presented in this review do not support the use of intraperitoneal local anaesthetics.

Other hypothesis of reducing peritoneal damage during laparoscopic surgery is to keep the peritoneal surface moist by changing the condition of the gas for pneumoperitoneum. Applying CO_2 at body temperature and humidified condition is close to the homeostatic condition of the peritoneal cavity which is thought to be more physiologic and less damaging to the peritoneal cavity. Future studies need to elucidate this hypothesis [33].

In conclusion, based on the findings in this review, PRM using a pressure of 40 cmH_2O can be recommended as a simple and cost-effective method to reduce SP after laparoscopy for benign gynaecological disease. However, it is not possible to make a definite conclusion concerning the clinical effects and larger well-designed trials are needed to investigate the most appropriate technique.

References

1. Yuen PM, Mak TW, Yim SF, Ngan Kee WD, Lam CW, Rogers MS et al (1998) Metabolic and inflammatory responses after laparoscopic and abdominal hysterectomy. Am J Obstet Gynecol 1:1–5
2. Ferrari MM, Berlanda N, Mezzopane R, Ragusa G, Cavallo M, Pardi G (2000) Identifying the indications for laparoscopically assisted vaginal hysterectomy: a prospective, randomised comparison with abdominal hysterectomy in patients with symptomatic uterine fibroids. BJOG 5:620–625
3. Olsson JH, Ellstrom M, Hahlin M (1996) A randomised prospective trial comparing laparoscopic and abdominal hysterectomy. Br J Obstet Gynaecol 4:345–350
4. Bijen CB, Vermeulen KM, Mourits MJ, de Bock GH (2009) Costs and effects of abdominal versus laparoscopic hysterectomy: systematic review of controlled trials. PLoS One 10:e7340
5. Phelps P, Cakmakkaya OS, Apfel CC, Radke OC (2008) A simple clinical maneuver to reduce laparoscopy-induced shoulder pain: a randomized controlled trial. Obstet Gynecol 1115:1155–1160
6. Alexander JI (1997) Pain after laparoscopy. Br J Anaesth 3:369–378
7. Dobbs FF, Kumar V, Alexander JI, Hull MG (1987) Pain after laparoscopy related to posture and ring versus clip sterilization. Br J Obstet Gynaecol 3:262–266
8. Tsai HW, Chen YJ, Ho CM, Hseu SS, Chao KC, Tsai SK et al (2011) Maneuvers to decrease laparoscopy-induced shoulder and upper abdominal pain: a randomized controlled study. Arch Surg 12:1360–1366
9. Dixon JB, Reuben Y, Halket C, O'Brien PE (2005) Shoulder pain is a common problem following laparoscopic adjustable gastric band surgery. Obes Surg 8:1111–1117
10. Benhamou D, Narchi P, Mazoit JX, Fernandez H (1994) Postoperative pain after local anesthetics for laparoscopic sterilization. Obstet Gynecol 5:877–880
11. Callesen T, Hjort D, Mogensen T, Schouenborg L, Nielsen D, Reventlid H et al (1999) Combined field block and i.p. instillation of ropivacaine for pain management after laparoscopic sterilization. Br J Anaesth 4:586–590
12. Johnson N, Onwude JL, Player J, Hicks N, Yates A, Bryce F et al (1994) Pain after laparoscopy: an observational study and a randomized trial of local anesthetic. J Gynecol Surg 3:129–138
13. Kaufman Y, Hirsch I, Ostrovsky L, Klein O, Shnaider I, Khoury E et al (2008) Pain relief by continuous intraperitoneal nebulization of ropivacaine during gynecologic laparoscopic surgery—a randomized study and review of the literature. J Minim Invasive Gynecol 5:554–558
14. Ozer Y, Tanriverdi HA, Ozkocak I, Altunkaya H, Demirel CB, Bayar U et al (2005) Evaluation of a local anaesthesia regimen using a subphrenic catheter after gynaecological laparoscopy. Eur J Anaesthesiol 6:442–446
15. Chou YJ, Ou YC, Lan KC, Jawan B, Chang SY, Kung FT (2005) Preemptive analgesia installation during gynecologic laparoscopy: a randomized trial. J Minim Invasive Gynecol 4:330–335
16. Sharami SH, Sharami MB, Abdollahzadeh M, Keyvan A (2011) Randomized clinical trial of the influence of pulmonary recruitment maneuver on reducing shoulder pain after laparoscopy. Eur J Pain Suppl 1:36
17. Swift G, Healey M, Varol N, Maher P, Hill D (2002) A prospective randomised double-blind placebo controlled trial to assess whether gas drains reduce shoulder pain following gynaecological laparoscopy. Aust N Z J Obstet Gynaecol 3:267–270
18. Shen CC, Wu MP, Lu CH, Kung FT, Huang FJ, Huang EY et al (2003) Effects of closed suction drainage in reducing pain after laparoscopic-assisted vaginal hysterectomy. J Am Assoc Gynecol Laparosc 2:210–214
19. Abbott J, Hawe J, Srivastava P, Hunter D, Garry R (2001) Intraperitoneal gas drain to reduce pain after laparoscopy: randomized masked trial. Obstet Gynecol 1:97–100
20. Suginami R, Taniguchi F, Suginami H (2009) Prevention of postlaparoscopic shoulder pain by forced evacuation of residual CO(2). JSLS 1:56–59
21. Ghezzi F, Cromi A, Siesto G, Uccella S, Boni L, Serati M et al (2011) Minilaparoscopic versus conventional laparoscopic hysterectomy: results of a randomized trial. J Minim Invasive Gynecol 4:455–461
22. Guido RS, Brooks K, McKenzie R, Gruss J, Krohn MA (1998) A randomized, prospective comparison of pain after gasless laparoscopy and traditional laparoscopy. J Am Assoc Gynecol Laparosc 2:149–153
23. Jackson SA, Laurence AS, Hill JC (1996) Does post-laparoscopy pain relate to residual carbon dioxide? Anaesthesia 5:485–487
24. Berberoglu M, Dilek ON, Ercan F, Kati I, Ozmen M (1998) The effect of CO_2 insufflation rate on the postlaparoscopic shoulder pain. J Laparoendosc Adv Surg Tech A 5:273–277
25. Lepner U, Goroshina J, Samarutel J (2003) Postoperative pain relief after laparoscopic cholecystectomy: a randomised prospective double-blind clinical trial. Scand J Surg 2:121–124
26. Kang H, Kim BG (2010) Intraperitoneal ropivacaine for effective pain relief after laparoscopic appendectomy: a prospective, randomized, double-blind, placebo-controlled study. J Int Med Res 3:821–832
27. Park YH, Kang H, Woo YC, Park SG, Baek CW, Jung YH et al (2011) The effect of intraperitoneal ropivacaine on pain after laparoscopic colectomy: a prospective randomized controlled trial. J Surg Res 1:94–100
28. Sherwinter DA, Ghaznavi AM, Spinner D, Savel RH, Macura JM, Adler H (2008) Continuous infusion of intraperitoneal bupivacaine after laparoscopic surgery: a randomized controlled trial. Obes Surg 12:1581–1586
29. Goldstein A, Grimault P, Henique A, Keller M, Fortin A, Darai E (2000) Preventing postoperative pain by local anesthetic instillation after laparoscopic gynecologic surgery: a placebo-controlled comparison of bupivacaine and ropivacaine. Anesth Analg 2:403–407
30. Kahokehr A, Sammour T, Srinivasa S, Hill AG (2010) Systematic review and meta-analysis of intraperitoneal local anaesthetic for pain reduction after laparoscopic gastric procedures. Br J Surg 1:29–36
31. Kahokehr A, Sammour T, Vather R, Taylor M, Stapelberg F, Hill AG (2010) Systemic levels of local anaesthetic after intra-peritoneal application—a systematic review. Anaesth Intensive Care 4:623–638
32. Uchiyama K, Tani M, Kawai M, Terasawa H, Hama T, Yamaue H (2007) Clinical significance of drainage tube insertion in laparoscopic cholecystectomy: a prospective randomized controlled trial. J Hepatobiliary Pancreat Surg 6:551–556
33. Ott DE (2004) The peritoneum and the pneumoperitoneum: a review to improve clinical outcome. Gynecol Surg 1:101–106

Staff perceptions of the effects of an integrated laparoscopic theatre environment on teamwork

Andreas Stavroulis · Alfred Cutner · Lih-Mei Liao

Abstract Laparoscopic surgery has now replaced traditional open surgery as the preferred method of intervention for many procedures. Although there are advantages of laparoscopic surgery to the patient, the technology puts additional strain on the surgical team. There are three aspects to the theatre environment that need to be considered: staff safety, patient safety and cost efficiency. We have previously published on the effect of the laparoscopic theatre environment on staff safety. To our knowledge, there are no data on the effect of integrated theatres on surgical teamwork. We therefore wished to determine staff perception of the effect that the integrated theatre environment had on their working interactions and behaviour in the operating room. This was a cross-sectional questionnaire survey. Twenty-seven theatre staff (nurses, consultants and trainees) working in a laparoscopic theatre were asked to complete a questionnaire. This included general demographics and their perception regards the theatre environment and team interaction. Visual analogue scores were used to compare the integrated and non-integrated theatres. Non-parametric statistical analysis was used. Overall the theatre team members had a strong preference for working in an integrated theatre environment. They felt that it resulted in greater efficiency, better teamwork and reduced stress levels. Differences were highly significant ($p<0.0001$). This is the first paper ever to look at the impact of the theatre environment on comfort and behaviour of medical and nursing staff involved in carrying out laparoscopic surgery. It is only by assessing these factors and the quality of the operating theatre environment that the true benefits of integrated theatres will be appreciated. This investment not only protects staff and patients but these data suggest that the improved behaviours may further enhance safety and also create greater efficiency resulting in cost savings.

A. Stavroulis (✉) · A. Cutner · L.-M. Liao
University London College Hospitals NHS Foundation Trust, 235 Euston Road, NW1 2BU London, UK
e-mail: stavroulis@btinternet.com

Keywords Staff perceptions · Integrated laparoscopic theatre environment · Teamwork

Background

Laparoscopy was first described by Kelling in 1901 [1]. The introduction of laparoscopic appendectomy in 1983 transformed it from a diagnostic tool to a therapeutic intervention [2]. Further development has seen laparoscopic surgery replacing traditional open surgery as the preferred method of intervention in many clinical situations [3–5]. More recent technological advances have led to improved visualisation and greater precision and accuracy [6].

The avoidance of an abdominal incision is associated with reduced post-operative pain and wound complications and a more acceptable cosmetic result. Early mobilisation has sped up recovery and reduced the length of hospital stay [5, 7, 8] with attendant advantages for cost control [9]. On the other hand, the technology could put additional strain on the surgical team. Open surgery has a high degree of freedom and surgeons work in line with their visual axis. There is a three-dimensional direct vision and direct tactile feedback. There is no need for monitors, accessory equipment like gas insufflators or extra wiring. During laparoscopic surgery, there are two-dimensional vision and a loss of depth perception to some extent as well as a fulcrum effect with tremor enhancement. There are only 4 degrees of freedom and the major limitation is that the view is not the under control of the surgeon. The increased technological complexity and sometimes poorly adapted equipment for the laparoscopic theatre environment have increased the potential risks to the surgical team [10].

The laparoscopic integrated theatre is a superior operating environment in which the laparoscopic equipment and multiple flat-screen monitors are permanently installed to be operational on demand inside the theatre. The equipment is installed in columns attached to a ceiling-mounted suspension system that facilitates versatile positioning away from the monitors. All the wiring is concealed inside the suspension system and led out through the ceiling. The laparoscopic equipment can be remotely controlled by the operating surgeon or by the circulating nurse using a touch panel at a control station. It links together, via an interface, all surgical equipment including the room and camera lights, gas insufflator and diathermy machine.

There are three aspects to the theatre environment that need to be considered: staff safety, patient safety and cost efficiency. We have previously published on the effect of the laparoscopic theatre environment on staff safety [10].

The airline industry has demonstrated that teamwork can have a positive effect on safety outcomes [11]. There is also strong evidence coming from industry and commerce that the physical work environment can affect staff motivation and ability to effectively carry out their jobs [12].

There is increasing interest within the health care sector in the relationships between teamwork and patient safety. The audit commission carried out a review of operating theatres in the UK in 2003 and emphasised the importance of teamwork rather than just individual expertise [13]. The entire team must work in harmony towards a safe and cost-effective system. Integrated operating theatres are expensive to install and the question of the impact of integrated theatres on teamwork and safety is of interest to stakeholders and service users. Such an assessment would inevitably be complex and require ongoing research. One way to begin a line of inquiry in the topic is to evaluate staff perceptions of the effect that the integrated theatre environment had on interactions and behaviour in the operating room. This was the focus of our pilot study.

Methods

This is a cross-sectional survey, in which an opportunistic sample of theatre staff of different disciplines at a tertiary referral hospital completed a brief questionnaire that asked about their experience of integrated and non-integrated operating theatres. The inclusion criteria were work experiences in both types of theatres. The study sample comprised nine theatre nurses, nine consultants and nine trainees.

Table 1 Demographics

	Median age (IQR)	Males (%)
Nurses	41 (34, 48.5)	44.4
Trainees	38 (32.5, 39.5)	77.8
Consultants	44 (42, 50)	66.7

Table 2 Preference for working in an integrated theatre

	Integrated theatre, median (IQR) for all three groups together	Non-integrated theatre, median (IQR) for all three groups together
Satisfaction/preference overall	9 (9, 10)	4 (3, 6)
Overall efficiency/theatre efficiency	9 (8, 10)	5 (3, 6)
Positive theatre team behaviour/ teamwork	9 (7, 10)	5 (5, 7)
Stress level	2 (1, 2)	7 (6, 8)

The questionnaire included demographic information: age, gender, years of theatre work experience, years and current percentage of work in an integrated theatre, level of laparoscopic surgery (minor, intermediate and advance) and level of assistance (main surgeon or assistant).

The participants were asked to rate on a number of items from 1 (poor) to 10 (excellent). The nurses were asked questions to compare their experience in working in an integrated versus non-integrated theatre. These included their everyday tasks as well their interaction with the medical team, their perception of teamwork, stress and overall satisfaction.

The consultants were asked to compare their experience in both theatre settings. The questions were addressing their attitude towards the rest of the team members, their stress, their satisfaction as well as their overall performance and efficiency.

For the trainees, in addition to the above, they were asked to comment on the support and therefore the training they had in the two theatre settings.

Statistical methods (data analysis)

The main perception questions that the participants were asked consisted of responses that ranged from 1 (poor) to 10 (excellent) satisfaction levels. The numerical ratings were treated as interval data. Pairwise comparisons were made for each group's responses between integrated and not integrated theatre with the use of the non-parametric Wilcoxon-Sign test.

Table 3 Nurses' answers

	p value	Integrated theatre, median (IQR)	Non-integrated theatre, median (IQR)
Efficiency at start of day	0.018	10 (8, 10)	6 (3. 5,7)
Efficiency at end of day	0.018	9 (8, 10)	6 (4, 7)
Interaction with medics	0.017	9 (8, 10)	6 (5, 8.5)
Interaction with nurses	0.017	10 (8.5, 10)	7 (6, 9)

Table 4 Trainees' answers

	p value	Integrated theatre, median (IQR)	Non-integrated theatre, median (IQR)
Positive scrub nurse behaviour	0.020	8 (5.5, 9.5)	5 (4.5, 5.5)
Positive circulating staff behaviour	0.018	8 (7, 9)	5 (4, 6)
Positive consultant behaviour	0.049	8 (7.5, 9.5)	5 (3.5, 8.5)
Ability to perform tasks well	0.008	9 (8, 9.5)	6 (3, 7)

A non-parametric test was chosen over a parametric one due to the very small number of participants, i.e. nine pairs for each group. Due to this same reason, medians and IQRs (interquartile ranges) were used to summarise the data. Percentages were used for categorical variables. For those questions that were applicable to all three groups the responses for all 27 subjects were combined. Within group differences for these variables were also checked for significance.

Findings

The demographic characteristics of the staff are shown in Table 1. The complexity of laparoscopic surgery that the consultants were involved in were graded by them as minor (10 %), moderate (20 %) and major (70 %).

Overall the theatre team members indicated an overriding preference for working in an integrated theatre environment. They reported that it had resulted in greater efficiency, better teamwork and reduced stress levels. The median values and interquartile ranges are shown in Table 2. Differences were highly significant ($p<0.0001$). Within group differences were also significant for each of these variables.

The nurses were also asked about efficiency at the start and the end of each working day as this reflects the effort required to prepare and shut down the theatre environment when it is to be used for laparoscopic surgery. Interactions with medical and nursing staff in both theatre environments were also assessed. Results are shown in Table 3. All differences were significant.

The trainees were asked additional questions regarding the behaviour of specific team members in both of the theatre environments and regarding their ability to perform their own tasks adequately. All their responses were significantly in favour of the integrated theatre (Table 4).

The consultants felt that behaviour and performance was enhanced by the integrated theatre (Table 5). The only variable on which there was no significant difference was consultants' impression of the degree of helpfulness of the person manipulating the lower end during the operation.

Table 5 Consultants' answers

	p value	Integrated theatre, median (IQR)	Non-integrated theatre, median (IQR)
Positive scrub nurse behaviour	0.011	9 (8, 10)	4 (3.5, 6.5)
Positive circulating staff behaviour	0.024	8 (7, 9.5)	4 (3.5, 6.5)
Surgical performance	0.012	9 (8.5, 9.5)	7 (3, 7.5)
Helpfulness of main assistant	0.041	8 (6.5, 9.5)	6 (5, 8)
Helpfulness of bottom assistant	0.334	7 (5.5, 8)	6 (5, 7)

Conclusion

This is an exploratory study that aimed to gather information about the perceptions of theatre staff of the impact of the theatre environment on the work experiences of themselves and their colleagues involved in laparoscopic surgery. It is the first paper addressing the impact of integrated theatres.

A number of weaknesses limit the capacity to conclude from the pilot data. The number in each staff group was small. However, the small numbers differences were highly significant. A further weakness lies in the use of unvalidated visual analogue scales although these are widely used in medical research. There are also potentially confounding variables, e.g. the levels of difficulty of surgery carried out in the two theatre environments, and technical errors during surgery that could have influenced staff perceptions about the two theatre environments being compared.

However, the results fell into a consistent pattern of discriminatory responses in staff perceptions of the two physical work settings. This overriding pattern strongly suggests the need for further research in the impact of theatre environments on staff experiences and the attendant consequences on performance, safety and satisfaction. Further research should involve larger samples from multi centres.

It is only by assessing these factors and the quality of the operating theatre environment that the true benefits of integrated theatres will be appreciated. This investment not only protects staff and patients but these data suggest that the improved behaviours may further enhance safety and also create greater efficiency resulting in cost savings.

Acknowledgment We would like to acknowledge Eirini Koutoumanou (BSc MSc GradStat MPhil/PhD student Teaching Fellow Centre for Paediatric Epidemiology and Biostatistics, Institute of Child Health, UCL 30 Guilford Street, London, WC1N 1EH) for the statistical analysis.

Conflict of interest Andreas Stavroulis and Lih-Mei Liao have no conflicts of interest or financial ties to disclose. Alfred Cutner has received funding from Storz for lectures and education purposes.

References

1. Kelling G (1901) Die Tamponade der Speiseroehre und des magens mit beigsamen instrumenten. Verdhandlungen der Gesellschaft Deutscher Naturtorscher und Aerzte, vol 73. Vogel verlag, Leipzig, pp 117–119
2. Semm K (1983) Endoscopic appendectomy. Endoscopy 15:59–64
3. Togas T, Ahmed S (1999) Surgical management of ectopic pregnancy. Clin Obstet Gynecol 42(1):31–38
4. Berci G, Sackier JM, Paz-Partlow M (1991) Emergency laparoscopy. Am J Surg 161(3):332–335
5. Warren O, Kinross J, Parasceva P, Darzi A (2006) Emergency laparoscopy—current best practice. World J Emerg Surg 1:24
6. Gitsch E, Vytiska-Binstorfer E, Skodler W (1990) Various effects of abdominal and vaginal hysterectomy in benign diseases. Eur J Obstet Gynecol Reprod Biol 36:259–63
7. Theodoros DT, John NB (2006) Laparoscopy and oncology: where do we stand today? Ann N Y Acad Sci 997(1)
8. Arnold PA, Karen W (2009) Evolving role and current state of robotics in minimally invasive gynecologic surgery. J Minim Invasive Gynaecol 16(3):291–301
9. Paraiso MF (2006) Laparoscopic Burch colposuspension and the tension-free vaginal tape procedure. Curr Opin Obstet Gynecol 18(4):385–390
10. Cutner A, Stavroulis A, Zolfaghari N (2012) Risk assessment of the ergonomic aspects of laparoscopic theatre. Gynecological Surgery 10(2):99–102
11. Hamman W (2004) The complexity of team training: what we have learned from aviation and its applications to medicine. Qual Saf Health Care 13(Suppl 1):i72–i79
12. Gensler (2008) 2008 US Workplace Survey. http://www.gensler.com/uploads/documents/2008_Gensler_Workplace_Survey_US_09_30_2009.pdf. Accessed 29 Apr 2013
13. Operating Theatres (2003) A Bulletin for Health Bodies. http://archive.audit-commission.gov.uk/auditcommission/sitecollectiondocuments/AuditCommissionReports/NationalStudies/TheatresAHP.pdf. Accessed 29 Apr 2013

LiquiBand® Surgical S topical adhesive versus sutures for the closure of laparoscopic wounds

Haider Jan · Natasha Waters · Pat Haines · Andrew Kent

Abstract Cyanoacrylate adhesives offer the surgeon and patient an alternative to subcuticular suturing. LiquiBand® Surgical S (LBSS) is a new formulation with a blend of monomeric *n*-butyl and 2-octyl cyanoacrylates. In this study, the effectiveness, safety, and clinical utility of LBSS was compared to Vicryl™ sutures for the closure of laparoscopic incisions. This was a prospective randomized study of LBSS skin adhesive versus Vicryl™ sutures for the topical closure of laparoscopic surgical incisions. Subjects were asked to return at 2 weeks postsurgery to report complications and adverse events. Wounds were evaluated for apposition and cosmesis using a modified Hollander Wound Evaluation Scale (HWES). The Shapiro–Wilk test of normality was done. Independent-samples T test, Mann Whitney U test, and chi-square test were used to compare variables between the two wound closure methods. A total of 114 subjects participated in this trial completing all aspects of the study. Fifty-five subjects received sutures for topical wound closure, with 59 subjects receiving LBSS. Surgeons were found to be satisfied with 100 % of all applications using the LBSS device. One hundred percent of wounds closed with sutures and 98.9 % wounds closed with LBSS achieving an optimal HWES of 0. There was no statistical difference in cosmesis or complications for either method. Closure with LBSS was significantly faster by a mean of 2 min. LiquiBand® Surgical S is as good as sutures for the closure of laparoscopic wounds in terms of cosmesis and complications with the added benefit of being significantly faster.

Keywords LiquiBand® Surgical S · Vicryl · Randomized trial · Laparoscopy

H. Jan (✉) · N. Waters · P. Haines · A. Kent
Royal Surrey County Hospital NHS Foundation Trust,
Egerton Road, Guildford, Surrey GU2 7XX, UK
e-mail: hjan@me.com

Background

Throughout history, various exotic materials have been used to close surgical wounds. Leather has been used as far back as 1100 BC [1]. Woven horse hair, cotton, and linen are examples of natural fibers used in sutures; in fact, silk is still used today. With the evolution of advancing technology, arrays of synthetic polymeric threads have replaced natural fibers for the majority of purposes with Vicryl™ (Ethicon, Kirkton, Scotland) absorbable sutures becoming one of the most popular. Cyanoacrylate adhesives offer the surgeon and patient an alternative to suturing wounds. They offer a fast and less traumatic closure for appropriately selected wounds and typically do not require the use of local anesthesia [2]. These adhesives are commonly used for the closure of topical skin incisions and trauma-induced lacerations in areas of low skin tension [3]. Numerous potential advantages have been reported for both surgeons, healthcare system providers, and patients compared to conventional surgical wound closure techniques, including faster closure time, good cosmesis, non-invasive, less tissue trauma, no requirement for secondary dressing, ease of bathing, and no requirement for suture or staple removal [4]. Additionally, they spontaneously slough off in a short time period of time (5–10 days), thereby not requiring clinician removal [5]. These unique benefits have resulted in a significant increase in both the use and acceptance of the product within the medical community.

LiquiBand® Surgical S (Advanced Medical Solutions, Plymouth, UK) is a new formulation with a blend of monomeric *n*-butyl and 2-octyl cyanoacrylates. The blend combines the fast setting wound closure properties of the butyl-cyanoacrylates with the more flexible liquid wound dressing capabilities of the slower setting octyl-cyanoacrylates. It is indicated for the closure of clean and easily approximated incisions or trauma-induced lacerations, used in conjunction with but not in place of deep dermal stitches. The applicator features a narrow cannula and flow control tip for precise wound closure that can be removed to reveal an integrated foam pad for applying a broad occlusive wound dressing (Fig. 1). It has sufficient volume of octyl-blend monomer to close and protect wounds up to 8–10 cm in length.

In this study, the effectiveness, safety, and clinical utility of LiquiBand® Surgical S (LBSS), formerly marketed as LiquiBand® Laparoscopic, was compared to sutures (Vicryl™) for the closure of laparoscopic incisions. The two devices were evaluated for time to complete wound closure, user and patient satisfaction with closure, cosmesis, and complication rates following the use of either device.

Methods

This was a prospective randomized study of LBSS skin adhesive versus suture for the topical closure of laparoscopic surgical incisions. Female patients 18 years and older, scheduled for laparoscopic surgery, and willing to return for a 2-week follow-up visit were invited to participate in this trial. Exclusion criteria included known sensitivity to cyanoacrylates, wounds under high tension, pregnancy or breastfeeding, or the presence of a disease or condition that interferes with wound healing such as diabetes mellitus. The protocol and informed consent received regional ethics committee approval and study subjects provided full consent prior to participating in any study-related procedures.

Subjects were randomly assigned to receive either LBSS or sutures for topical wound closure of laparoscopic incisions. A random number generator determined the assignment to either LBSS or sutures at time of surgery. The sutures used were 3-0 Vicryl™ and a subcuticular method of dermal closure was used. Due to the inherent differences between the two closure methods, it was not possible for the surgeon, study subjects, or evaluator to be masked from the knowledge of the randomized treatment assignments.

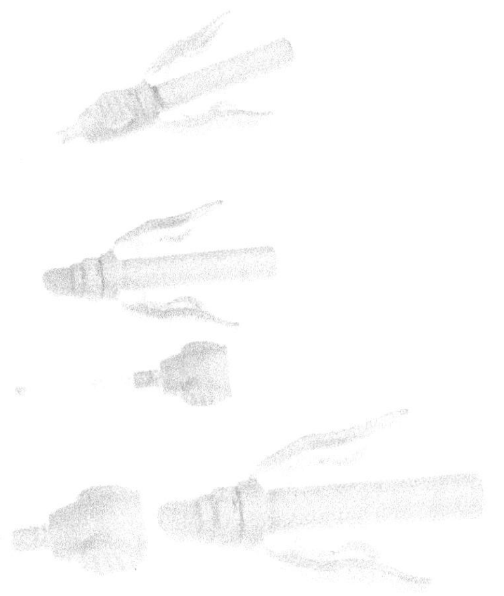

Fig. 1 The LiquiBand® Surgical S device

All enrolled study subjects, regardless of randomized device assignment, received the same preoperative cleansing routine as per hospital standard operating procedures. It involved a chlorhexidine alcohol mix. Additionally, hemostasis was achieved prior to any wound closure and study surgeons were instructed to use each study device according to their respective instructions for use.

Closure technique

LBBS was applied to a clean, dry wound with careful use of tissue forceps to obtain skin edge approximation and tissue aversion. We avoided having instruments or gloved fingers coming into contact with freshly applied adhesive as they can become stuck to the skin. Once the edges of the incision were adherent and opposed, the fine tip of LBSS device was removed and an oval dressing of the glue spread over the wound. This adheres to the glue in the wound edge and spreads the tension forces over a greater area as well as providing a waterproof dressing.

In the group that had sutures used, the following technique was used: The needle was inserted deep to the subcutaneous layer of the skin and pierced the subcutaneous fascia just underneath the skin. Once removed from one side of the wound, it was then inserted subcutaneously on the opposite skin surface and removed deep to the subcutaneous plane. The suture was tied using a surgical knot that was buried deep to the subcutaneous layer.

The surgeons taking part in the study were all senior gynecologists of consultant or subconsultant level with greater than 10 years experience in gynecological surgery. Along with subject demographics including subject age and body mass index (BMI), the length (in millimeter) of each incision requiring closure, and whether the incision required deep tissue suture was captured at wound closure.

The primary outcome measure of the study was to show a reduction in the time taken to close laparoscopic port site skin wounds with LBBS when compared with wounds closed with were 3-0 Vicryl™ using a subcuticular method.

Secondary outcome measures were as follows: Surgeons were asked to document whether they were satisfied or dissatisfied with the wound closure device and whether they found the device easy to use. Subjects were asked to return at 2 weeks postsurgery at which time any applicable wound complications (erythema, edema, pain, inflammation, discharge, odor, and dehiscence) were recorded along with any reported adverse events. Wounds were evaluated for apposition (<50, 50–99, and 100 %), and also for cosmesis using a modified Hollander Wound Evaluation Scale (HWES) [6]. The HWES was modified to a five-point scale with one point assigned to any of the following observed wound appearances; step off borders, contour irregularities, margin separation, edge inversion, and excessive distortion. A HWES of 0 indicated an optimal wound appearance, with each point between 0 and 5 indicating a less adequate appearance of the wound. The same evaluator also rated wound appearance as either acceptable or unacceptable. Study subjects were asked to rate their satisfaction with their wound appearance as either satisfied or dissatisfied.

Sample size and power calculation

The sample size was calculated to detect a 50 % reduction in wound closure time from 240 s with sutures to 120 s, with a standard deviation of 120 s, with tissue adhesive at a two-tailed significance level of 0.05 with a power of 95 %. Allowing for a dropout rate of 30 %, 163 wounds were needed in each of the two treatment arms.

Statistical methods

Data was analyzed in SPSS. The Shapiro–Wilk test of normality was done for the continuous variables including age, BMI, length of incision, number of incisions, and closure time in seconds.

Independent samples *T* test was used to compare normally distributed data and Mann–Whitney *U* test used to compare non-normally distributed data. A chi-square test was used to compare the nominal data including the difference between the dressings used, the wound infection rate, the complication rate, and satisfaction rate. A *p* value of 0.05 was used as the critical level for determining statistical significance.

Findings

A total of 152 subjects were enrolled in this study between 14 August 2009 and 2 April 2012 with 126 subjects completing all study-related procedures by 17 April 2012. Twenty-six subjects did not complete the study and were terminated due to voluntary withdrawal, not meeting inclusion/exclusion criteria, or being lost to follow-up. Twelve subjects were omitted from data analysis due to missing or incomplete data points, resulting in a total of 114 subjects used in the data analysis. Of the 114 subjects assessed, 55 subjects received sutures for topical wound closure, with 59 subjects receiving LBSS (Table 1). The subjects were well matched for both age and BMI with no significant differences between the two groups (Table 1). Pre-existing medical conditions for study subjects (14.7 % of subjects assigned with sutures and 6.8 % for LBSS) included eczema, psoriasis, active infection, and previous surgical site infection. Subjects from either treatment group had a median of three incisions closed with a total number of 167 incisions closed by sutures and 178 by LBSS. There was no significant difference in wound length between each group ($p=0.775$). The time taken to close wounds using LBSS was found to be significantly faster ($p<0.001$) than by sutures (Fig. 2). The median closure time for LBSS (approximately 78 s) was around two and a half times faster than closure by suture (approximately 210 s), with a difference between the medians of approximately 2 min 20 s. Following surgery, dressings (Opsite®, Smith and Nephew Inc.) were applied to the majority of wounds closed with sutures (92.2 %), while most wounds closed by LBSS (94.9 %) required no dressings after application.

Surgeons were found to be satisfied with 100 % of all applications using the LBSS device and also found the device easy to use for all wound closures. Surgeons were also found to be satisfied with 100 % of the wounds closed with subcuticular stitching.

At the 2-week visit, wounds were assessed by an evaluator for apposition and cosmesis (Table 2). Most wounds achieved apposition of >50 % with 18.6 % wounds closed by sutures and 18.5 % wounds closed by LBSS resulting in 100 % apposition which was not statistically significant ($p=0.906$). Only one wound closed by LBSS resulted in apposition of <50 %. High levels of cosmesis were also reported for all wounds regardless of closure device with no statistical significance between them ($p=0.17$). One hundred percent of wounds closed with sutures and 98.9 % wounds closed with LBSS achieved an optimal HWES of 0. Further inspection of wound sites closed with LBSS found that the adhesive had sloughed off either partially or completely from most sites (94 %), with 6 % of sites still retaining an intact adhesive layer. The adhesive typically remained intact for 5–7 days. All wounds were evaluated as acceptable by the evaluator at the 2-week visit with 100 % of subjects of both treatment groups satisfied by the appearance of their wounds.

Adverse events expected in this trial were complications typically experienced from wound closure following surgery and restricted to the site of treatment. Complications were assessed at the 2-week visit and included assessments at the wound site for erythema, edema, inflammation, odor, pain, and dehiscence (Table 3). There was no significant difference in complication rates ($p=0.956$). Of the 178 wounds closed with LBSS, a total of 39 wounds (21.9 %) reported complications and of the 167 wounds closed with sutures; the incidence of complications was 38 (22.8 %). Erythema was the most reported complication with 29 cases reported for each wound closure method (approximately 75 % of the reported complications for both treatment groups). The next most common complication was pain or tenderness at the wound site with six cases reported for both LBSS and sutures. Other complications reported were one case of edema from sutures, one case of

Table 1 Demographics and Wound incision characteristics

	Sutures	LBSS	*p* value
Number of subjects	55	59	N/A
Mean age of subjects (SD)	45.4 (10.1)	41.7 (11)	0.06
Median BMI of subjects (SD)	25	24	0.52
Medical history			N/A
Total pre-existing, *n* (% subjects), by type	8 (14.7)	4 (6.8)	
Eczema	3 (5.5)	2 (3.4)	
Psoriasis	2 (3.7)	0	
Active infection	1 (1.8)	0	
Previous SSI	2 (3.7)	2 (3.4)	
Total number of incisions	167	178	N/A
Median length of incisions (SD)	5	5	0.78
Median no. incisions per subject (min/max)	3	3	0.85
Dressing used post closure, *n* (% of wounds)			Yates chi-square
None	13 (7.8)	169 (94.9)	$p<0.0001$
Opsite®	154 (92.2)	9 (5.1)	
Status of tissue adhesive, *n* (% wounds)	N/A		N/A
Intact		10 (6)	
Completely sloughed off		63 (38.2)	
Partially sloughed off		92 (55.8)	
Median closure time per subject, in seconds (SD)	210	78	$p<0.0001$

inflammation from LBSS, two cases of drainage/discharge from sutures, one from LBSS, and one case each of odor and dehiscence for LBSS. All complications reported were minor in nature and resolved without further treatment. No serious adverse incidents were reported throughout the duration of the study. Not all fields for the status of the tissue adhesive were at 2 weeks were completed. Thirteen wound evaluations were incomplete. The percentage calculated was based on the 165 completed not the 178 total wounds. The trial ended once the number of patients required was reached.

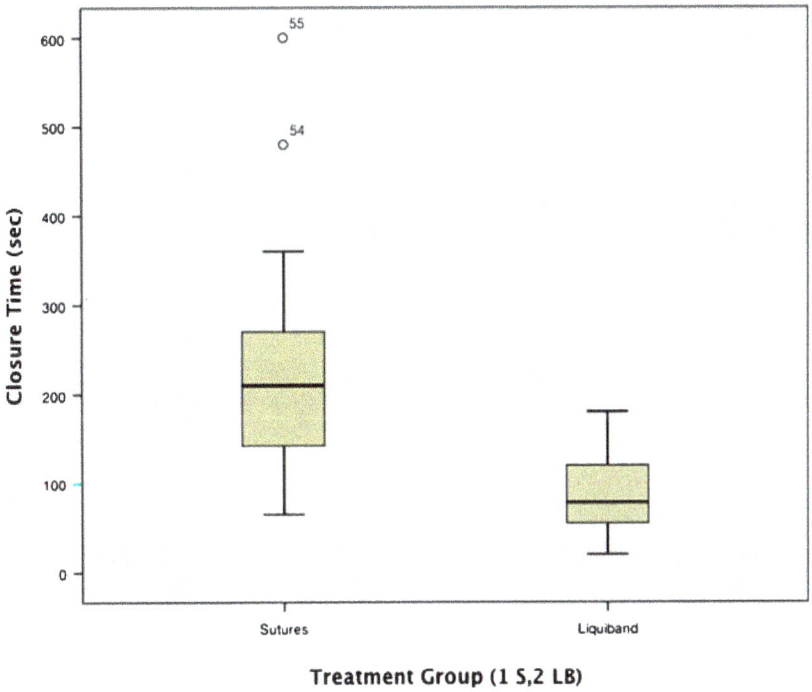

Fig. 2 Comparison of closure times between the 2 groups

Table 2 Two-week follow-up visit

		Sutures	LBSS	*p* Value
Assessed by evaluator	Apposition	*N* (%)	*N* (%)	Yates chi-square
	100 %	31 (18.6)	33 (18.5)	$p=0.906$
	50–99 %	136 (81.4)	144 (80.9)	
	<50 %	0 (0)	1 (0.6)	
	MHWES (% score=0)	100	98.9	0.17
	Overall appearance (% acceptable)	100	100	N/A
	Patient satisfaction with wound appearance (%)	98.9	100	N/A

Discussion

The use of cyanoacrylates for tissue adhesion was first described in 1959. Although it was very effective, the degradation products had significant tissue toxicity [7]. Through time, newer products have emerged without tissue toxicity including LiquiBand® Surgical S. It contains a 90 % *n*-butyl and 10 % 2-octylcyanoacrylate blend. The *n*-butyl cyanoacrylate dries faster but potentially a more brittle glue, while the 2-octyl cyanoacrylate is more flexible but takes longer to dry. Various studies have demonstrated the effectiveness of 2-octyl cyanoacrylate [8–12] and *n*-butyl cyanoacrylate [13] to subcuticular stitching for the closure of laparoscopic wounds. This study is the first reported using a combination of both monomers in the literature.

There was no significant difference in cosmesis or complication rates in the use of LBSS as compared to subcuticular stitches for the closure of laparoscopic wounds. This makes it a realistic and useful alternative to sutures. Surgeons were very happy with the application particularly with the very quick drying time and excellent wound apposition.

The high surgical satisfaction is likely due to the fact that this form of closure is very easy to use. The placement of the tissue adhesive is a simple procedure, less technically demanding than placement of subcutaneous sutures. The learning curve is extremely rapid and is described to require the use of a glue with at least three incisions [11]. This could easily be achieved in one or two cases. One key note to all users is that the surgeon must avoid placing adhesive directly in the wound, in the deeper layers, as it will create a barrier, affect tissue healing, and will extrude through the wound [10].

Patient satisfaction was very high which is in part aided by the ease of bathing immediately after surgery, with no need to replace the dressings, and lack of requirement for suture or staple removal [4]. The lack of requirement for secondary dressing was apparent in this study and consistent with other cyanoacrylate studies in the literature [4].

The material costs of LBBS are higher than those for sutures and dressings. The NHS cost of LiquiBand® Surgical S is £13.45 per device as compared to the cost of a single 3-0 vicryl of £2.11 together with and Opsite dressings cost of £0.28 each per wound. In addition, patients are often given extra dressings to take home to replace after bathing.

However, when the total closure costs of material expenses and operating room time are considered, LBBS closure is more economical than suture closure. This study demonstrated that the time taken to close wounds using LBSS was consistently faster than using sutures with an average saving of 2 min per patient. Routine use extrapolated to 105 cases a week would potentially free up 210 min a week equating to freeing up a half day operating list per week. In addition, it has been estimated that theater time costs approximately US$30 per minute in the US and £20 per minute in the UK [14]. This can provide a substantial cost reduction based on the time saved [11].

Table 3 Complications at 2-week follow-up visit

		Device		p-value
		Sutures	LBSS	
	Total no. complications (% of total incisions)	38 (22.8)	39 (21.9)	Yates chi-square $p=0.956$
Incidence, *N* (% of complications per device)	Erythema	29 (76.3)	29 (74.3)	
	Edema	1 (2.6)	0	
	Pain or tenderness	6 (15.8)	6 (15.4)	
	Inflammation	0	1 (2.6)	
	Discharge/drainage	2 (5.3)	1 (2.6)	
	Odor	0	1 (2.6)	

Additional cost saving can be taken into account when comparing LBBS to non-absorbable sutures. With LBBS, there is no need for appointments to be made to remove any suture material [15], although this is not a factor with dissolvable subcuticular sutures.

Other potential benefits include a reduction in the risk of allergic reactions associated with sutures [16] and the fact no needles are required essentially eliminates the risk of needle stick injury for wound closure [16, 17].

LiquiBand® Surgical S is as good as sutures for the closure of laparoscopic wounds in terms of cosmesis and complications with the added benefit of being significantly faster to apply and provides an immediate impermeable dressing.

Conflict of interest Funding of the study was provided by Advanced Medical Solutions (Plymouth) Ltd. Western Wood Way, Langage Science Park, Plympton, Plymouth, Devon PL7 5BG, England. Advanced Medical Solutions (Plymouth) Ltd funded the presentation of the paper at a national conference. The authors report no other conflicts of interest.

References

1. Majno G (1975) The healing hand: man and wound in the ancient world, 1st edn. Harvard University Press, Cambridge, MA
2. Coulthard P, Esposito M, Worthington HV, van der Elst M, van Waes OJF, Darcey J (2010) Tissue adhesives for closure of surgical incisions. Cochrane Database Syst Rev CD004287
3. Farion K, Osmond MH, Hartling L, Russell K, Klassen T, Crumley E, Wiebe N (2002) Tissue adhesives for traumatic lacerations in children and adults. Cochrane Database Syst Rev CD003326
4. Chow A, Marshall H, Zacharakis E, Paraskeva P, Purkayastha S (2010) Use of tissue glue for surgical incision closure: a systematic review and meta-analysis of randomized controlled trials. J Am Coll Surg 211:114–125
5. Tajirian AL, Goldberg DJ (2010) A review of sutures and other skin closure materials. J Cosmet Laser Ther 12:296–302
6. Hollander JE, Singer AJ, Valentine S, Henry MC (1995) Wound registry: development and validation. Ann Emerg Med 25:675–685
7. Penoff J (1999) Skin closures using cyanoacrylate tissue adhesives. Plastic Surgery Educational Foundation DATA Committee. Device and Technique Assessment. Plast Reconstr Surg 103:730–731
8. Romero P, Frongia G, Wingerter S, Holland-Cunz S (2011) Prospective, randomized, controlled trial comparing a tissue adhesive (Dermabond™) with adhesive strips (Steri-Strips™) for the closure of laparoscopic trocar wounds in children. Eur J Pediatr Surg 21:159–162
9. Jallali N, Haji A, Watson CJE (2004) A prospective randomized trial comparing 2-octyl cyanoacrylate to conventional suturing in closure of laparoscopic cholecystectomy incisions. J Laparoendosc Adv Surg Tech A 14:209–211
10. Sebesta MJ, Bishoff JT (2004) Octylcyanoacrylate skin closure in laparoscopy. JSLS 8:9–14
11. Matin SF (2003) Prospective randomized trial of skin adhesive versus sutures for closure of 217 laparoscopic port-site incisions. J Am Coll Surg 196:845–853
12. Maartense S, Bemelman WA, Dunker MS, de Lint C, Pierik EGJM, Busch ORC, Gouma DJ (2002) Randomized study of the effectiveness of closing laparoscopic trocar wounds with octylcyanoacrylate, adhesive papertape or poliglecaprone. Br J Surg 89:1370–1375
13. Dowson CC, Gilliam AD, Speake WJ, Lobo DN, Beckingham IJ (2006) A prospective, randomized controlled trial comparing n-butyl cyanoacrylate tissue adhesive (LiquiBand) with sutures for skin closure after laparoscopic general surgical procedures. Surg Laparosc Endosc Percutan Tech 16:146–150
14. Ciechanowicz S, Wilson N (2011) Delays to operating theatre lists: observations from a UK centre. IJH. doi:10.5580/e82
15. Osmond MH, Klassen TP, Quinn JV (1995) Economic comparison of a tissue adhesive and suturing in the repair of pediatric facial lacerations. J Pediatr 126:892–895
16. Singer AJ, Quinn JV, Hollander JE (2008) The cyanoacrylate topical skin adhesives. Am J Emerg Med 26:490–496
17. Rosin D, Rosenthal RJ, Kuriansky J, Brasesco O, Shabtai M, Ayalon A (2001) Closure of laparoscopic trocar site wounds with cyanoacrylate tissue glue: a simple technical solution. J Laparoendosc Adv Surg Tech A 11:157–159

24

Leiomyomatosis peritonealis disseminata as a possible result of laparoscopic myomectomy

Martina Ribič-Pucelj · Branko Cvjetićanin · Vesna Šalamun

Abstract Between 2008 and 2010, four patients were treated for leiomyomatosis peritonealis disseminata, three were symptomatic and in one pelvic tumor was found during a routine pelvic examination. All four patients were in reproductive age and had never used any hormonal medication. Possible etiological factors were analyzed. The only common feature we found in these patients was laparoscopic myomectomy (in one additional laparoscopic supracervical hysterectomy 1 year after the first procedure) performed 3–11 years previously. Laparoscopy confirmed multiple myoma-like tumors and was converted to laparotomy in two patients; in the two patients, the tumors were removed laparoscopically. Laparoscopic myomectomy with morcellation could be an etiological factor for leiomyomatosis peritonealis disseminata. In selected cases and in experienced hands, the disease can be treated laparoscopically.

Keywords Leiomyomatosis peritonealis disseminata · Unclear etiology · Potential risk factor · Laparoscopic myomectomy

Introduction

Leiomyomatosis peritonealis disseminata (LPD) is a rare, usually benign tumor, and varying in size and number of smooth muscle cells that grow along the subperitoneal surface and can mimic a disseminated malignancy. The condition was first described in 1952 by Wilson and Peale [1]. LPD is usually discovered incidentally during a cesarean section or laparotomy for unrelated reasons or when searching for the cause of nonspecific pain or menorrhagia related to uterine myomas. Its etiology is poorly understood. This condition has mostly been described in case reports; therefore, different possible etiological factors have been proposed for its occurrence. They can be divided into hormonal, subperitoneal mesenchymal stem cells, metaplasia, genetic, or iatrogenic [2]. Increasing number of reports on LPD as a complication of laparoscopic myomectomy and morcellation support the iatrogenic theory [2–4], according to which small pieces of a myoma remaining after morcellation and their subsequent growth are supposed to be etiological factors.

Moreover, possible underlying factors have also been investigated. Several treatment modalities have been proposed such as discontinuation of hormonal medication, medical treatment, and surgery.

Patients and methods

Laparoscopic myomectomy was introduced at our department in 1997 and laparoscopic supracervical hysterectomy (LASH) in 2000. Four patients with LPD were treated at the department between 2008 and 2010, the longest time interval since the initial procedure was 7 years. Three patients were symptomatic; one abdominal tumor was detected by transabdominal ultrasound examination done for unrelated reasons.

Informed consent was obtained from all patients for being included in the study.

Case 1

A 37-year-old woman, para 1, presented at the department 3 years after laparoscopic removal of a 10-cm myoma. She complained of abdominal pain lasting 2 months. Abdominal ultrasound scan and MRI revealed multiple tumors measuring from 1 to 4 cm in the abdominal cavity. Diagnostic laparoscopy revealed a uterine myoma and several myoma-like tumors in the rectosigmoid colon, appendix, and omentum and was

M. Ribič-Pucelj (✉) · B. Cvjetićanin · V. Šalamun
Department of Obstetrics and Gynecology, University Medical Centre Ljubljana, Šlajmerjeva 3, SI-1000 Ljubljana, Slovenia
e-mail: martina.ribic@gmail.com

converted to laparotomy. Total hysterectomy with bilateral adnexectomy, appendectomy, and omentum resection were performed; on the request of a general surgeon, bowel resection was performed as well. Due to enlarged lymph nodes along the iliac vessels, lymphadenectomy was also performed, but frozen sections of the tumors and lymph nodes did not confirm malignancy.

Case 2

A 36-year-old woman, para 1, presented to the gynecologist who performed laparoscopic removal of a 10-cm myoma 6 years earlier for recurrent menorrhagia. Bimanual examination revealed an enlarged uterus of irregular shape, whereas abdominal and transvaginal ultrasound revealed tumors with sonographic characteristics of myomas. The patient was admitted to the hospital for hysterectomy. Laparoscopy revealed a 6-cm myoma on the anterior abdominal wall which was removed. On further exploration of the small pelvis and abdominal cavity, four myoma-like tumors 1 to 3 cm in size were found in the rectosigmoid colon and two small subserous myomas on the uterus. Laparoscopy was converted to laparotomy which further revealed three 2 mm myoma-like tumors and a myoma also in the abdominal fascia at the suprapubic trocar site. Biopsy and frozen sections excluded malignancy. The tumors were removed; the uterus and the adnexa were not.

Case 3

A 50-year-old patient, para 1, referred to the gynecologist who performed laparoscopic myomectomy 7 years earlier and laparoscopic supracervical hysterectomy without adnexectomy for recurrent myomas 6 years ago. She was asymptomatic but the transabdominal ultrasound examination performed for an unrelated reason detected a 7×6 cm large tumor in the small pelvis. A transvaginal ultrasound confirmed the tumor with ultrasonographic characteristics of a myoma. The preoperative diagnosis was a recurrent myoma on the cervical stump, but to evaluate the true nature of the tumor, laparoscopy was performed. The cervical stump was found normal, but behind it were two myomas measuring 5 and 4 cm large, three small myomas measuring 2 cm arising from the rectosigmoid colon were detected, and another one, 4 cm large arising was located retroperitoneally above the right tube. Biopsy and frozen sections excluded malignancy. Myomas were removed laparoscopically. Because of the patient's age, bilateral oophorectomy was performed as well despite apparently functional ovaries.

Case 4

A 50-year-old woman, para 2, was referred to the department for a 5-cm tumor in the pelvis behind the cervix. The transperitoneal involvement of the colon was excluded by colonoscopy as requested by the general practitioner. The patient underwent laparoscopic myomectomy and tubal sterilization 11 years earlier. She never missed her annual gynecological examination, but the tumor was first detected at the last visit only. She reported discomfort in the small pelvis lasting about 3 months. Preoperative diagnosis, based on bimanual examination and transvaginal ultrasound scan, was a cervical myoma. Laparoscopy revealed a 5-cm myoma-like tumor in the subperitoneal space of the rectum and 5 and 4 cm nodules on the sigmoid colon. All tumors were removed laparoscopically. The final pathologic diagnosis—benign myoma agreed with frozen section biopsy.

None of the four patients was ever taking any hormone therapy.

The tumors removed at primary surgery were diagnosed by the pathologist as benign myomas and described as densely cellular spindle-shaped smooth muscle tumors in all four patients. Histological description of LPD nodules was completely identical.

There were no intra- or postoperative complications. Currently, all patients are symptom free and no recurrence has been registered (follow-up period from 2 to 5 years).

Tumors were removed laparoscopically using electric morcellator; the defects on the site of enucleation were peritonized, after which the abdominal cavity was extensively washed performed to remove any remaining small particles.

Discussion

LPD is most prevalent in women of reproductive age, particularly in those subjected to altered hormonal milieu, such as prolonged use of oral contraceptives [5, 6], hormonal replacement therapy [7], pregnancy [8], estrogen secreting tumors [9], and ovarian stimulation [10]. Al-Tahib and Tulandi encountered 132 of LPD in the English literature, 113 were described in premenopausal women, 7 in postmenopausal women, 6 in males, 1 in a horse, 1 in a fetus, and 4 were not classified [2].

None of our four patients was exposed to increased exogenous or endogenous estrogen concentrations. The only common factor was previous laparoscopic myomectomy done with the aid of electric morcellator. Laparoscopic myomectomy or laparoscopic supracervical hysterectomy with morcellation has been reported as a possible cause of LPD in recently published papers [2, 11–15]. Therefore, multiple tumors in the abdominal cavity should raise suspicion of LDP in patients with a previous history of laparoscopic myomectomy or LASH. Tumors are usually detected in symptomatic patients or at regular checkups with imaging techniques such as ultrasound, CT, or MRI [16–18]. The reports on the use of these techniques in LPD are rare because many reports are old and because many LPD cases were usually found incidentally at laparotomy for unrelated reasons. Regardless of the sensitivity and specificity of imaging techniques, the differential diagnosis between malignant and benign nature of the disease can be made only by biopsy and histological evaluation, particularly if we take into account that LPD can mimic peritoneal carcinomatosis [19, 20] or can be complicated, although extremely rarely, by sarcomatous transformation [21, 22], and that the treatment of malignancy is significantly different from that of a benign disease.

To evaluate the nature of preoperatively diagnosed tumors and the extent of the disease, we performed diagnostic laparoscopy and intraoperative frozen sections of myoma-like tumors to exclude malignancy in all four patients before taking the decision on the type of treatment. Spontaneous regression of LPD has been reported after discontinuation of hormone therapy, such as oral contraceptives or after pregnancy [23, 24]. Reports on medical treatment are rare, a successful treatment of LPD with the aromatase inhibitor anastrazole and with gonadotropin-releasing hormone agonists has been reported [25, 26]. Surgical treatment of LPD is usually the method of choice, particularly in symptomatic patients with no history of exogenous hormonal therapy, but there is no consensus on the type of the surgical procedure, although hysterectomy with oophorectomy is suggested in women with completed child-bearing. Hysterectomy with oophorectomy was performed in one of our four patients and oophorectomy in one, whereas ovaries were left in place in two patients, although it is still debatable whether ovaries should be removed or not. The purpose of oophorectomy is to deprive patients from estrogen stimulus which is supposed to play the most important role in tumor growth. Unfortunately, this theory cannot explain the occurrence of LPD in postmenopausal women [27–29], in women after abdominal hysterectomy [22, 30], and in men [31]. The same is true of the procedures of the bowel. Bowel resection is rarely indicated because tumors usually involve the subserosa only and rarely cause bowel obstruction, a rare indication is obstruction of the small bowel [32].

Looking back, we may conclude that the extremely radical procedure applied in our first case was unnecessary, but it was the general surgeon's decision due to lack of knowledge and experience with the disease of both the general surgeon and the gynecologist, as this was the first case they met within their carrier. Due to frequent involvement of the bowel, the general surgeon and oncologist are usually the first to meet with the disease and they may not be always familiar with its nature, although a minimally invasive approach in the treatment of LPD was reported and proposed already in 1994 by Krueczynsky [33]. Among all the cases treated surgically, laparoscopic approach was used in two only [12, 33]; in all others, laparotomy was performed. In cases 3 and 4, we removed tumors laparoscopically. Surgery was performed by gynecologists experienced in advanced laparoscopic surgery such as pelvic and paraaortic lymphadenectomy and bowel and urinary tract endometriosis. In our experience, the laparoscopic approach is safe and feasible, although the procedure can be time-consuming in case of multiple tumors, but not extremely demanding because the encapsulated nodules grow subperitoneally and do not invade the lumen of the adjacent organs.

An increasing number of reports on laparoscopic myomectomy with morcellation suggest morcellation as a possible cause of the development of LPD. Small particles of the minced tissue remaining in the abdominal cavity grow to become LPD under exposure to steroid hormones and growth factors. The only common factor that could be pointed out in the four cases here presented was laparoscopic myomectomy and no other previously mentioned potential risk factor in their previous history. Regarding thousands of laparoscopic myomectomies and LASHs performed all over the world, over 2,500 at our department only, the occurrence of LPD as a complication of myomectomy is rare. In addition to the particles that remained in the abdominal cavity and the iatrogenic theory, there must be some underlying etiological factors in these women. Some authors have suggested the genetic theory and abnormalities of chromosomes X, 8, 12, and 17 [13]; the hormonal theory explains the occurrence of LPD with proliferation of subcelomic submesenchymal cells and their differentiation into myoblasts, myofibroblasts, and fibroblasts under estrogen stimulation [34]. The diagnosis is usually based only on histological evaluation confirming benign myoma, whereas immunohistochemical evaluation has been rarely reported. Danikas and co-workers explained the occurrence of LPD in postmenopausal women with the presence of LH receptors [35], Butnor and co-workers found progesterone receptor activity in pre- and post-menopausal women as well [24], Takeda and co-workers found progesterone receptors positive in leiomyomas that were histologically almost identical to the myoma at primary surgery [12], and Ruscalleda and co-workers found negative estrogen and positive progesterone receptors [17].

Conclusion

Despite the above mentioned theories, the etiology of the occurrence of LPD remains unclear. The iatrogenic theory is supported by increasing number of reports on LPD as a complication of laparoscopic surgery with morcellation. Because small particles of minced tissue remaining in the peritoneal cavity after morcellation are supposed to be much more frequent as is the occurrence of LPD, these procedures are probably only a co-factor for LPD development and further research is required to find possible underlying factors. LPD occurs only rarely, but due to increasing number of laparoscopic myomectomies and LASHs, the number of cases is expected to increase; therefore, physicians faced with LPD must be familiar with the disease. If surgery is indicated and malignancy excluded, minimally invasive surgical approach is, according to our experience, feasible and safe, but should be performed by surgeons skilled in advanced laparoscopic procedures.

Conclusion for practice

LPD is a rare condition, the etiology of which is unknown; laparoscopic myomectomy and morcellation can be a possible risk factor for LPD. Extensive washing of the abdominal cavity at the end of the procedure is proposed to reduce the risk of the occurrence of LPD.

Conflict of interest The authors report no conflicts of interest. The authors alone are responsible for the contents and writing of the paper.

References

1. Wilson JR, Peale AR (1952) Multiple peritoneal leiomyoma associated with a granulose-cell tumor of the ovary. Am J Obstet Gynecol 64:204–208
2. Al-Talib A, Tulandi T (2010) Pathophysiology and possible iatrogenic cause of leiomyomatosis peritonealis disseminata. Gynecol Obstet Invest 69:239–244
3. Hilgar WS, Magrina JE (2008) Removal of pelvic leiomyomata and endometriosis 5 years after laparoscopic supracervical hysterectomy. Obstet Gynecol 108:772–774
4. Kumar S, Sharma JB, Verma D et al (2008) Disseminated peritoneal leiomyomatosis: an unusual complication of laparoscopic myomectomy. Arch Gynecol Obstet 278:93–95
5. Dallenbach C, Miklaw H, Dallenbach FD et al (1989) Disseminated peritoneal leiomyomatosis: a rare disease picture. Geburtshilfe Frauenheilkd 49:201–204
6. Wise LA, Palmer JR, Harlow BL et al (2004) Reproductive factors, hormonal contraception, and risk of uterine leiomyomata in African-American women: a prospective study. Am J Epidemiol 159:113–123
7. Heinig J, Neff A, Cirkel U, Klockenbusch W (2003) Recurrent leiomyomatosis peritonealis disseminata after hysterectomy and bilateral oophorectomy during combined hormonal replacement therapy. Eur J Obstet Gynecol Reprod Biol 111:216–218
8. Izadi-Mood N, Azordegan N (2003) Disseminated peritoneal leiomyomatosis: a case report. Arch Iran Med 6:216–218
9. Drake A, Dhundee J, Buckley CH et al (2001) Disseminated leiomyomatosis peritonealis in association with estrogen secreting ovarian fibrothecoma. Br J Obstet Gynaecol 108:661–664
10. Deering S, Miller B, Kopelman J et al (2000) Recurrent leiomyomatosis peritonealis disseminata exacerbated by in vitro fertilization. Am J Obstet Gynecol 182:725–726
11. Epstein JH, Nejat EJ, Tsai T (2009) Parasitic myomas after laparoscopic myomectomy: case report. Fertil Steril 91(3):13–14
12. Takeda A, Mori M, Sakai K et al (2007) Parasitic peritoneal leiomyomatosis diagnosed 6 years after laparoscopic myomectomy with electric morcellation: report of a case and review of the literature. J Minim Invasive Gynecol 14:770–775
13. Miyake T, Enomoto T, Ueda Y et al (2009) A case of disseminated peritoneal leiomyomatosis developing after laparoscope-assisted myomectomy. Gynecol Obstet Invest 67:96–102
14. Osterzensky A (1997) Uterine leiomyoma particle growing in an abdominal wall incision after laparoscopic retrieval. Obstet Gynecol 89:853–854
15. Paul PG, Koshy AK (2006) Multiple peritoneal parasitic myomas after laparoscopic myomectomy and morcellation. Fertil Steril 85:492–493
16. Guarigilia L, Conte M (1996) Sonographic findings in a case report of benign leiomyomatosis peritonealis disseminata. Acta Obstet Gynecol Scand 75:804–805
17. Ruscalleda N, Eixarch E, Pages M et al (2006) Leiomyomatosis peritonealis disseminata. Eur Radiol 16:2879–2882
18. Demir MK (2007) Disseminated peritoneal leiomyomatosis: magnetic resonance imaging and differential diagnosis. Australasian Radiol 51:B268–B271
19. Altinok G, Usubütün A, Küçükali T et al (2000) Disseminated peritoneal leiomyomatosis. A benign entity mimicking carcinomatosis. Arch Gynecol Obstet 264:54–55
20. Ramesh L, Edozien LC (2005) Not all disseminated intra-abdominal lesions are malignant: a case of leiomyomatosis peritonealis disseminata. J Obstet Gynecol 25:409
21. Fulcher AS, Szucs RA (1998) Leiomyomatosis peritonealis disseminata complicated by sarcomatous transformation and ovarian torsion: presentation of two cases and review of the literature. Abdom Imaging 23:640–644
22. Sharma P, Chaturvedi KU, Gupta R et al (2004) Leiomyomatosis peritonealis disseminata with malignant change in a postmenopausal woman. Gynecol Oncol 95:742–745
23. Düe W, Pickartz H (1989) Immunohistological detection of estrogen and progesterone receptors in disseminated peritoneal leiomyomatosis. Int J Gynecol Pathol 46–53
24. Butnor K, Burchette JL, Robboy SJ (1999) Progesterone receptor activity in leiomyomatosis peritonealis disseminata. Int J Gynecol Pathol 18:259–264
25. Takeda T, Masuhara K, Kamiura S (2008) Successful management of a leiomyomatosis peritonealis disseminata with an aromatase inhibitor. Obstet Gynecol 112(2 Pt 2):491–493
26. Hales HA, Petrerson CM, Jones PK, Quinn JD (1992) Leiomyomatosis disseminate treated with a gonadotropin-releasing hormone agonist. Am J Obstet Gynecol 167:515–516
27. Komatsu M, Tsuchya S, Kuroda T (1996) Leiomyomatosis peritonealis disseminata occurring in a postmenopausal woman: report of a case. Jpn J Surg 26:700–703
28. Strinić T, Prusac-Kuzmić I, Eterović D et al (2000) Leiomyomatosis peritonealis disseminata in a postmenopausal woman. Arch Gynecol Obstet 264:97–98
29. Nigojević S, Kapural L, Scukanec-Spoljar S et al (1997) Leiomyomatosis peritonealis disseminata in a postmenopausal woman. Arch Gynecol Obstet Scand 26:893–894
30. Rajab KE, Aradi AN, Datta BN (2000) Postmenopausal leiomyomatosis peritonealis disseminata. Int J Gynecol Obstet 68:271–272
31. Yamaguchi T, Imamura Y, Yamamoto F et al (2003) Leiomyomatosis peritonealis disseminata with malignant change in a man. Radiographics 53:179–185
32. Ghosh K, Dorigo O, Bristow R, Berek J (2000) A radical debulking of leiomyomatosis peritonealis disseminata from colonic obstruction: a case report and review of the literature. J Am Coll Surg 191:212–215
33. Krueczynsky D, Merz E, Knapstein PG (1994) Minimal invasive therapie bei peritoneal leiommyomatose. Geburtshilfe Frauenheilkd 167:181–183
34. Tavassoli FA, Norris HJ (1982) Peritoneal leiomyomatosis (leiomyomatosis peritonealis disseminata): a clinicopathologic study of 20 cases with ultrastructural observations. Int J Gynecol Pathol 1:59–74
35. Danikas D, Goudas VT, Rao CV et al (2000) Luteinizing hormone receptor expression in leiomyomatosis peritonealis disseminata. Obstet Gynecol 95:1000–1011

25

Aberrant obturator vessels in minimally invasive pelvic lymph node dissection

Latchesar S. Tantchev · Grigor A. Gorchev · Slavcho T. Tomov · Zdravka V. Radionova · Angelika S. Velkova

Abstract The presence of aberrant obturator vessels, arising from the external iliac circulatory system and their lesion during a surgical intervention in the area, may lead to bleeding, which is difficult to control. For a period of 5 years, 133 endoscopic bilateral pelvic lymph node dissections in patients with cervical cancer were performed, and the present aberrant vessels were registered and filmed. Aberrant obturator vessels were present in 58 cases (43.6 %). Eight obturator arteries and 58 obturator veins, branches of the external iliac vascular system, were visualized. Arterial type of obturator variation was found in one (0.07 %) case, venous type—in 50 (37.5 %), and combined (arterial and venous) type—in seven (5.26 %), out of all patients. Of the observed aberrant obturator arteries, three were found to arise from the inferior epigastric artery, and five from the external iliac artery. Of all available 73 veins, 51 (70 %) drained directly into the external iliac vein and 22 (30 %) in the inferior epigastric vein. The frequency of the aberrant obturator veins was 27.44 % ($n=73$), and of the arteries—3 %, related to the investigated pelvic halves ($n=266$). The presence of aberrant obturator vessels is a relatively common anatomic variation, important for the clinical practice.

Keywords Aberrant obturator vessels · Corona mortis · Pelvic lymph node dissection

Background

Vascular anastomoses, between the obturator and the external iliac arterial and venous systems, are observed in surgical interventions in the obturator and inguinal region. The lesion of the variant obturator vessels may lead to bleeding, which significantly deteriorates the view to the operative field and can seriously impede the surgical team in performing the required intervention. Minimally invasive surgical techniques allow clear visualization of the pelvic structures under optic magnification and require manipulation in bloodless environment. Knowing the anatomical variations of these vascular anastomoses, their protection or selective transection are essential for the smooth course of the retroperitoneal pelvic lymph node dissection.

Materials and methods

The present study includes 133 patients diagnosed with cervical cancer, assessed preoperatively with FIGO stage 1b1. Laparoscopically assisted radical hysterectomy and pelvic lymph node dissection was carried out in 52 patients (from January 2007 to May 2008), and robot-assisted radical hysterectomy and pelvic lymph node dissection in the remaining 81 (from May 2008 to December 2011). All robotic and laparoscopic lymphadenectomies were accomplished by one surgical team, using the same operative methods. Upon resection of the round ligaments, the parietal peritoneum was opened laterally from the infundibulopelvic ligament. The proximal border of the pelvic lymph node dissection was the bifurcation of the common iliac artery and vein, and the distal border was the junction of the deep circumflex iliac vein with the external iliac vein. The inferior epigastric artery (IEA) and the inferior epigastric vein (IEV) were visualized. The superficial and the deep lymphatic chains were removed followed by isolation of the obturator nerve.

The clinical data of the patients in the two groups is presented in Table 1. There were no significant differences between the two groups ($p>0.05$), except the lower mean age of the patients in the laparoscopic group ($p=0.001$).

All surgical interventions were recorded and the available vascular obturator variations were registered in the course of

L. S. Tantchev (✉) · G. A. Gorchev · S. T. Tomov · Z. V. Radionova · A. S. Velkova
Gynecologic Oncology Clinic, Medical University—Pleven, Georgi Kochev Str. 8a, 5800 Pleven, Bulgaria
e-mail: l_tantchev@yahoo.com

Table 1 Characteristics of the patients in laparoscopic and robotic group

	Laparoscopic group	Robotic group
Age	40.5±9.9	44.0±11.2
BMI	24.02 kg/m^2 (±5.03)	24.51 kg/m^2 (±6.11)
Average number of extirpated lymph nodes	11.1±5.1(range 3–25)	11.4±7.0 (range 4–36)
Cases with metastatic lymph nodes (pN1) (FIGO IIIB)	6 (11.5 %)	15 (18.5 %)
Histology	47 (90.3 %)—squamous cell carcinoma	72 (88.8 %)—squamous cell carcinoma
	5 (9.6 %)—adenocarcinoma	9 (11.1 %)—adenocarcinoma

operation. The records were reviewed later, appropriate images were processed and by using a graphical editor, frames of the basic types of obturator vascular variations were selected. Standard statistical methods were used for data description.

Findings

In most of the cases the obturator vascular bundle was located caudally under the obturator nerve, belonging to the internal iliac vascular system. Aberrant obturator vein (AOV) draining into the external iliac vein (EIV) or the IEV was frequently visualized (43.6 %, n=58). In some cases, the vein anastomosed with the obturator vein, a branch of the internal iliac vein. Aberrant obturator artery (AOA), arising either from the external iliac artery (EIA), or the IEA, running caudally and medially, to enter with the obturator nerve the canal of the same name, were less often seen (6 %, n=8). To systematize the cases with vascular variation, a classification proposed by Rusu et al. was used to define three major types of aberrant obturator variations—arterial, venous, and combined [1]. An aberrant obturator vessel was present in 58 cases (43.6 %). There were no significant differences between the robotic and the laparoscopic group, regarding the incidence of the arterial (FET p= 0.092) and venous (χ^2, 2.81; p=0.094) obturator anastomoses.

Aberrant obturator artery

The presence of AOA was registered in 6 % (n=8) of the cases. In all the cases, the variation was unilateral. In seven of the cases with AOA, AOV was also present. In half of the patients with arterial obturator variation, the artery was located on the right side, and in the remaining four, on the left side. Of the AOAs found, three arose from the IEA (Fig. 1) and five from the EIA (Fig. 2).

Aberrant obturator vein

Aberrant obturator vein was identified significantly more often than AOA—in 43.6 % (n=58). In 52 % (n=30) of the cases, the variation was observed on the right side, in 22 % (n=13) on the left side, and in 26 % (n=15) in both pelvic halves.

Seventy-three aberrant obturator veins were found in all studied patients (n=133). In one case, there were two AOV on the right side, one draining into the external iliac vein, and the other in the inferior epigastric vein (Fig. 3). From the available 73 AOV, 51 (70 %) drained directly into EIV (Fig. 4) and 22 (30 %) in the IEV (Fig. 5). The frequency of AOV related to the studied pelvic halves (n=266) was 27.44 % (n=73).

Types of aberrant obturator variations

The frequency of the aberrant obturator vessels, divided into three main types and associated subtypes by a number of cases (n=133), is presented in Table 2. In two of the cases, venous anastomoses, between aberrant obturator venous vessel, draining into the external iliac system, and a vessel draining into the internal iliac vein, were dissected (Figs. 6 and 7). Combined arterial and venous type is presented in Figs. 8, 9, and 10.

Discussion

There is a terminological diversity in defining the atypical vessels in the obturator area. Some authors define as obturator any vessel entering the obturator canal, regardless of its origin,

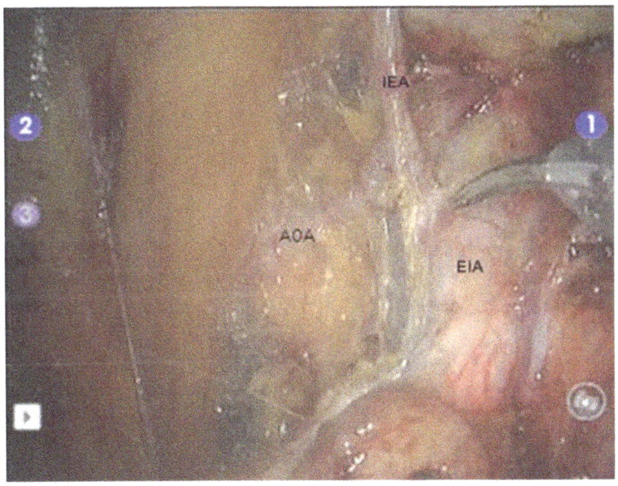

Fig. 1 The proximal part of the inferior epigastric artery (*IEA*) is skeletonized and the separation of the aberrant obturator artery (*AOA*) from it is visualized (*right side*)

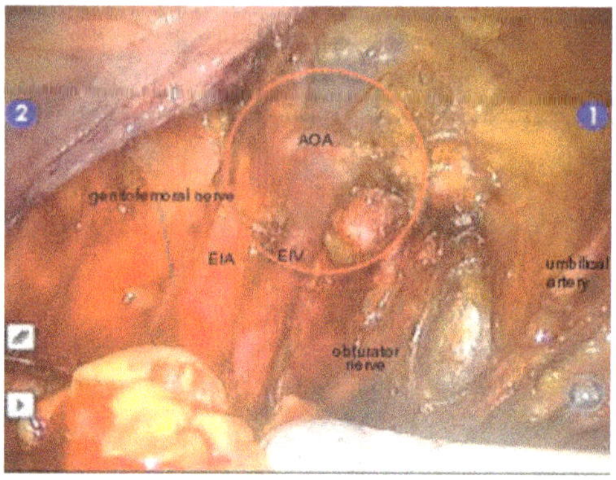

Fig. 2 Aberrant obturator artery (*AOA*) separates from the external iliac artery (*EIA*) between the proximal 2/3 s and distal 1/3 and directs medially and caudally to the obturator canal (*left side*)

irrespective of its drainage [2–4]. Von Lanz and Wachsmuth term the veins passing through the obturator canal and draining into the external iliac system, "vv. comitantes" [5]. Berberoğlu et al. term accessory obturator artery/vein any anatomical variant of an obturator vessel, arising from the external iliac system [6]. Other authors prefer the term aberrant obturator vessel, used to denote any abnormal deviation [7–9]. Rusu et al. perceive the accessory as additional to another existing obturator vein, respectively artery [1]. According to them, in the absence of another obturator vessel, the only one available is the obturator artery, respectively vein, regardless of its origin and drainage. The term "aberrant obturator artery, respectively vein", describes the atypical course of the blood vessel and in this sense, an obturator vessel can be aberrant, whether arising either from the external iliac circulatory system, or entering atypically the obturator canal.

Due to conceptual differences in terminology, "aberrant obturator artery/vein" was used. The term was used to denote any vessel passing through the obturator canal and connected to the external iliac system. The obturator vessels below the obturator nerve were not always completely dissected, and it was impossible to determine whether the vessel was accessory

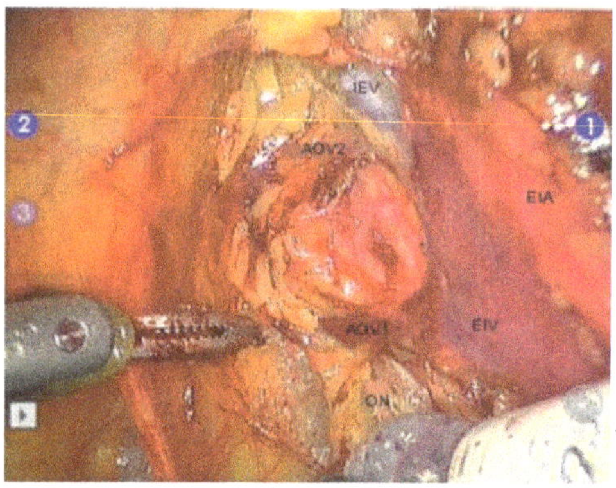

Fig. 3 Two aberrant obturator veins on the right drain in the inferior epigastric vein (*IEV*) (*AOV1*) and the external iliac vein EIV (*AOV2*), respectively (*right side*)

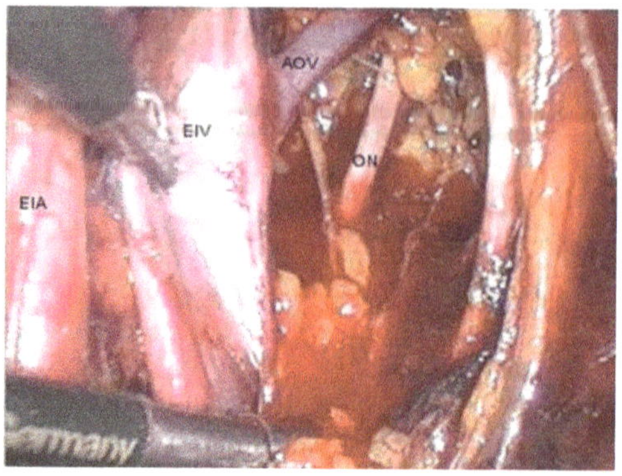

Fig. 4 Aberrant obturator vein (*AOV*) draining in the external iliac vein (*EIV*) (*left side*)

in relation to another obturator vessel. The risk of inducing bleeding when skeletonizing the vessels in this area may impede the therapeutic and diagnostic procedure. Atypical location of the obturator nerve, artery, and vein, in relation to another one in the fossa, was not considered as aberrant obturator vessel.

The anatomical variations of the obturator vessels are an interdisciplinary problem, concerning different areas of medicine. There is a significant amount of research articles considering this topic. Some of them consider only variants of the arterial obturator vessels [10–18]. Other studies discuss the presence of venous aberrant obturator vessels as well [1, 3, 4, 6, 8, 9, 19–23].

In most of the publications, data is from cadaver dissections [1, 4, 9, 11, 14, 18–24]. In vivo results are presented only in three papers [6, 8, 13] and a case report [15]. Two of the studies are endoscopic, in operative treatment of inguinal hernias. Karakurt et al. study AOA angiographically only in the right pelvic half [13]. Berberoglu et al., apart from a group with cadaver dissection, study a group with endoscopic extraperitoneal dissection in patients with inguinal hernia [6].

No publications concerning aberrant obturator vessels in laparoscopic or robotic transperitoneal iliac lymph node dissection are available in the literature. There were no differences between the robotic and the laparoscopic approach

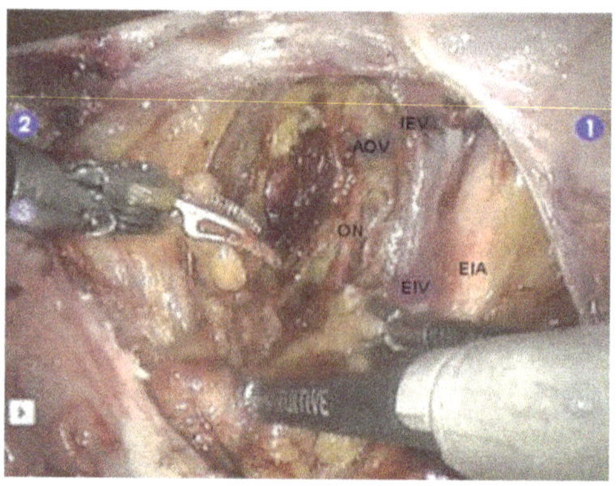

Fig. 5 Aberrant obturator vein (*AOV*) draining in the inferior epigastric vein (*IEV*) (*right side*)

Table 2 Frequency of the basic types of aberrant obturator vessels

	N	% of the cases with aberrant obturator vessel ($n=58$)	% of all cases ($n=133$)
Arterial type	1	1.72	0.07
OA arises from EIA	0	–	–
OA arises from IEA	1	1.72	0.07
Venous type	50	86.20	37.50
OV drains in EIV	31	53.44	23.30
OV drains in IEV	11	18.96	8.27
Venous anastomosis between OV and EIV	2	3.44	1.50
Venous anastomosis between OV and IEV	0	–	–
OV drains in EIV+OV drains in IEV	1	1.72	0.07
OV drains in EIV+venous anastomosis between OV and EIV	3	5.17	2.25
OV drains in EIV+venous anastomosis between OV and EIV	1	1.72	0.07
OV drains in IEV+venous anastomosis between OV and IEV	1	1.72	0.07
Arterial and venous variation	7	12.06	5.26
OA arises from EIA+OV drains in EIV	3	5.17	2.25
OA arises from EIA+OV drains in IEV	0	–	–
OA arises from IEA+OV drains in EIV	2	3.44	1.50
OA arises from IEA+OV drains in EIV	2	3.44	1.50
Total	58	100	43.60

OA obturator artery, *OV* obturator vein; *EIA* external iliac artery, *EIV* external iliac vein, *IEA* inferior epigastric artery, *IEV* inferior epigastric vein

regarding the frequency of the obturator vascular variants. This is most likely due to the lack of considerable differences in the basic patient characteristics, as well as to the fact that all interventions were performed by one team using one and the same technique.

In all cited articles, the data is based on the number of pelvic halves. Due to the fact that our study was totally clinical and the pelvic lymph node dissection performed was bilateral in all 133 cases, we processed the data in relation to the total number of patients as well.

In our opinion, determining the frequency of the anatomical variation by the number of patients studied is as important, as determining its type and frequency by pelvic halves. In the course of the study, it was found that the classification of obturator variations, used by Rusu et al., suited our purposes [1]. The approach we adopted to calculate the frequency of the AOA/AOV types hindered the juxtaposition of data. Therefore, we calculated the frequency, not only by the number of cases, but also by the absolute number of aberrant obturator vessels in pelvic halves.

Aberrant obturator artery was found in eight cases (6 %), distributed by four, in both pelvic halves. The frequency of AOA reported is 3 %, related to 266 pelvic halves. The frequency of AOA ranged from 5.5 % [9] to 65 % [1] in the cited literature. According to Berberoglu et al., the AOA frequency is 8 %, which is similar to our observations [6].

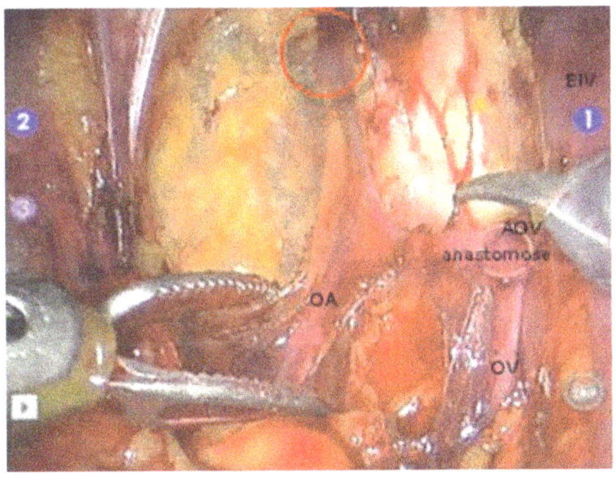

Fig. 6 Venous anastomosis between the obturator (*OV*) and aberrant obturator veins (*AOV*), draining in the internal iliac vein and the external iliac vein (*EIV*), respectively (*right side*)

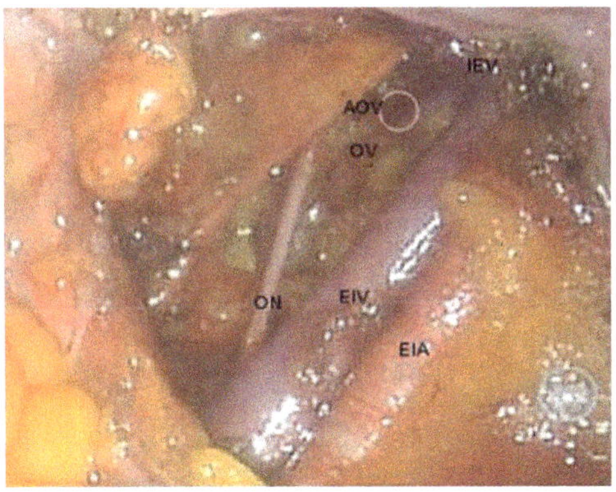

Fig. 7 Venous anastomosis between the obturator vein (*OV*) and the inferior epigastric vein (*IEV*) (*right side*)

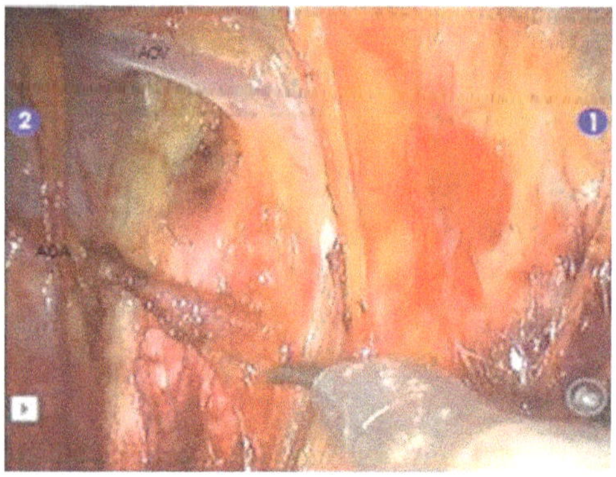

Fig. 8 Aberrant obturator artery arising from the external iliac artery (*EIA*) and aberrant obturator vein (*AOV*) draining in the external iliac vein (*EIV*) (*left side*)

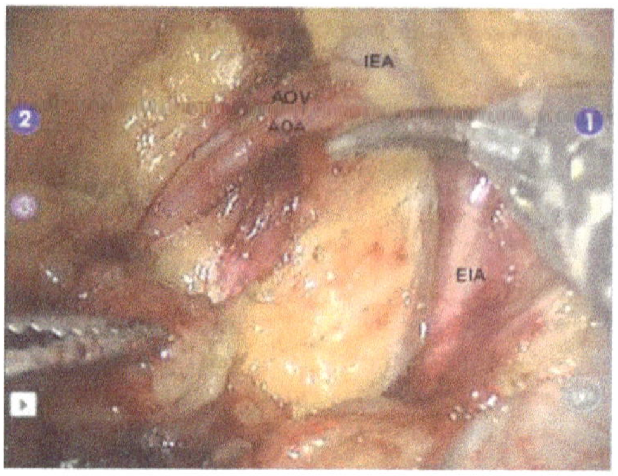

Fig. 10 Aberrant obturator artery (*AOA*) and aberrant obturator vein (*AOV*) originating from the inferior epigastric artery (*IEA*) run in parallel and drain in the inferior epigastric vein (*IEV*), respectively (*right side*)

Sarikcioglu et al. observe arterial variation more often (10 %) [4]. Other authors register AOA significantly more frequently than us (20–30 %) [8, 23, 25–27].

Of the visualized eight AOA, five originated from IEA, and three directly from EIA. The data presented by most of the authors [1, 10–12, 17] are in favor of AOA's origin from IEA. According to others, AOA is most commonly a branch of EIA [24, 26]. Sarikcioglu et al. have not found any case of AOA originating from IEA [4], while according to M. Berberoglu et al., the frequency of AOA from either IEA or EIA is equal [6].

Bergman et al., in a review article, state that the unilateral presence of AOA, branch of EIA, is comparable in frequency to the bilateral variation [10]. We observed AOA unilaterally only. Another conclusion made by the authors, is that the cases with unilateral AOA, branch of IEA, are equally distributed in both pelvic halves. Our observations confirm a similar distribution pattern of AOA in the left and right pelvic halves.

Papers concerning the venous obturator variations are considerably fewer than the arterial studies, a tendency that is in dissonance with the frequency of the arterial and venous variation. Moreover, some authors even accept the existence of AOV as normal rather than an exception. Berberoglu et al. have found AOV in 96 % of the cases they studied [6]. We

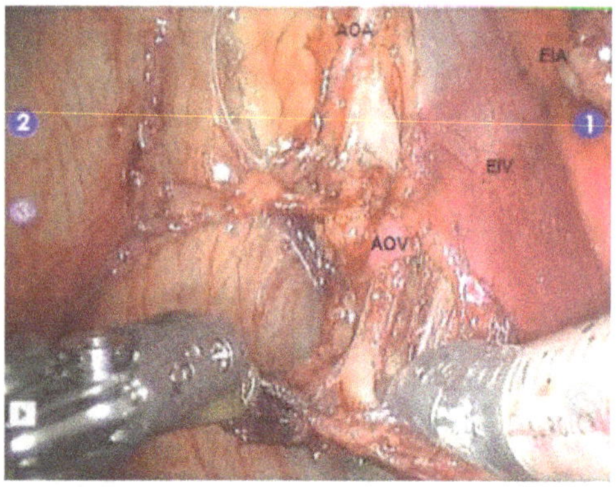

Fig. 9 Aberrant obturator artery arising from the inferior epigastric artery (*IEA*) and aberrant obturator vein (*AOV*) draining in the external iliac vein (*EIV*) (*right side*)

calculated the total number of AOV (73), related to 233 pelvic halves 27.44 %, in order to compare our results with those of the cited authors. Our results are similar to those of Missankov et al. (26 %), Sarikcioglu et al. (20.37 %), and Lau et al. (27 %) [4, 8, 24]. In 15 (25.8 %) of the 58 cases identified with AOV, the variation was bilateral. Okcu et al. also found bilateral obturator venous variation in 25 % of the cases [23].

In most of the patients, AOV was visualized only unilaterally (43/74, 13 %), as more frequently, AOV was found in the right side ($n=30$), and only in 13 in the left. However, Namking et al. observed approximately equally often venous variation in both pelvic halves [22]. In over half of the cases, AOV was found to drain into EIV ($n=51/69.86$ %). Rusu et al. reported that in the pelvises they dissected, AOV was found to drain significantly more often in IEV than in EIV [1]. Other papers, describing the location of influx of AOV were not found in the available literature.

In the patients operated ($n=133$), a venous type of obturator variation was observed most often—in 37.50 % of the cases, while the arterial type was seen in only one case (0.07 %). The data of Rusu et al. are quite different from ours. Most often, they observed a combined (arterial+venous) type of obturator variation (40 %), and most rarely a venous type (15 %) [1]. This difference is due to the high frequency of aberrant obturator arteries in their study, unlike the ones identified in our study.

Explanation for the presence of variants of obturator arterial and venous vessels could be sought in the embryonic development of the vascular network. Definitive aberrant obturator artery is formed as a result of uneven growth of anastomoses between the external and internal iliac artery, which are connected in between by variations of the regional organogenesis. Two critical periods are distinguished in the morphogenesis of the anastomoses between the iliac arteries: renal and gonadal obstruction [27]. Obturator vessels are formed relatively late to participate in the blood supply of the lower limb. This could explain the diversity of origin and the relatively high frequency of anatomical variations.

According to Arey and Fitzgerald, vascular anomalies are due to an unusual selection of channels from the primary capillary plexus [28, 29]. The most appropriate channels widen, while others atrophy and disappear, thus providing the means of branching of the arterial and venous system.

Conclusion

Pelvic lymph node dissection is a basic procedure for staging and treatment of malignant gynecological diseases. The presence of aberrant obturator vessels is a relatively common anatomic variation, important for the clinical practice. Timely proceeding with the complex oncological therapy is made possible by the absence of complications in the course of surgical intervention and fast recovery of the patient. Last, but not least, the modern minimally invasive techniques, with detailed review of the retroperitoneal anatomy in vivo, may serve for educational purposes in the field of pelvic surgery.

Acknowledgments All procedures followed were in accordance with the ethical standards of the responsible committee on human experimentation (institutional and national) and with the Helsinki Declaration of 1975, as revised in 2008.

Conflict of interest On behalf of all authors, the corresponding author states that there is no conflict of interest.

References

1. Rusu MC, Cergan R, Motoc AG, Folescu R, Pop E (2010) Anatomical considerations on the corona mortis. Surg Radiol Anat 32(1):17–24
2. Naguib NN, Nour-Eldin NE, Hammerstingl RM, Lehnert T, Floeter J, Zangos S, Vogl TJ (2008) Three-dimensional reconstructed contrast-enhanced MR angiography for internal iliac artery branch visualization before uterine artery embolization. J Vasc Interv Radiol 19:1569–1575
3. Saraiya PV, Chang TC, Pelage JP, Spies JB (2002) Uterine artery replacement by the round ligament artery: an anatomic variant discovered during uterine artery embolization for leiomyomata. J Vasc Interv Radiol 13(9 Pt 1):939–941
4. Sarikcioglu L, Sindel M, Akyildiz F, Gur S (2003) Anastomotic vessels in the retropubic region: corona mortis. Folia Morphol (Warsz) 62:179–182
5. von Lanz T, Wachsmuth W (1938) Practical anatomy, first volume/fourth part [in German]. Springer, Berlin
6. Berberoğlu M, Uz A, Ozmen MM, Bozkurt MC, Erkuran C, Taner S, Tekin A, Tekdemir I (2001) Corona mortis: an anatomic study in seven cadavers and an endoscopic study in 28 patients. Surg Endosc 15(1):72–75
7. Dargent DF (1999) Laparoscopic techniques for gynecologic cancer: description and indications. Hematol Oncol Clin North Am 13:1–19
8. Lau H, Lee F (2003) A prospective endoscopic study of retropubic vascular anatomy in 121 patients undergoing endoscopic extraperitoneal inguinal hernioplasty. Surg Endosc 17:1376–1379
9. Pungpapong SU, Thum-umnauysuk S (2005) Incidence of corona mortis; preperitoneal anatomy for laparoscopic hernia repair. J Med Assoc Thai 88(Suppl 4):S51–S53
10. Bergmark K, Avall-Lundqvist E, Dickman PW, Henningsohn L, Steineck G (1999) Vaginal changes and sexuality in women with a history of cervical cancer. N Engl J Med 340:1383–1389
11. Biswas S, Bandopadhyay M, Adhikari A, Kundu P, Roy R (2010) Variation of origin of obturator artery in Eastern Indian population—a study. J Anat Soc India 59(2):168–172
12. Braithwaite J (1952) Variations in origin of the parietal branches of the internal iliac artery. J Anat 86:423–430
13. Karakurt L, Karaca I, Yilmaz E, Burma O, Serin E (2002) Corona mortis: incidence and location. Arch Orthop Trauma Surg 122:163–164
14. Kawai K, Honma S, Koizumi M, Kodama K (2008) Inferior epigastric artery arising from the obturator artery as a terminal branch of the internal iliac artery and consideration of its rare occurrence. Ann Anat 190(6):541–548
15. Ebraheim NA, Liu J, Lee AH, Patil V, Nazzal MMS, Sanford CG (2008) Obturator artery disruption associated with acetabular fracture: a case study and anatomy review. Injury Extra 39(2):44–46
16. Pai MM, Krishnamurthy A, Prabhu LV, Pai MV, Kumar SA, Hadimani GA (2009) Variability in the origin of the obturator artery. Clinics (Sao Paulo) 64(9):897–901
17. Pick JW, Anson B, Ashley FL (1942) The origin of the OBA artery. Am J Anat 70:317–343
18. Sañudo JR, Roig M, Rodriguez A, Ferreira B, Domenech JM (1993) Rare origin of the obturator, inferior epigastric and medial circumflex femoral arteries from a common trunk. J Anat 183(Pt 1):161–163
19. Ersoy M, Sagsoz N, Bozkurt MC, Apaydin N, Elhan A, Tekdemir I (2004) Important anatomical structures used in paravaginal defect repair: cadaveric study. Eur J Obstet Gynecol Reprod Biol 112(2):206–213
20. Gilroy AM, Hermey DC, DiBenedetto LM, Marks SC Jr, Page DW, Lei QF (1997) Variability of the obturator vessels. Clin Anat 10(5):328–332
21. Nagabhooshana S, Vollala V, Rodrigues V, Bhat S, Pamidi N, Lobo S (2008) Anatomical variation of obturator vessels and its practical risk: a case report from an anatomic study. J Vasc Bras 7(3):275–277
22. Namking M, Woraputtaporn W, Buranarugsa M, Kerdkoonchorn M, Chaijarookhanarakq W (2007) Variation in origin of the obturator artery and corona mortis in Thai. Siriraj Med J 59:12–15
23. Okcu G, Erkan S, Yercan HS, Ozic U (2004) The incidence and location of corona mortis: a study on 75 cadavers. Acta Orthop Scand 75:53–55
24. Missankov AA, Asvat R, Maoba KI (1996) Variations of the pubic vascular anastomoses in black South Africans. Acta Anat (Basel) 155:212–214
25. Bergman RA, Thompson SA, Afifi AK (1984) Catalog of human variation. Urban & Schwarzenberg, Baltimore, pp 124–125
26. Jakubowicz M, Czarniawska-Grzesińska M (1996) Variability in origin and topography of the inferior epigastric and obturator arteries. Folia Morphol (Warsz) 55:121–126
27. Petrenko VM (2000) Development of the obturator artery in human prenatal ontogenesis. Morfologiia 118(4):51–53
28. Arey LB (1963) The development of peripheral blood vessels. In: Orbison JL JL, Smith DE (eds) The peripheral blood vessels. Williams and Wilkins, Baltimore, pp 1–16
29. Fitzgerald MJT (1978) Human embryology. Harper International, New York, pp 38–56

26

A hybrid technique of combined conventional and robotic-assisted laparoscopy for staging and debulking of early, advanced, and recurrent ovarian, fallopian tube, and primary peritoneal cancer

Farr R. Nezhat · Susan S. Khalil · Tamara N. Finger · Patrick F. Vetere

Abstract This study aims to describe a hybrid laparoscopic and robotic-assisted laparoscopic technique to access all four abdominal quadrants during pelvic procedures. This technique was utilized in the surgical management of select cases that included early, advanced, and recurrent ovarian, fallopian tube, and peritoneal cancer. A retrospective analysis of a prospectively maintained database was used to extract cases that this surgical method was utilized in. This included 20 patients that underwent 21 surgical procedures using this hybrid technique of conventional laparoscopy and robotic-assisted laparoscopy. Ten were early stage, and 11 were advanced and/or recurrent (six advanced, five recurrent). In the early-stage group, mean age was 42.3 years (range, 29–55), average BMI was 32.1 kg/m^2 (range, 17–65 kg/m^2), mean blood loss was 212.5 ml (range, 50–1,000 mL), operating room time (ORT) was 306.1 min (range, 87–639), and average length of stay (LOS) was 1.6 days (range, 1–2). There were no intraoperative complications and two grade 1 postoperative complications. Of the 11 for advanced and/or recurrent disease, mean age was 63.9 years (range, 39–92), average BMI was 29.7 kg/m^2 (range, 22.1–37.2), mean blood loss was 129.1 ml (range, 20–400), ORT was 238 min (range, 103–477), and LOS was 3.8 days (range, 1–17). There were no intraoperative complications. Three cases had postoperative grade 1–3 complications. There was one second look, nine cytoreductions to no visible disease, and 1 to <0.5 cm. Use of this hybrid technique, combining conventional laparoscopy and the present robotic platform, is effective in the surgical management of early, advanced and recurrent ovarian, fallopian tube, and peritoneal cancer in accessing all four abdominal quadrants with pelvic surgery.

F. R. Nezhat
Division of Gynecologic, Oncology and Minimally Invasive Surgery, Department of Obstetrics and Gynecology, Columbia University, New York, NY 10019, USA

F. R. Nezhat (✉)
Department of Obstetrics and Gynecology, St. Luke's-Roosevelt Medical Center, 10th Floor, 1000 10th Avenue, New York, NY 10019, USA
e-mail: fnezhat@chpnet.org

F. R. Nezhat
e-mail: frn2103@columbia.edu

F. R. Nezhat · S. S. Khalil · T. N. Finger
Division of Minimally Invasive Surgery, Department of Obstetrics and Gynecology, St. Luke's-Roosevelt Medical Center, New York, NY, USA

F. R. Nezhat · P. F. Vetere
Division of Minimally Invasive Gynecologic Surgery, Department of Obstetrics and Gynecology, Winthrop University Hospital, Mineola, NY, USA

Keywords Hybrid technique · Conventional laparoscopy · Robotic-assisted laparoscopy · Ovarian cancer Staging and Cytoreduction

Introduction

Advances in minimally invasive surgical techniques now make it feasible to accomplish comprehensive surgical staging, using conventional or robotic-assisted laparoscopy in select patients [1]. The present computer enhanced telesurgery (Intuitive Surgical, Sunnyvale, CA, USA), called robot-assisted surgery, was approved by the Food and Drug Administration for gynecological surgery in 2005 and has been increasingly applied to complex gynecologic procedures, such as surgical staging for gynecologic malignancies including endometrial, cervical, and ovarian cancers [2–5].

Limitations exist with the present robotic platform for staging and cytoreduction in ovarian cancer. Once the robot is docked for pelvic surgery, it is more difficult to access the upper abdomen, without having to undock and reposition the robot, or add additional ports to be able to perform the procedure. The Society of Gynecologic Oncology's consensus statement on robotic-assisted surgery commented on its utility in ovarian cancer as poorly suited for advanced ovarian cancer due to its limitation, with conventional port placement for pelvic surgery, in gaining upper abdominal access [6].

In the USA, ovarian cancer will affect approximately 22,280 women in 2012 with 15,500 estimated deaths. Currently, the lifetime risk of developing ovarian cancer in the USA is approximately 1 in 70 with more than 65 % given the diagnosis of advanced stage disease [7]. The standard treatment of ovarian cancer includes upfront surgery with intent to properly diagnose, stage, and to achieve maximal cytoreduction preferably to no visible disease followed by taxanes and platinum-based combination chemotherapy in majority of cases [8]. Traditionally, a comprehensive surgical staging procedure for ovarian, fallopian tube, and primary peritoneal cancers include total abdominal hysterectomy, bilateral salpingo-oophorectomy, peritoneal washings, biopsies of adhesions and peritoneal surfaces, omentectomy, and retroperitoneal lymph node sampling from the pelvic and para-aortic regions through a generous vertical midline laparotomy incision.

There have been attempts to strategize the utility of the robot for such cases in order to gain upper abdominal access without difficulty. Magrina et al. described their technique for approaching debulking procedures in patients with epithelial ovarian cancer that require upper abdominal access and for infrarenal aortic lymphadenectomy. This method involves undocking the robotic arms, then rotating the operating table 180°, insertion of additional ports, and then redocking [5, 9].

We describe our surgical method, a hybrid technique, in which both conventional laparoscopy and the robot are utilized in gynecologic malignancies in all four abdominal quadrants and the pelvic cavity. This surgical technique and its use in select patients with early and advanced ovarian cancer will be described for laparoscopic management of both pelvic and upper abdominal disease.

Materials and methods

A retrospective analysis of a prospectively maintained database was performed to extract select cases where this hybrid technique combining conventional laparoscopy (CL) and robotic-assisted laparoscopic surgery (RALS) was utilized. These cases included early, advanced, and recurrent ovarian, fallopian tube, and peritoneal cancer. Institutional review board approval was obtained and data was collected from two urban university affiliated community hospitals. All patients underwent preoperative evaluation including history, physical examination, medical assessment, computed tomography imaging of the chest or abdomen and pelvis, or positron emission tomography scan, and tumor marker assays, and were counseled extensively preoperatively and appropriate informed consent was obtained. Patients with significant perioperative morbidity who were not candidates for any surgical procedures, either laparoscopy or laparotomy, or who had significant metastatic disease involving chest or solid organs, such as liver, were excluded. The same board-certified gynecologist oncologist, assisted by a minimally invasive gynecological surgical fellow and resident performed the surgeries. Early stage disease included patients that were in stages I to II. This group also included patients referred for restaging after prior ovarian cystectomy or oophorectomy. Advanced disease was classified as International Federation of Gynecology and Obstetrics stages III to IV. Postoperative complications were graded using the Memorial Sloan-Kettering Cancer Center severity grading system [10].

Technique

Under general endotracheal anesthesia, the patients were positioned in dorsal lithotomy position, bilateral sequential compression devices were placed on both lower extremities and arms were padded and tucked. Egg crate foam was also placed across the chest to protect patients and they were secured to the operating table with tape or a gel pad underneath them. They were draped in a sterile manner, and given preoperative antibiotic prophylaxis with 1–2 g of cefazolin or 80 mg or gentamycin and 900 mg of clindamycin if they were allergic to penicillin. A Foley catheter was inserted into the bladder, and a uterine manipulator was placed if the uterus was in situ. An incision is made in either the left upper quadrant or 4–5 cm above the umbilicus, using a Veress needle to introduce carbon dioxide gas and establish pneumoperitoneum. After adequate pneumoperitoneum is obtained, a 5 or 8 mm primary port is inserted into the left upper quadrant. If pneumoperitoneum is established supraumbilically, then a 12-mm trocar and sleeve are introduced into the supraumbilical port. After assessing the abdominopelvic cavity, either a 10- or 12-mm port is introduced into the right upper quadrant or two 8-mm robotic ports are introduced 8–10 cm lateral to the umbilicus bilaterally (Fig. 1). Further peritoneal inspection is performed by conventional laparoscopy and peritoneal washings or aspiration of existing ascites are obtained and sent for cytology. Decision to proceed with laparoscopic/robotic-assisted surgical or laparotomy staging or debulking was made based on the extent of the disease and patients comorbidity for lengthy operation. In advanced stages, the goal was to achieve cytoreduction to preferably no visible or at least <1 cm disease either via robotic-assisted laparoscopy, conventional laparoscopy, or laparotomy.

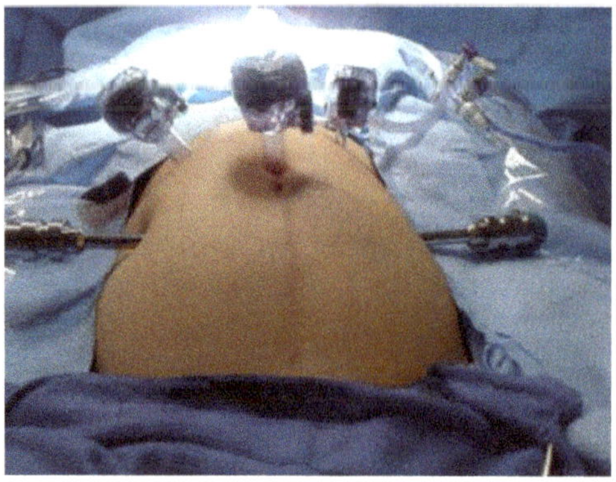

Fig. 1 Port placement

Thorough four-quadrant abdominopelvic cavity evaluation was performed by inserting additional ports, when necessary, to implement the choice of treatment. If surgical debulking to no visible disease is not possible, then biopsies are taken and salpingo-oophorectomy is performed if feasible [11, 12]. The procedure is terminated and the patient is given neoadjuvant chemotherapy to achieve higher rate of optimal cytoreductive surgery and decrease morbidity [13]. The patient is then reoperated on after reducing the load of the disease, which has been shown in randomized trials not to compromise oncological outcomes. Only patients in whom this hybrid technique was utilized were included in this study.

If disease is present in the upper abdomen and pelvis, surgery begins with conventional laparoscopy to perform an omentectomy and upper abdominal debulking (Fig. 2). This is performed via use of the supraumbilical port for the camera and ports for introduction of instruments. The surgeon stands between the patient's legs with two assistants on either side of the

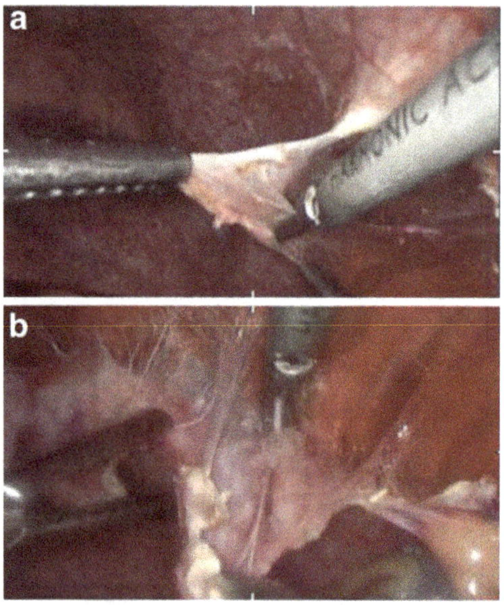

Fig. 2 **a** Diaphragmatic stripping of peritoneum with grasper and Harmonic scalpel (Ethicon Endosurgery, Cincinnati, OH, USA). **b** Diaphragmatic stripping showing stripped-away peritoneum and the underlying muscle fibers

patient and an additional monitor placed towards the patient's head. A combination of various conventional laparoscopic instruments such as the Harmonic shears, the 5- or 10-mm LigaSure™ (Covidien, Boulder, CO) or other blood vessel sealant devices including surgical clips and staples can be used. The infracolic omentum is transected from the transverse colon and the gastrocolic omentum is transected all the way towards the spleen and stomach by coagulating and transecting the short gastric vessels. The specimen(s) is removed confined to a laparoscopic bag. Metastatic lesions noted on the hepatic flexure or transverse colon are mobilized. Using a combination of Harmonic shears (Ethicon Endo-Surgery, Cincinnati, OH, USA), PlasmaJet (Plasma Surgical Limited, Oxfordshire, UK), and bipolar electrocoagulation, all diaphragmatic lesions are removed in the form of stripping, ablation, and coagulation (Fig. 2a,b). This same approach can be applied if there is no upper abdominal disease and only infracolic omentectomy is performed as part of surgical staging for presumed early ovarian cancer.

Any abdominal and pelvic adhesions which interfere with proper application of the robotic platform are lysed using conventional laparoscopy. After the upper abdominal portion is performed, the robotic apparatus is side docked on the patient's left side, using the supraumbilical port for the camera and the bilateral robotic 8-mm ports. The posterior parietal peritoneum over the right common iliac is incised and retroperitoneal dissection is completed cephalad to above inferior mesenteric artery. We use the electrosurgical spatula or scissors as a cutting modality and bipolar forceps for achieving hemostasis. The left and right upper assist ports are utilized for introduction of ancillary instruments for traction, tissue removal, as well as suction and irrigation. After para-aortic lymphadenectomy is completed, pelvic lymphadenectomy, hysterectomy, bilateral salpingo-oophorectomy, and any pelvic tumor debulking are performed (Fig. 3). The same

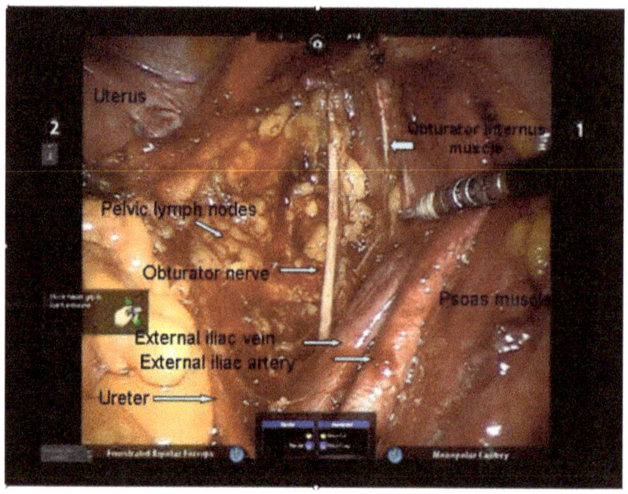

Fig. 3 Right pelvic sidewall exposing the iliac vessels and obturator fossa for robotic-assisted laparoscopic pelvic lymphadenectomy

instrumentation utilized is as before, or at times, standard blood vessel sealing devices such as the LigaSure(Covidien, Boulder, CO, USA), etc. can be employed for ligation of the infundibular ligaments and performing hysterectomy. If access to the para-aortic lymph nodes above the inferior–mesenteric artery is not possible using the robotic platform setup, this portion of the operation is performed using a conventional laparoscopic approach after undocking the robot or the camera is moved from supraumbilical port to the right upper quadrant one. After the uterus is transected, it is removed from the vagina along with the omentum and any other specimens, which are confined to a laparoscopic specimen bag. The vaginal cuff is closed in two layers. After complete hemostasis is achieved, the robotic apparatus is undocked.

Bowel resections can be performed with conventional laparoscopy and robotically using the appropriate port and robot placement. In case of the need for mid-abdominal debulking, such as appendectomy or ileocecal resection, mobilization of the bowel is performed using the robotic platform, and appendectomy or bowel resection is performed using a stapling device introduced in the right upper abdominal port. Anastomosis can be performed either in situ or extracorporeally by extending the supraumbilical incision after pelvic tumor debulking and undocking the robot. This approach can be utilized for segmental transverse colon resection and reanastomosis to achieve optimal cytoreduction to no visible disease. For rectosigmoid colon resection and anastomosis, we use a 12-mm port in the right lower abdomen for introduction of the stapling device. This is especially true for a bulky lesion involving the rectosigmoid colon. Using a laparoscopic 60 mm GIA stapler, a rectosigmoid resection can be performed proximally and distally. Once the proximal sigmoid colon is appropriately mobilized, this end can be brought out through a widened incision in the right lower quadrant, lower middle incision, or transvaginally along with the specimen. An anvil can then be placed and secured with a purse string suture. The anvil and proximal sigmoid colon is then brought back into the pelvis and an end-to-end anastomosis can be performed with an end-to-end anastomosis stapler passed through the rectum. Once the device is properly activated, it is important to test the integrity of the anastomosis. This can be accomplished by clamping the proximal colon with a bowel grasper, filling the pelvis with saline, and insufflating the rectum with air while observing laparoscopically. The anastomosis can be alternatively or additionally examined by filling the rectum with indigo carmine and observing for leakage. Cystoscopy is routinely performed to ensure that there is no damage to the bladder or ureters. Ports are removed and port sites are closed in a routine manner.

In the case of recurrences that occur primarily in the upper abdomen, debulking can be performed with the robotic apparatus. In this situation, after exploratory laparoscopy and peritoneal washings are performed using conventional laparoscopy, the robot is side docked from above the patient on the right side using the same port placement as above (Fig. 1) and instrumentation is as described previously.

Results

There were 20 women that underwent 21 surgical procedures for the management of early, advanced, and recurrent ovarian, fallopian tube, or peritoneal cancer using our hybrid technique of conventional laparoscopy and RALS. There were 10 surgical procedures performed for early stage disease and 11 for advanced and/or recurrent disease (six advanced and five recurrent). The early group consisted of three cases that were stage IA (Table 1; cases 1–3), six that were stage IC (Table 1; cases 4–9), and one case that was stage IIC (Table 1, case 10). The advanced and recurrent group consisted of seven cases that were advanced, with six cases that were stage IIIC (Table 2: cases 1,2,3,5,7 and 11), one case that was stage IV (Table 2: case 4). The remainder in this group had recurrent disease (Table 2: cases 6,8,9, 10). There were no conversions to laparotomy in either group.

Of the 10 surgeries for early stage disease, the mean age was 42.3 years (range, 29–55), average BMI was 32.1 kg/m^2 (range, 17–65 kg/m^2), average estimated blood loss (EBL) was 212.5 ml (range, 50–1,000 mL), surgical time was 306.1 min (range, 87–639), and average length of stay (LOS) was 1.6 days (range, 1–2). In this group, the surgical procedures performed included five hysterectomies, eight oophorectomies, one cystectomy, eight omentectomies, five pelvic lymph node dissections (average, 10.3; range, 5–18), four para-aortic lymph node dissections (average, 8.6; range, 3–12), four appendectomies, and seven upper abdominal and diaphragmatic biopsies. None of these patients were upstaged after surgical and pathological staging.

There were no intraoperative complications or intraoperative transfusions, and two grade 1 postoperative complications. One patient was readmitted on postoperative day 9 with a wound infection. The other was readmitted with fever of unknown origin that resolved with IV antibiotics.

Three patients in this group underwent fertility sparing surgery (Table 1; cases 6, 8, and 9) [14]. In the first case listed (Table 1), the para-aortic lymphadenectomy was performed laparoscopically as there was difficulty with adequate visualization when the robotic apparatus was docked. Four patients in the early ovarian cancer group had prior surgical intervention and presented for restaging (Table 1; cases 3, 5, 8, and 9). Two patients in this group did not have an omentectomy (Table 1; cases 2 and 6). Case 2 was a double primary that was initially staged for endometrial cancer with final pathology that showed ovarian cancer as a second primary. Case 6 presented for restaging, after prior left salpingo-oophorectomy and staging.

Table 1 Early stage ovarian cancer cases

Case	Age	BMI	Procedure: Laparoscopic	Procedure: Robotic	Pathology	EBL	ORT	LOS	Complications
1	52	17	Infracolic omentectomy, para-aortic lymphadenectomy, diaphragmatic biopsy, right upper abdominal peritoneal biopsy, peritoneal washings	LAVH, left oophorectomy, pelvic lymphadenectomy, appendectomy, peritoneal biopsies	Grade 3 serous carcinoma of the fallopian tube	200	n/a	2	None
2	53	21	Exploratory laparoscopy, peritoneal washings	Pelvic and para-aortic lymphadenectomy, hysterectomy, BSO	Grade 3 endometrioid adenocarcinoma of the ovary	150	366	2	None
3	54	40	Infracolic omentectomy, peritoneal biopsies, diaphragmatic biopsy and upper abdominal peritoneal biopsies, peritoneal washings	Lysis of extensive small bowel and pelvic adhesions, bilateral pelvic lymphadenectomy, peritoneal biopsies, total hysterectomy	Grade 3 serous carcinoma of the ovary	150	361	2	Admission on POD#21 for FUO
4	38	25	Infracolic omentectomy, appendectomy, upper abdominal peritoneal biopsies, peritoneal washings	Para-aortic lymphadenectomy, pelvic lymphadenectomy, hysterectomy, LSO, peritoneal biopsies	Mucinous low malignant potential tumor of the ovary	100	338	2	Wound infection
5	55	27	Upper abdominal peritoneal biopsies, peritoneal washings	Infracolic omentectomy, hysterectomy, LSO	Serous low malignant potential tumor of the ovary	50	178	1	None
6	34	23	Upper abdominal biopsies, peritoneal washings	Pelvic and para-aortic lymphadenectomy, RSO, peritoneal biopsies, lysis of pelvic adhesions	Grade 3 mucinous adenocarcinoma of the ovary	125	271	1	None
7	30	53	Infracolic omentectomy, peritoneal washings	Right ovarian cystectomy, resection of pelvic endometriosis, appendectomy, myomectomy, peritoneal biopsies	Serous low malignant potential tumor of the ovary	50	87	1	None
8	29	22	Infracolic omentectomy, resection of diaphragmatic lesions, peritoneal biopsies, peritoneal washings	Resection of pelvic lesions, LSO, peritoneal biopsies, LOA	Grade 2 immature ovarian teratoma	200	172	1	None
9	31	28	Infracolic omentectomy, diaphragmatic biopsies, upper abdominal peritoneal biopsies, peritoneal washings	LSO, resection of pelvic lesions and endometriosis, pelvic and para-aortic lymphadenectomy, peritoneal biopsies, LOA	Grade 2 endometrioid adenocarcinoma of the ovary	100	343	1	None
10	47	65	Infracolic omentectomy	Radical hysterectomy, BSO, tumor debulking, resection of endometriosis, appendectomy, peritoneal biopsies, , extensive LOA	Grade 1 endometrioid adenocarcinoma of the ovary	1000	639	3	None

BMI body mass index, *EBL* estimated blood loss, *ORT* operating room time, *LOS* length of stay, *LAVH* laparoscopic-assisted vaginal hysterectomy, *BSO* bilateral salpingo-oophorectomy, *LSO* left salpingo-oophorectomy, *D&C* dilation and curettage, *POD* postoperative day, *LOA* lysis of adhesions

Table 2 Advanced and recurrent ovarian cancer cases

Case	Age	BMI	Disease status	Procedure: Laparoscopic	Procedure: Robotic	Procedure: Other	Pathology	Status of cytoreduction	EBL	ORT	LOS	Complications
1	92	24.7	Advanced	Total omentectomy, lysis of extensive adhesions, enterolysis	Hysterectomy, BSO, pelvic tumor debulking	Cystoscopy	Grade 3 serous carcinoma of the fallopian tube	Optimal to no visible disease	200	362	2	None
2	54	37.2	Advanced	Total omentectomy, lysis of pelvic and upper abdominal adhesions	Hysterectomy, BSO, resection of pelvic implants	Cystoscopy	Grade 3 serous carcinoma, primary peritoneal	Optimal to no visible disease	100	306	2	None
3	50	36.2	Advanced	Total omentectomy, upper abdominal tumor debulking including tumor of hepatic flexure, and transverse colon, diaphragmatic stripping and ablation, appendectomy	Hysterectomy, BSO, pelvic tumor debulking, metastatic lymph node debulking	Cystoscopy, sigmoidoscopy	Grade 3 serous carcinoma of the ovary	Optimal to no visible disease	20	103	3	None
4	75	29.3	Advanced	Total omentectomy, diaphragmatic biopsy	Hysterectomy, BSO, resection of pelvic tumor metastasis, anterior and posterior cul de sac tumor debulking and culdectomy, resection of rectal tumor	Cystoscopy, sigmoidoscopy, inguinal lymph node dissection	Grade 3 serous carcinoma of the ovary	Optimal to no visible disease	400	477	6	None
5	70	27	Advanced	Supracolic omentectomy, upper abdominal and diaphragmatic debulking	Tumor debulking of anterior cul-de-sac and rectosigmoid, hysterectomy, LOA, enterolysis, peritoneal biopsies	Cystoscopy sling procedure	Grade 3 serous carcinoma of the ovary	Optimal to no visible disease	150	454	17	Bowel perforation
6	55	29.1	Recurrent	Aspiration of ascites, lysis of adhesions, enterolysis	Appendectomy, para-aortic lymphadenectomy, tumor debulking		Grade 3 clear cell carcinoma of the ovary	Optimal to no visible disease	100	252	1	None
7	53	32.9	Recurrent	Diaphragmatic biopsy (second look)	Pelvic and para-aortic lymphadenectomy, lysis of adhesions, peritoneal biopsies.	Cystoscopy	Grade 3 serous carcinoma of the ovary	N/A	100	226	2	None
8	39	25	Recurrent	Peritoneal biopsies, diaphragmatic biopsy, aspiration of ascites, upper abdominal tumor and diaphragmatic tumor debulking	Pelvic tumor debulking, lysis of adhesions.	Cystoscopy, sigmoidoscopy, insertion of IP port	Grade 1 mucinous adenocarcinoma of the ovary	Optimal to less than 0.5 cm	100	317	3	port-site cellulitis, peritoneal vaginal fistula

Table 2 (continued)

Case	Age	BMI	Disease status	Procedure: Laparoscopic	Procedure: Robotic	Procedure: Other	Pathology	Status of cytoreduction	EBL	ORT	LOS	Complications
9	70	35.4	Recurrent	Omentectomy, appendectomy	Lysis of extensive pelvic adhesions, upper vaginectomy, pelvic tumor debulking, peritoneal biopsies	Cystoscopy	Grade 3 serous carcinoma of the ovary	Optimal to no visible disease	100	212	1	None
10	63	27.5	Recurrent	Lysis of severe upper abdominal adhesions, resection of porta hepatis mass, cholecystectomy, supracolic omentectomy	Pelvic and para-aortic lymphadenectomy, lysis of adhesions, peritoneal biopsies	Cystoscopy	Grade 3 serous carcinoma of the ovary	Optimal to no visible disease	50	322	3	None
11	82	22.1	Advanced	Infracolic omentectomy	Hysterectomy, BSO, bilateral pelvic lymphadenectomy, appendectomy	Cystoscopy	Grade 3 serous carcinoma of the ovary	Optimal to no visible disease	100	238	2	None

BMI body mass index, *EBL* estimated blood loss, *ORT* operating room time, *LOS* length of stay, *BSO* bilateral salpingo-oopherectomy, *IP port* intraperitoneal port, *FIGO* International Federation of Gynecology and Obstetrics

Among the 11 cases operated for advanced and/or recurrent ovarian cancer, the mean age was 63.9 years (range, 39–92), average BMI was 29.7 kg/m^2 (range, 22.1–37.2), EBL was 129.1 ml (range, 20–400), operating room time was 238 min (range, 103–477), and LOS was 3.8 days (range, 1–17). In this group, surgical procedures consisted of six hysterectomies, five oophorectomies, eight omentectomies, three pelvic lymph node dissections (average, 10.7; range, 4–18), three para-aortic lymph node dissections (average, 5; range, 1–9), four appendectomies, five diaphragmatic biopsies, four upper abdominal debulking or diaphragmatic debulking, and one resection of a porta hepatis mass (Table 2; case 10; Fig. 4). Five patients had received neoadjuvant chemotherapy (Table 2; cases 2, 3, 4, 5, and 11). Of the 11 procedures, there was one second look (Table 2, case 7), 9 were cytoreduced to no visible disease and 1 to less than <0.5 cm. There were no intraoperative complications.

There were three postoperative complications; two were grade 1 and one was grade 3. Two complications (both grade 1) occurred in the same patient; one being port-site cellulitis and the other a peritoneal vaginal fistula. Both were managed conservatively with antibiotic therapy and observation. The peritoneal vaginal fistula was revealed by leakage of peritoneal ascites. The other patient was reoperated on postoperative day 3 for a sigmoid colon perforation which required reoperation and was discharged home on day 17 (Table 2; case 5). This case was the only Intensive Care Unit admission in both early and advanced groups.

Of all the patients operated on, there were no trocar site metastases within the follow-up period. However, one patient developed trocar metastasis beyond 30 days postoperatively and had recurrent intraperitoneal disease.

Discussion

Laparoscopy offers multiple advantages over laparotomy such as better visualization, smaller incisions, shorter hospital

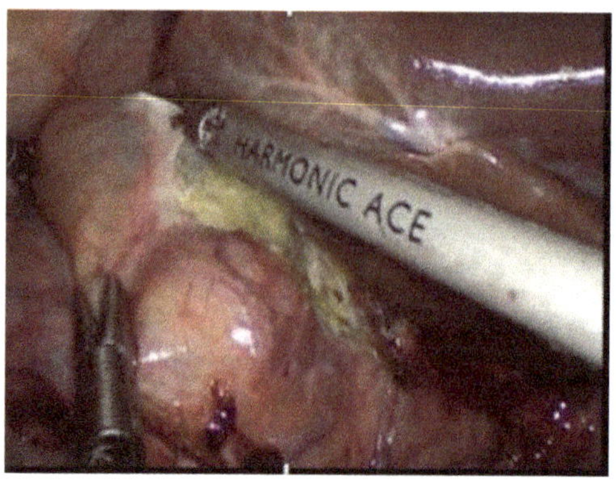

Fig. 4 Porta hepatis mass attached to the gallbladder that has been resected laparoscopically, with cholecystectomy

stays, decreased blood loss, less need for analgesics, more rapid recovery, and shorter interval to chemotherapy and radiation when indicated. In the assessment of an adnexal mass and early-stage ovarian cancer, laparoscopy can be both diagnostic and therapeutic. The combination of laparoscopic visualization and frozen section analysis is the most reliable method for the detection of malignancy [15]. Once malignancy is diagnosed, comprehensive surgical staging can be performed laparoscopically, which has been shown to be feasible, safe, and accurate in tumors of low malignant potential and invasive early-stage disease [16–19]. Furthermore, in select cases of localized disease, it can be used to perform fertility-sparing surgical staging [14].

Minimally invasive surgery has emerged as an option in the management of advanced or recurrent ovarian cancer with multiple applications that have been presented in the literature [5, 20–22]. This includes a triage tool for resectability, primary and secondary cytoreduction, second-look evaluation, and placement of intraperitoneal catheters for chemotherapy [23].

In the early 1990s, the pioneers of laparoscopic surgery applied minimally invasive surgical techniques to gynecologic cancers for the staging of early and select cases of advanced or recurrent ovarian cancer cytoreduction [24, 25]. Since that time, the role of minimally invasive surgery in gynecologic oncology has been continuously expanding and has even been further applied to other disease sites in the female genital tract.

The advent of computer enhanced telesurgery or robotic-assisted surgery has seemingly presented itself as a new alternative to conventional laparoscopy. It offers the benefits of improving the learning curve associated with conventional laparoscopy, and other additional features, such as optimal visualization and a wider range of motion for more precise surgical manipulation. Yet, this innovation currently presents with limitations in the surgical management of patients with malignancy. Conventional laparoscopy offers a better understanding of the status of the disease, while robotic-assisted laparoscopy presents as an innovation in offering precise surgical motion and visualization of the disease process. However, this comes at the cost of some key elements required with surgical management, which are possible with conventional laparoscopy.

One such limitation is the lack of haptics, which may lead to missing tumor entirely or the ability to discern between normal tissue and tissue that is involved with carcinoma. Further limitations are in accessing all four abdominal quadrants simultaneously in one surgical setting and completing comprehensive surgical evaluation and treatment for patients with ovarian malignancy. This hybrid technique is presented to overcome these challenges, and the limited manipulation that exists with robotic-assisted surgery with the current platform. This is particularly true with limitations encountered when manipulating bulky tumor and tissue, such as that of the rectosigmoid with the present robotic platform and instruments.

The hybrid technique described offers advantages that are inherent to conventional laparoscopy for management of ovarian cancer. One limitation is the need for a second setup of a conventional laparoscopy in addition to the robotic platform. In our experience, it is customary to use this setup as an adjunct to robotic-assisted surgery. Conventional laparoscopy is used for port placement, in preparation of robotic-assisted laparoscopic surgery, thus making this setup not an additional component. Thus, using this method offers an extension of the use of conventional laparoscopy, while retaining the same port setup for pelvic surgery and utilizing conventional laparoscopy to operate cephalad to the pelvis.

Another inherent benefit is that conventional laparoscopy can also be used as an initial checkpoint in triaging for resectability based on the extent of disease and surgeon experience with robotic-assisted surgery versus other conventional methods. The conventional laparoscopy setup can also be further utilized after completion of robotic-assisted surgery to survey the abdomen and pelvis for any potential injury caused by the robotic instruments not detected due to the blind spot of the robotic camera and lack of haptics. Studies are lacking with innovative methods or strategies to counter this limitation of upper abdominal access with pelvic surgery when using the robotic platform. With advanced laparoscopic skills, this method facilitates the limitations of the robotic platform. An added advantage of using this method is enhanced visualization of surgical planes that require fine dissection in the pelvis due to prior surgery or disease involvement in the pelvis. In the upper abdomen, conventional laparoscopic methods can be utilized for limited disease, with this as the initial portion of the surgery, thus reducing surgeon fatigue (of the primary surgeon).

This technique also extends to novice surgeons who are aided by tactile feedback that conventional laparoscopy extends. However, it has its limitations in more challenging skills that are more easily afforded with robotic assistance (i.e., suturing, controlling bleeding, etc.). In comparison to other described techniques for accessing the upper abdomen, this method is less cumbersome and can be used in settings with residency and fellowship training programs that have bedside assistants who are less experienced. One complication reported with use of the alternate technique of placing the robot tower at the patient's head was conversion to laparotomy in order to access bleeding from the descending branch of the inferior mesenteric artery that could not be reached by the bedside assistant or the surgeon [9]. The access afforded in operating cephalad with use of this technique is not hindered in our experience. This technique has widespread application for use, and is versatile with the level of experience required by surgical assistants.

Minimally invasive surgical staging, more specifically cytoreductive surgery, are time-consuming procedures that are associated with surgeon fatigue that ensues with the course of the procedure. This method offers the benefit of conventional laparoscopy at the beginning of the case followed by the robotic-assisted portion of the procedure, which can help in the reduction of surgeon fatigue during the course of these lengthy procedures. This is an added benefit when the skill of an expert laparoscopist is needed for challenging initial portions of the procedure in the upper abdomen and then for more difficult portions with pelvic disease site affection in the latter portion of the procedure.

One issue that has to be addressed is the cost-effectiveness of the initial investment in the robotic platform relative to the cost of performing laparotomy, conventional laparoscopy, or robotic hybrid technique. Although only well-designed randomized studies will be able to adequately address this issue, presently, it is rather difficult to establish such a study in early and advanced ovarian cancer. In Wright et al. [26], the cost of robotic-assisted radical hysterectomy was least expensive comparative to laparotomy and even laparoscopy, due to shorter hospital stay. We believe that the use of this modality will allow more patients to be managed by a minimally invasive approach and thus reduce the number of laparotomies.

In summary, minimally invasive surgical techniques are consistently furthered from conventional laparoscopy to computer-enhanced telesurgery (also known as robotic surgery), and eventually to more compact devices that provide greater surgical precision with versatility in accessing all four abdominal quadrants more readily. Our technique serves as an interim improvisation to counter the limitations that exist with the present robotic platform.

Successful maximum cytoreductive interperitoneal metastatic disease in advanced ovarian cancer has been associated with the best outcomes [23]. However, this technique is not always possible and it carries significant morbidity. In randomized clinical trials, neoadjuvant chemotherapy followed by cytoreductive surgery has been shown much more effective in decreasing morbidity without compromising oncological outcomes [13]. Another benefit of neoadjuvant chemotherapy is that by reducing the bulky tumor, the chance of achieving optimal cytoreductive surgery by minimally invasive approach is greatly increased.

It has been our experience that using this hybrid technique, of a combination of conventional laparoscopy and the present robotic platform has been effective in the management of early, advanced, and recurrent ovarian, fallopian tube and peritoneal cancer while gaining the advantages of both technical approaches.

Conflict of interest The authors declare that there are no conflicts of interest.

References

1. Sternchos J, Finger T, Mahdavi A, Nezhat F (2013) Laparoscopic management of ovarian, fallopian tube and primary peritoneal cancer. In: Nezhat C, Nezhat F, Nezhat C (eds) Nezhat's video-assisted and robotic-assisted laparoscopy and hysteroscopy, 4th edn. Cambridge University Press, Cambridge, pp 508–525
2. Nezhat FR, Shoma D, Liu C, Chuang L, Zakashansky K (2008) Robotic radical hysterectomy versus total laparoscopic radical hysterectomy with pelvic lymphadenectomy for treatment of early cervical cancer. JSLS 12:227–237
3. Cho JE, Nezhat FR (2009) Robotics and gynecologic oncology: review of the literature. J Minim Invasive Gynecol 16(6): 669–681
4. Lim PC, Kang E, Park DH (2011) A comparative detail analysis of the learning curve and surgical outcome for robotic hysterectomy with lymphadenectomy versus laparoscopic hysterectomy with lymphadenectomy in treatment of endometrial cancer: a case-matched controlled study of the first one hundred twenty-two patients. Gynecol Oncol 120:413–418
5. Magrina JF, Zanagnolo V, Noble BN et al (2011) Robotic approach for ovarian cancer: perioperative and survival results and comparison with laparoscopy and laparotomy. Gynecol Oncol 121(1):100–105
6. Ramirez PT, Adams S, Boggess JF, Burke WM, Frumovitz MM, Gardner GJ, Havrilesky LJ, Holloway R, Lowe MP, Magrina JF, Moore DH, Soliman PT, Yap S (2012) Robotic-assisted surgery in gynecologic oncology: a Society of Gynecologic Oncology consensus statement. Developed by the Society of Gynecologic Oncology's Clinical Practice Robotics Task Force. Gynecol Oncol 124(2):180–184
7. Siegel R, Deepa N, Ahmedin AJ (2012) Cancer statistics 2012. Cancer J 62(10):10–29
8. Katz VL, Lentz GM, Lobo RA, Gershenson DM (2007) Comprehensive gynecology, 5th edn. Elsevier, Philadelphia
9. Magrina JF, Long JB, Kho RM et al (2010) Robotic transperitoneal infrarenal aortic lymphadenectomy. Int J Gynecol Cancer 20(1):184–187
10. Dindo D, Demartines N, Clavien PA (2004) Classification of surgical complications: a new proposal with evaluation in a cohort of a 6336 patients and results of a survey. Ann Surg 240: 205–213
11. Nezhat FR, Denoble SM, Cho JE, Brown DN, Soto E, Chuang L, Gretz H, Saharia P (2012) The safety and efficacy of video laparoscopic surgical debulking of recurrent ovarian, fallopian tube, and primary peritoneal cancers. JSLS 16:511–518
12. Nezhat FR, DeNoble SM, Liu CS, Cho JE, Brown DN, Chuang L, Gretz H, Saharia P (2010) The safety and efficacy of laparoscopic surgical staging and debulking of apparent advanced stage ovarian, fallopian tube, and primary peritoneal cancers. JSLS 14: 155–168
13. Vergote I, Tropè C, Amant F et al (2010) Neoadjuvant chemotherapy or primary surgery in stage IIIC and IV ovarian cancer. N Engl J Med 363:943–953
14. Finger T, Nezhat F (2013) Robotic-assisted fertility sparing surgery for early ovarian cancer. JSLS (in press)
15. Nezhat F, Nezhat C, Welander CE, Benigno B (1992) Four ovarian cancers diagnosed during laparoscopic management of 1011 women with adnexal masses. Am J Obstet Gynecol 167: 790–796
16. Liu CS, Nagarsheth NP, Nezhat FR (2009) Laparoscopy and ovarian cancer: a paradigm change in the management of ovarian cancer? J Min Inv Gynecol 16(3):250–262

17. Park JY, Bae J, Lim MC, Lim SY, Seo SS, Kang S et al (2008) Laparoscopic and laparotomic staging in stage I epithelial ovarian cancer: a comparison of feasibility and safety. Int J Gynecol Cancer 18:1202–1209
18. Tozzi R, Kohler C, Ferrara A, Schneider A (2004) Laparoscopic treatment of early ovarian cancer: surgical and survival outcomes. Gynecol Oncol 93:199–203
19. Nezhat FR, Ezzati M, Chuang L, Shamshirsaz AA, Rahaman J, Gretz H (2009) Laparoscopic management of early ovarian and fallopian tube cancers: surgical and survival outcome. Am J Obstet Gynecol 200(1):e1–e6
20. Nezhat FR, Datta MS, Lal N (2008) Laparoscopic cytoreduction for primary advanced or recurrent ovarian, fallopian tube, and peritoneal malignancies. Gynecol Oncol 108:S60
21. Fanning J, Yacoub E, Hojat R (2011) Laparoscopic-assisted cytoreduction for primary ovarian cancer: success, morbidity and survival. Gynecol Oncol 123:47–49
22. Krivak TC, Elkas JC, Rose GS, Sundborg M, Winter WE, Carlson J, MacKoul PJ (2005) The utility of hand-assisted laparoscopy in ovarian cancer. Gynecol Oncol 96:72–76
23. Nezhat F, Lavie O (2013) The role of minimally invasive surgery in ovarian cancer. Int J Gynecol Cancer 23(5):782–783
24. Querleu D, Leblanc E (1994) Laparoscopic infrarenal para-aortic lymph node dissection for restaging of carcinoma of the ovary or fallopian tube. Cancer 73:1467–1471
25. Amara DP, Nezhat C, Teng N, Nezhat F, Nezhat C, Rosati M (1996) Operative laparoscopy in the management of ovarian cancer. Surg Laparoscop Endosc 6:38–45
26. Wright JD, Herzog TJ, Neugut AI et al (2012) Comparative effectiveness of minimally invasive and abdominal radical hysterectomy for cervical cancer. Gynecol Oncol 127:11–17

Lipomesosalpinx: a rare possible missed tubal factor of infertility

Atef Darwish

Abstract This study aims to estimate the proportion of significant mesosalpingeal adipose tissue condensation (lipomesosalpinx, at least of a caliber similar to the ampulla of the ipsilateral tube regardless of well-defined or poorly defined margins) among infertile women subjected to diagnostic laparoscopy. This study is a cross-sectional study set at a specialized endoscopic center. All infertile women scheduled for diagnostic/therapeutic laparoscopy during the period between July 1994 and December 2012 was included in this study. Interventions used were preoperative hysterosalpingography, transvaginal ultrasonography, as well as body mass index for all cases. Laparoscopic documentation of a significant mesosalpingeal condensation of adipose tissue as well as histopathologic assessment of the adipose tissues in some cases was observed. The main outcome measures included number of cases with unilateral or bilateral lipomesosalpinx. Significant lipomesosalpinx was diagnosed in 145 (5.7 %) out of 2,563 cases examined by laparoscopy. In all but seven cases, lipomesosalpinx was seen bilaterally (99.7 %). There was insignificant correlation between those cases and high body mass index when compared to the rest of the cases. Infertility was unexplained by laparoscopy in 621 cases (24.3 %) while laparoscopy diagnosed etiologic factors in 1, 942 (75.7 %) cases. Lipomesosalpinx was seen in 46 (7.4 %) and 79 (3.9 %) of the unexplained and explained cases, respectively, without a statistically significant difference ($P-0.48$). Despite being a rare laparoscopic finding, significant lipomesosalpinx should be reported and documented as a possible missed tubal factor of infertility. Whether to treat lipomesosalpinx or not, bilaterally or unilaterally and by which means, require further studies with proper second-look laparoscopy.

A. Darwish
Woman's Health University Center, Assiut University, Assiut, Egypt

A. Darwish (✉)
Department of Obstetrics & Gynecology, Woman's Health University Hospital, 71111 AssiutP.O. Box: (1)Assiut, Egypt
e-mail: atef_darwish@yahoo.com

Keywords Lipomesosalpnix · Laparoscopy · Infertility · Tubal factor

Introduction

There is a general consensus among gynecologists that tubal patency at hysterosalpingography (HSG) is quite assuring about tubal factor and they proceed to investigate other factors or advise patients to try assisted reproduction. Actually, the fallopian tube is a complex paired organ, not a simple tubing. The classic tubal factors include post-inflammatory peritubal adhesions and prominal or diatal tubal occlusion [1] which can be easily diagnosed by most gynecologists based on HSG. Other rare tubal diseases are seldom investigated. For instance, salpingitis isthmica nodosa which is a nodular swelling of the isthmic segment of the fallopian tube are rarely reported [2]. Anatomically, mesosalpinx is defined as the part of the broad ligament enclosing a fallopian tube forming its mesentery. Histologically, it is formed of a thin layer of squamous epithelium and a small amount of loose areolar connective tissue [3, 4]. It contains sympathetic ganglia and plexuses [5]. Laparoscopically, mesosalpinx is a thin vascular layer without evident fat in most cases.

Unexplained infertility is a real challenge for gynecologists. It is idiopathic in the sense that its cause remains unknown even after an infertility work-up, usually including semen analysis in the man and assessment of ovulation and fallopian tubes in the woman [6]. In Assiut, we believe that diagnostic laparoscopy is an integral step of the diagnostic work-up of any infertile couple before saying the term "unexplained". With time, interest to discover minute lesions that may affect fertility increased at our institution [7]. In practice, we observe some fatty tissue condensation in the mesosalpinx in some cases that deserve studying why it is present in some women. To make this study valuable, we considered mesosalpingeal adipose tissue significant if its caliber was at least similar or exceeds the caliber of the ampulla of the ipsilateral fallopian tube regardless of the appearance of its borders. The tested hypothesis is a significant lipomesosalpinx that would hinder tubal motility and would be a cause of infertility. This study aims to estimate the proportion of significant mesosalpingeal adipose tissue condensation (lipomesosalpinx) among infertile women subjected to diagnostic/operative laparoscopy.

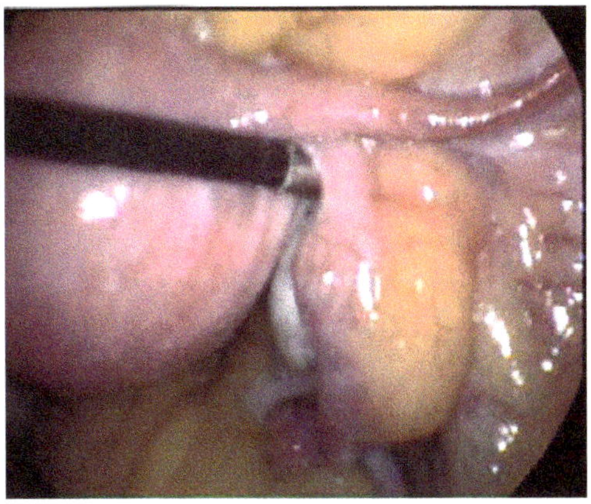

Fig. 1 Laparoscopic appearance of lipomesosalpinx

Patients and methods

This study was conducted between July 1996 and December 2012 at the Endoscopic Unit of the Woman's Health University Hospital, Assiut University, Egypt. It was approved by the institutional review board (IRB) of the Faculty of Medicine. All patients gave a clear written consent to participate in this study. It prospectively comprised 2,563 infertile patients submitted to video-assisted laparoscopy for diagnostic or operative purposes (Table 1). Preoperative metric body mass index (BMI) estimation and transvaginal ultrasonography (TVS) were done as a routine for all of the cases. Metric BMI is calculated as weight in kilograms divided by height in meters squared. Meticulous evaluation of HSG was made to identify tubal shape and patency whenever available. At laparoscopy, a thorough visualization of the mesosalpinx for evidence of adipose tissue condensation was reported. We considered mesosalpingeal adipose tissue significant if its caliber was at least similar or exceeds the caliber of the ampulla of the ipsilateral fallopian tube (Fig. 1). In all cases, using tubal chromopertubation, tubal patency was assessed and the relationship of the mass to the tubal lumen was recorded. Moreover, observation of the range of mobility of the tubes to the Douglas pouch was reported.

Table 1 Laparoscopic procedure for 2,563 cases

Laparoscopic finding	No (%)
Diagnostic (normal findings)	621 (24.3)
Operative (abnormal findings)	1942 (75.7)
Ovarian drilling for polycystic ovaries	523 (20.4)
Salpingectomy for hydrosalpinx	165 (6.4)
Oophorectomy for a benign ovarian mass	46 (1.7)
Adhesiolysis	344 (13.4)
Cystectomy of ovarian cyst	298 (11.6)
Myomectomy	29 (1.1)
Miscellaneous	587 (22.9)

More one than procedure was required in 50 cases

Based on the recommendations of the IRB, only unilateral excision or lysis of significant lipomesosalpinx was performed even if it was seen bilaterally in an otherwise normal genital tract anatomy at laparoscopy. Since it is a preliminary study, ethics recommended if any intervention should be unilateral until clear results of better bilateral excision of lipomesosalpinx with second-look laparoscopies. The side of the tube that will be operated upon was recorded. If this fatty condensation is pedunculated, it was excised with a bipolar scissors. If nonpedunculated but localized, a small microsurgical incision of the mesosalpinx was made followed by extraction of the adipose tissue with a fine-grasping forceps. The mesosalpingeal defect was then coagulated with bipolar forceps. Sutures or monopolar diathermy were not used in any case to minimize the risk of peritubal adhesions or tubal damage. On the other hand, if the adipose tissue mass was diffuse and ill-defined, it was coagulated as far as possible from the fallopian tube utilizing a 3-mm bipolar needle till complete melting of the adipose tissue. In most cases, histopathologic examination of the adipose tissue biopsy (Fig. 2) was done.

Copious peritoneal washing was done followed by leaving about 1 L of lactated Ringer's solution intraperitoneally. All the laparoscopic findings were correlated with the preoperative TVS findings. The X^2 test was used to compare the studied groups. For each comparison, $P>0.05$ was considered not significant, while $P\leq 0.05$ was considered significant.

Results

This study included 2,563 infertile patients submitted to diagnostic or operative laparoscopy (Table 1). They were in the child-bearing period with a mean age of 24.5 years and mean parity of 1. Preoperatively, TVS was done for all cases that failed to detect any paraovarian echogenic condensation in all cases. Body mass index was calculated for all cases. Its mean was 29.4 with statistically insignificant correlation to lipomesossalpinx ($P=0.12$). Significant lipomesosalpinx

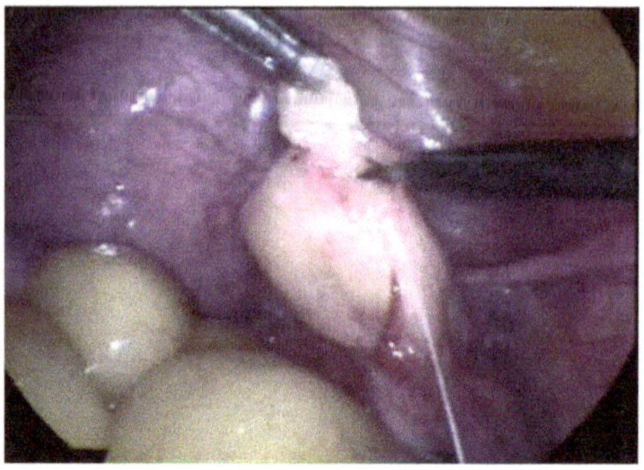

Fig. 2 Biopsy taking of lipomesosalpinx

was diagnosed in 145 cases (5.7 %). In all but seven cases, lipomesosalpinx was diagnosed bilaterally (99.7 %). Infertility was unexplained by laparoscopy in 621 cases (24.3 %) while the cause of infertility could be explained in 1,942 (75.7 %) of the cases. Lipomesosalpinx was diagnosed in 46 cases (7.4 %) and 79 (3.9 %) in both groups respectively without statistically significant difference (P=0.48). Biopsy of lipomesosalpinx revealed a normal adipose tissue in all cases. Surgical management of lipomesosalpinx was done, but data were excluded according to the aim of this study.

Discussion

Tubal factor infertility accounts for nearly one quarter of all cases of infertility [8]. The fallopian tubes may be abnormal in structure or function. Structural disorders can block the fallopian tubes. They include tubal scarring or blockage most commonly from pelvic infections, prior abdominal surgeries, and endometriosis. Practically, many gynecologists are reluctant when reporting on diagnostic laparoscopy. Some perform a single-puncture intraumbilical procedure that neglects an auxiliary portal for proper grasping of the adnexa and thorough evaluation of the ovarian fossa. Most of them comment on tubal patency only and neglect tubal morphology, size, length, and proximity to the pouch of Douglas. Rarely, they comment on the mesosalpinx and Wolffian duct remnants. This study directs attention towards more concentration on some factors that would affect tubal motility and commonly missed by gynecologists. Previously, some authors reported on hydatid of Morgagni as a cause of unexplained infertility (UI) [9]. Likewise, an old study diagnosed fimbrial agglutinations (25 %), accessory tubes (13 %), accessory ostia (10 %), phimoses (13 %), and sacculations (7 %) more in the infertile women [10]. Tubal abnormalities would affect the prognosis of natural pregnancy as well as laparoscopic gamete intrafallopian transfer [11]. At our institution, we consider tubal sacculations, diverticulae, convolutions, phimosis, or fimbrial agglutination as laparoscopic criteria of subtle tubal endometriosis specially if seen with other typical or atypical endometriotic tubal or peritoneal lesions. Proper endoscopic training would eliminate all these mistakes that would affect diagnosis as well as therapy.

Mesosalpingeal lesions include paratubal cyst [7], leiomyosarcoma of the broad ligament [12], choristoma of the heterotopic adrenal tissue [13], primary fallopian tube carcinoma [14], or lipoma of the broad ligament [15]. Preciously, among 1,853 cases subjected to laparoscopy, we succeeded to diagnose a paratubal or paraovarian cyst in 118 patients (15.7 %) [7]. Fat condensation in the mesosalpinx is not described in textbooks on histology, pathology, or even endoscopic surgery as far as I know. Due to our interest in missed factors of infertility, we tried to study the clinical significance of lipomesosalpinx. To be practical, we excluded cases with small amounts of adipose tissue that would not be expected to affect tubal motility. In this study, preoperative TVS failed to diagnose lipomesosalpinx in all cases. Fallopian tubes are not usually visualized on a routine transvaginal sonographic examination unless outlined by fluid. However, the interstitial segment may be identified on TVS as an echogenic line arising from the endometrial canal and extending through the uterine wall. When surrounded by intraperitoneal fluid, the remaining segments of the fallopian tubes are commonly seen as tubular structures extending between the uterus and the ovaries. Fallopian tubes are best visualized on sonography when thickened or fluid-filled as a result of pelvic inflammatory disease, torsion, ectopic pregnancy, or tumors [15]. Nevertheless, we still recommend performing TVS routinely prior to laparoscopy to detect important findings like paraovarian cysts [7] and more importantly intrauterine lesions that would make concomitant hysteroscopy a mandatory step.

Despite similarity of the histopathologic appearance of lipomesosalpinx to any adipose tissue in the body, failure to prove any correlation between lipomesosalpinx and obesity would support screening for lipomesosalpinx in all infertile women.

To date, there is no uniform definition for UI [6]. With the marvelous advancement in illumination and magnification, endoscopy would add a lot for the diagnostic work-up for cases with UI. The findings of this and our previous [7] studies would support the central role of dual endoscopy (combined laparoscopy and hysteroscopy) in all cases of infertility despite not being clearly stated by most of the infertility-interested societies when defining UI. One of the promising and attractive options for evaluation of subtle tubal and mesosalpingeal lesions is hydrolaparoscopy which offers a comparable accuracy to laparoscopy in 96.1 % of cases [16].

Despite being described for a long time [17], the impact of fatty condensation of the mesosalpinx on fertility is not yet studied so far; this is the first study in English literature to address this point and to report it in 5.7 % of infertile women. Lipomesosalpinx would theoretically affect tubal motility and more importantly leads to failure to reach the pouch of Douglas for ovum pick up despite being a patent tube. Nevertheless, the results of this study failed to prove a positive correlation between lipomesosalpinx and unexplained infertility. This calls for a larger sample-sized multicentric study. The main value of this study is to direct attention to mesosalpingeal lesions that would affect fertility. Despite being a rare laparoscopic finding, lipomesosalpinx should be reported and documented as a missed tubal factor of infertility. Whether to treat lipomesosalpinx or not, bilaterally or unilaterally and by which means, require further studies with proper second-look laparoscopy.

Informed consent All procedures followed were in accordance with the ethical standards of the Responsible Committee on Human Experimentation (institutional and national) and with the Helsinki Declaration of 1975 as revised in 2000 (5). Informed consent was obtained from all patients for being included in the study.

References

1. Gomel V, Taylor PJ, Yuzpe A, Roux J (1986) Laparoscopy and hysteroscopy in gynecologic practice. Year Book, Chicago
2. Chawla N, Kudesia S, Azad S, Singhal M, Rai SM (2009) Salpingitis isthmica nodosa. Indian J Pathol Microbiol 52(3):434–435
3. Kessel R (1998) Medical histology. Oxford University Press, London, p 486
4. Gartner LP, Hiatt JL (2007) Color textbook of histology, 3rd edn. Elsevier, New York, pp 477–78
5. Weiss L, Greep RO (1977) Histology, 4th edn. McGraw-Hill, New York, p 920
6. Ray A, Shah A, Gudi A, Homburg R (2012) Unexplained infertility: an update and review of practice. Reprod Biomed Online 24(6):591–602
7. Darwish AM, Amin AM, Mohammad SA (2003) Laparoscopic management of paratubal and paraovarian cysts. J Soc Laparoendosc Surg 7(2):101–106
8. Child T (2013) Optimising the management of patients with infertility. Practitioner 257(1759):19–22, 2–3
9. Rasheed SM, Abdelmonem AM (2011) Hydatid of Morgagni: a possible underestimated cause of unexplained infertility. J Obstet Gynecol Reprod Biol 158(1):62–66
10. Yablonski M, Sarge T, Wild RA (1990) Subtle variations in tubal anatomy in infertile women. Fertil Steril 54(3):455–458
11. Fakih H, Marshall J (1994) Subtle tubal abnormalities adversely affect gamete intrafallopian transfer outcome in women with endometriosis. Fertil Steril 62(4):799–801
12. Kolusari A, Ugurluer G, Kosem M, Kurdoglu M, Yildizhan R, Adali E (2009) Leiomyosarcoma of the broad ligament: a case report and review of the literature. Eur J Gynaecol Oncol 30(3):332–334
13. Janovski NA (1966) Choristoma of heterotopic adrenal tissue in mesosalpinx. Obstet Gynecol 28(3):380–382
14. Huang WC, Yang SH, Yang JM (2005) Ultrasonographic manifestations of fallopian tube carcinoma in the fimbriated end. J Ultrasound Med 24(8):1157–1160, quiz 1161–2
15. Benjaminov O, Atri M (2004) Sonography of the abnormal fallopian tube. AJR Am J Roentgenol 183(3):737–742
16. Ezedinma NA, Phelps JY (2012) Transvaginal hydrolaparoscopy. JSLS 16(3):461–465
17. Lockyer C (1919) Lipoma of the broad ligament. Proc R Soc Med 12(Obstet Gynaecol Sect):195–199

28

Options on fibroid morcellation

Hans Brölmann · Vasilios Tanos · Grigoris Grimbizis · Thomas Ind · Kevin Philips · Thierry van den Bosch · Samir Sawalhe · Lukas van den Haak · Frank-Willem Jansen · Johanna Pijnenborg · Florin-Andrei Taran · Sara Brucker · Arnaud Wattiez · Rudi Campo · Peter O'Donovan · Rudy Leon de Wilde · On behalf of the European Society of Gynaecological Endoscopy (ESGE) steering committee on fibroid morcellation

Abstract In laparoscopy, specimens have to be removed from the abdominal cavity. If the trocar opening or the vaginal outlet is insufficient to pass the specimen, the specimen needs to be reduced. The power morcellator is an instrument with a fast rotating cylindrical knife which aims to divide the tissue into smaller pieces or fragments. The Food and Drug Administration (FDA) issued a press release in April 2014 that discouraged the use of these power morcellators. This article has the objective to review the literature related to complications by power morcellation of uterine fibroids in laparoscopy and offer recommendations to laparoscopic surgeons in gynaecology. This project was initiated by the executive board of the European Society of Gynaecological Endoscopy. A steering committee on fibroid morcellation was installed and

H. Brölmann (✉)
Department of Gynaecology, VU University Medical Centre, de Boelelaan 1117, 1181HV Amsterdam, The Netherlands
e-mail: h.brolmann@vumc.nl

V. Tanos
Department of Obstetrics and Gynaecology, Aretaeio Hospital, St George's Medical School, Nicosia University, Nicosia, Cyprus
e-mail: v.tanos@aretaeio.com

G. Grimbizis
Department of Obstetrics and Gynecology, Aristotle University of Thessaloniki, Thessaloniki, Greece

T. Ind
Department of Gynaecological Oncology, Royal Marsden Hospital, London, UK

K. Philips
Spire Hull and East Riding Hospital, London, UK

T. van den Bosch
Catholic University Leuven, Leuven, Belgium

S. Sawalhe
Donauisar Klinikum Deggendorf-Dingolfing-Landau, Deggendorf, Germany

L. van den Haak · F.-W. Jansen
Leiden University Medical Centre, Leiden, The Netherlands

J. Pijnenborg
Elisabeth-twee steden Hospital, Tilburg, The Netherlands

F.-A. Taran · S. Brucker
Department for Women's Health, University Hospital Tuebingen, Eberhard Karls University, Tübingen, Germany

A. Wattiez
IRCAD, Strassburg, France

R. Campo
Leuven Institute for Fertility and Embryology (LIFE), Leuven, Belgium

P. O'Donovan
M.E.R.I.T. Centre, Bradford Royal Infirmary, Bristol, UK

R. L. de Wilde
Pius Hospital, Oldenburg, Germany

experienced ESGE members requested to chair an action group to address distinct clinical questions. Clinical questions were formulated with regards to the sarcoma risk in presumed uterine fibroids, diagnosis of sarcoma, complications of morcellation and future research. A literature review on the different subjects was conducted, systematic if appropriate and feasible. It was concluded that the true prevalence of uterine sarcoma in presumed fibroids is not known given the wide range of prevalences (0.45–0.014 %) from meta-analyses mainly based on retrospective trials. Age and certain imaging characteristics such as 'lacunes' suggesting necrosis and increased central vascularisation of the tumour are associated with a higher risk of uterine sarcoma, although the risks remain low. There is not enough evidence to estimate this risk in individual patients. Complications of morcellation are rare. Reported are direct morcellation injuries to vessels and bowel, the development of so-called parasitic fibroids requiring reintervention and the spread of sarcoma cells in the abdominal cavity, which may possibly or even likely upstaging the disease. Momentarily in-bag morcellation is investigated as it may possibly prevent morcellation complications. Because of lack of evidence, this literature review cannot give strong recommendations but offers only options which are condensed in a flow chart. Prospective data collection may clarify the issue on sarcoma risk in presumed fibroids and technology to extract tissue laparoscopically from the abdominal cavity should be perfected.

Keywords Leiomyoma uteri · Leiomyosarcoma · Endometrial stromal sarcoma · Laparoscopy · Morcellation · Power morcellation · Complication

Introduction

A uterine leiomyoma or myoma is a benign smooth muscle tumour of the myometrium and will be referred to in this article as fibroid. On April 17, 2014, the Food and Drug Administration (FDA) published a press release on the website where the use of laparoscopic power morcellation was 'discouraged' due to potential upstaging of uterine sarcoma [1]. The motive to do so was the case history of a patient with a presumed fibroid who underwent a laparoscopic hysterectomy and morcellation of the uterus. The fibroid turned out to be a sarcoma and at reintervention spread of the sarcoma in the abdominal cavity was present. The FDA reported a risk of a uterine sarcoma in patients with presumed fibroids of 0.28 % meta-analysing the data of 18 studies. As some way of morcellation has been used for a long time by gynaecologic surgeons to extract tissue from the vagina or the endoscopic openings in order to enable vaginal or laparoscopic surgery, the professional community was shocked and representatives of many scientific societies published their opinions on the matter [2–9]. A common statement was the lack of solid scientific data to reach strong recommendations with regard to the counselling of patients with fibroids on the issue to choose laparoscopic surgery with its established benefits or for laparotomy to escape the small risks related to morcellation of the fibroid.

This review looks at morcellation complications in cases of presumed fibroids. Although intra-abdominal spread of endometrial cancer, adenomyosis and even trophoblastic tissue by morcellation of the uterus has been reported, these issues will not be addressed in this paper as those diagnoses are less unexpected by their clinical features.

To explore the available literature, the subject will be divided into clinical questions:

- What is the risk of sarcoma in patients with a presumed fibroid
- How to diagnose a uterine sarcoma and distinguish it from a fibroid
- What are the complications of morcellation
- How to prevent morcellation complications
- What are the knowledge gaps
- Recommendations on clinical management in patients with fibroids

The objective of this article is to formulate and grade statements and recommendations on fibroid morcellation based on the level of available evidence. The grading of articles and recommendations was performed according to Eccles et al. [10] (Table 1). As statements can be based on several articles, they are treated as recommendations.

What is the risk of sarcoma in patients with presumed fibroid(s)

Uterine fibroids are a common disorder with an estimated incidence of 20–40 % in women during their reproductive years [11, 12]. In contrast, leiomyosarcoma of the uterus is a rare entity with an annual incidence quoted at 0.64/100,000 women [13]. According to a recently revised WHO classification of uterine sarcomas, the myometrial pure stromal sarcoma (leiomyoma, Smooth muscle Tumor of Unknown Potential [STUMP] and leiomyosarcoma) is to be distinguished from the endometrial stromal sarcoma (endometrial stromal nodule [ESN], the low-grade endometrial stromal sarcoma and the undifferentiated endometrial sarcoma). The carcinosarcoma or Mixed Müllerian Tumor (MMT) is classified as carcinoma. Excluding the MMT, leiomyosarcoma (LMS) accounts for 70 % and stromal sarcoma for 30 % of all uterine sarcomas [14]. Uterine sarcomas consist 2–7 % of all uterine malignancies. Reliable figures for the incidence of STUMP and cellular fibroids are poorly documented. In one article from a single institution over a period of 36 years, there were 18 cases of STUMP and 72 cases of uterine leiomyosarcoma (none of which had a prior diagnosis of

Table 1 Grading statements and recommendations [10]

Recommended grade	Evidence
A	Directly based on category I evidence
B	Directly based on: • Category II evidence, or • Extrapolated recommendation from category I evidence
C	Directly based on: • Category III evidence, or • Extrapolated recommendation from category I or II evidence
D	Directly based on: • Category IV evidence, or • Extrapolated recommendation from category I, II or III evidence
Good practice point	The view of the Guideline Development Group
NICE 2002	Recommendation taken from the NICE technology appraisal

Evidence category	Source
Ia	Systematic review and meta-analysis of randomised controlled trials
Ib	At least one randomised controlled trial
IIa	At least one well-designed controlled study without randomisation
IIb	At least one other type of well-designed quasi-experimental study
III	Well-designed non-experimental descriptive studies, such as comparative studies, correlation studies or case studies
IV	Expert committee reports or opinions and/or clinical experience of respected authorities

Adapted from Eccles M, Mason J (2001) How to develop cost-conscious guidelines. Health Technology Assessment 5 (16)

STUMP) in the hysterectomy specimens [15]. All cases of STUMP were registered as disease free after 5 years with only conservative management. Sarcomas spread usually by blood or lymphatic vessels. Five-year survival ranges from 17 to 55 %. Survival of patients with a LMS is strongly associated with the number of mitoses per 10 high power fields (×100 magnification): 1–4, 98 %; 5–9, 42 %; ≥10, 15 %. A LMS embedded and confined to the uterus that is removed 'en bloc' is associated with a better survival up to 83 % [14].

Methods

Two authors (TI, KP) performed a systematic review of the literature on prevalence of uterine sarcoma in patients after uterus surgery, mostly because of presumed fibroids. Searches were performed of Pubmed and Embase using the MESH terms "Fibroids and Sarcoma and uterine neoplasms", "Myomectomy and Complications". Further papers were obtained from the reference lists of papers reviewed. Two further papers were submitted for inclusions which were unpublished manuscripts [16, 17] (Ind et al. 2014, personal communication). Only papers with over 500 subjects were included to address the issues of publication bias in smaller series. Further analysis using the terms above and cross referencing with published reviews reference lists on this subject, but with the exclusion of review articles, letters and case reports from the analysis, 12 papers are left where the data seemed reliable and acceptable to help answer the question [8, 16–26]. All evidence finally reviewed has been retrieved from observational single arm cohort studies and is therefore level III evidence. The recommendations are therefore graded as Grade C.

Results

The overall risk of not previously presumed sarcomatous change in the uterus from all papers was 0.14 % (1 in 700). However, there were large differences between papers with figures varying from 0.49 % (1 in 204) [19] to 0.056 % (1 in 1,788) [16]. On average, papers that looked at myomectomy specimens gave a lower risk of sarcomatous change of 0.08 % (1 in 1,306) compared to those that looked at hysterectomy specimens where the overall pooled risk was 0.15 % (1 in 650). The risk appears to be age related with one study demonstrating a lower risk in patients under 45 years of age (Ind et al. 2014, personal communication).

Discussion

This meta-analysis, based largely on peer-reviewed articles and two submitted articles, shows a prevalence of 0.14 % which is lower than but within the range of similar literature reviews [1, 6]. In the current selection of studies, the small numbers (<500) were excluded. Recently presented data, submitted for publication, however show that including small trials brings the average reported prevalence of sarcoma down (Pritts E, 2014, personal communication).

Pritts et al. selected 131 articles with 29.877 patients operated for fibroids and found a sarcoma prevalence of 1:7,400 (0.014 %). They explain the large prevalence difference with the available literature by including more prospective trials (50 % half of which randomised trials) that lack the confounder of patient selection of retrospective trials. Also trials with smaller numbers were included increasing the power of the meta-analysis using Bayesian statistics to correct for small patient numbers. Although the large differences in prevalence undermine the credibility of all collected data on the prevalence of sarcoma in presumed fibroids, it is likely that the prevalence is much lower than recently reported. Prospective collection of multicentric data of contemporary patients may clarify the important issue of prevalence.

As the LMS has a similar clinical and diagnostic appearance to the leiomyoma in contrast to the endometrial stromal sarcoma, our interest is primarily to distinguish fibroids from LMS. The endometrial stromal sarcomas usually cause abnormal—non cyclic—uterine bleeding. But also LMS can present as a type 0—100 % protruding in the uterine cavity—causing abnormal uterine bleeding. In the current review, all kinds of sarcomatous changes were included in the meta-analysis, including STUMP's. This may have blurred the prevalence results. In particular including studies with laparoscopic supracervical hysterectomies, sometimes without the presumption of fibroids, will result in a lower reported prevalence. A difference in prevalence between studies where fibroids intended to be morcellated and the older (pathology) studies where all uteri and fibroids served as a denominator in the prevalence rate has also been demonstrated [27].

Data on age and prevalence does not allow the estimation of an accurate risk of sarcoma in the individual patient scheduled for fibroid surgery but they may be taken into account to define a low and intermediate risk group of patients. The paradox remains that as presumed fibroids are less prevalent in postmenopause, the highest (absolute) number of sarcomas is found in the fourth decade, although the incidence is still extremely low [23]. In one study, 18/21 sarcoma patients (86 %) were premenopausal [28]. The statements of this section are in Table 2.

Table 2 Statements on the prevalence of uterine sarcoma in presumed fibroids

Statements	Evidence
The incidence of leiomyosarcoma is 0.64/100,000 per year	
The prevalence of sarcoma in a presumed fibroid is 0.14 % (1:700) with a range from 0.49 % (1:204) to 0.014 % (1:7,400). This large range renders more prospective data collection necessary.	C
The risk of sarcoma in presumed fibroids is positively related to age, although the majority of sarcomas—in absolute numbers—will be in the fourth decade. Below the age of 40 sarcoma in a presumed fibroid is extremely rare.	C
Based on age, an accurate assessment of the risk of sarcoma in patients with presumed fibroids is not possible although a global estimation (intermediate risk versus low risk) could be made	C

How to distinguish a fibroid from a sarcoma by diagnostic tests

Even if an accurate distinction between fibroids and sarcomas by preoperative diagnostic test is not possible, potential specific characteristics of both disorders would enable the clinician to better predict the presence of sarcoma in a presumed fibroid and counsel patients likewise. Uterine sarcomas are characterised by the common oncologic features such as growth, necrosis and increased vascularity. However, these characteristics occur also in fibroids.

Although the focus of this overview is on fibroid morcellation, the same may be applicable to other therapeutic options such as selective uterine artery embolisation, fibroid ablation, hysteroscopic resection or medical treatment.

In this section, the evidence is reviewed as to the predictive value of imaging and other diagnostic tests in differentiating between a (benign) fibroid and a LMS of the uterus.

Methods

One of the authors (TvdB) performed a systematic Medline search of the literature in order to map the different diagnostic tests and their characteristics. The following search terms were used: "uterine leiomyosarcoma" [all fields], "diagnosis" [all fields], "ultrasonography" [all fields], "LDH" [all fields] or "LDH isoenzymes" [all fields] and "markers" [all fields]. After including cross references, 37 articles were available for further consideration [22, 28–64].

Imaging (US, MRI)

There are no pathognomonic features predicting a LMS on any imaging technique [29, 30, 36]. Rapid increase in size (within 3 months) has been reported in case reports of LMS [48, 59] but is generally not distinctive as it may occur in fibroids as well [22]. No growth—in 3 months—may be reassuring unless caused by GnRH [65, 66]. Not only can the uterine sarcoma be accompanied by fibroids responding to GnRH, but it may also be sensitive for estrogen deprivation itself due to its estrogen receptors. It has been reported in a group of 21 uterine sarcomas that all but one (95 %) was either solitary or in case of several myometrial lesions the largest [64]. Another study with ultrasound compared eight LMS and three STUMPs with 225 fibroids and reported that LMSs were significantly larger than other uterine smooth muscle tumours [35]. They were all solitary, and seven of eight lesions had a diameter ≥8 cm. Degenerative cystic changes were observed in four lesions, and increased peripheral and central vascularity was demonstrated in seven lesions. Sensitivity, specificity and positive predictive value of increased central and peripheral vascularity in the diagnosis of LMS were 100, 86 and 19 %, respectively. Combining other sonographic findings with marked central vascularity, the positive predictive value increased to 60 %, but sensitivity decreased to 75 %. 2D ultrasound Power Doppler (USPD) may be related to the nature of the tumour, with a peak systolic velocity having a sensitivity of 80 % for detecting sarcoma with a specificity of 97 %. No studies on sarcoma diagnosis have been published on vascular indices measured by 3D USPD.

Although LMS may have on ultrasound and MRI a similar appearance to fibroids [30, 36], a large >8 cm, solitary, oval-shaped, highly vascularised (peripheral and central) and irregular, heterogeneous myometrial tumour with central necrosis/degenerative cystic changes and absence of calcifications should raise the suspicion of a LMS [29, 30, 35, 41]. MR imaging is superior to CT scan to delineate the extent and to evaluate the tissue characteristics of the lesion [43]. MRI, especially the T2-weighted sequences, may help evaluating tumour extension in the uterus [47] and in differentiating between a leiomyoma and a LMS [51, 54]. In a small series, contrast enhancement after administration of gadolinium (Gd)-DTPA was detected in all 10 LMS, but absent in 28 of 32 uterine degenerated leiomyoma patients [39].

PET scan

Positron emission tomography has a place in the diagnostic armentarium of presumed fibroids. In PET scanning, a radionuclide (tracer) on a biologically active molecule is visualised. In imaging of fibroids, usually fluodeoxyglucose (FDG) is used, but also other molecules, such as deoxyfluorothymidine (FLT) or alphafluorobeta-estradiol (FES), have been reported. In general, the uptake of FDG in a fibroid is associated with the estrogen status, cellularity and the presence of malignancy [62]. One retrospective study compares different imaging techniques in the case of suspected uterine sarcoma. Of the five sarcomata, all were detected by FDG PET, four by dynamic MRI and two by PowerDoppler ultrasound [58]. FES may be more accurate in distinguishing LMS from fibroids than FDG, with an accuracy of respectively 93 and 81 % [67].

Serum markers (LDH and CA125)

In a prospective series of 227 patients, the total LDH and LDH isozyme type 3 were elevated in all 10 patients with LMS as compared with degenerated leiomyomas [39]. Elevated CA125 have been reported in patients with LMS, especially in advanced-staged LMS [44, 59]. In a series of 42 consecutive LMS, the values of preoperative serum CA125 were significantly higher in the uterine LMS group than those in the uterine leiomyoma group. However, there was significant overlapping of preoperative serum CA125 between the uterine leiomyoma group and early-stage uterine LMS which limits the clinical use [44].

Histology

The role of endometrial sampling without abnormal uterine bleeding in the detection of uterine sarcoma is not yet elucidated [68]. In a large series of 938 malignant tumours in hysterectomy specimens from a pathology laboratory, 142 specimens with sarcomas were found of which 72 (51 %) had endometrial sampling. In 62/72 (86 %), the sampling was positive for sarcoma. As preoperative abnormal uterine bleeding was not registered and analysed in this study, it is not clear which patients were selected for endometrial sampling. It may be assumed that abnormal uterine bleeding was the indication for endometrial sampling in sarcoma patients and not the presumed fibroid itself.

Also the role of image-guided *needle biopsies* is not completely clear. The predictive value of a negative biopsy might be expected to be low because of the large areas of necrosis, an excellent negative predictive value is reported using MRI-guided needle biopsies and Bell's classification on histology [31] with a cut-off level of 2 [45]. With this cut-off level, chosen not to miss malignancy, the sensitivity, specificity, positive and negative predictive values were 100, 98.6, 58 and 100.0 %, respectively. No data are found on the possible spread of sarcoma cells by multiple puncturing of the sarcoma. In breast cancer needle puncture, an increase of positive lymph nodes compared to breast tumours that were not punctured was found [69]. On the other hand, incisional biopsy of melanoma has no apparent effect on tumour spread [70]. Tulandi et al. [55] report on two cases of multiple transabdominal biopsies and frozen section before proceeding with morcellation.

Finally, it should be stressed that even the histological diagnosis of LMS on an intact hysterectomy specimen may be difficult because of locally differing diagnostic criteria [31, 38]. Statements on diagnosis of uterine sarcoma are listed in Table 3.

What are complications of morcellation?

A complication can be defined as an unintended and undesirable event following clinical management resulting in its adjustment or irreversible injury to the patient. Known complications are direct morcellation injuries where the activated morcellator injures intestines or blood vessels. Secondary to morcellation of fibroids, chips can implant on the peritoneum causing parasitic fibroids which may need further surgery. If a presumed fibroid appears to be a sarcoma (or other malignancy), any method of morcellation disrupts the integrity of the

Table 3 Statements on diagnostic tests for uterine sarcoma

Statements	Grade
There are no features predicting a leiomyosarcoma (LMS) on any imaging technique with certainty	C
A large (≥8 cm), solitary, oval-shaped, highly vascularised (peripheral and central) and irregular, heterogeneous myometrial tumour with central necrosis/degenerative cystic changes and absence of calcifications must raise the suspicion of a LMS	D
Rapid increase in size (within 3 months) has been reported in LMS but is generally not distinctive as it may occur in fibroids as well. No growth—in 3 months—may be reassuring unless in combination with GnRH	C
MRI with contrast enhancement may prove helpful in differentiating between LMS and fibroid	C
Total LDH and LDH isozyme 3 may help in differentiating between LMS and fibroid	C
CA125 may be elevated in advanced staged LMS but seems not useful in early stage LMS	C
Endometrial sampling in the detection of uterine sarcoma is indicated in abnormal uterine bleeding. Without abnormal uterine bleeding its role is unclear	D
Transcervical or transabdominal needle biopsy may prove of help in differentiating between LMS and a fibroid, although no data are available on spread of tumour cells caused by the biopsy needle	D

tumour, possibly upstaging the disease and affecting survival. In case of power morcellation, the centripetal forces of the cylindrical knife may add to the phenomenon of 'seeding' of tumour cells on the peritoneum. Finally, the fragmental state of the specimen due to morcellation may impair proper selection for histologic evaluation of that part of the tumour that is suspicious of malignancy. This might cause treatment delay. In this section, these complications will be discussed separately.

Direct morcellation injuries

In the field of gynaecology, the majority of symptomatic masses are represented by uterine fibroids. During operative laparoscopy, power morcellation is indispensable to remove large tissue fragments while the laparoscopy offers quicker recovery, less post-operative pain, fewer wound complications and less post-operative morbidity than open procedures. In addition, power morcellators shorten the time of surgery significantly. An 'electrical cutting device for laparoscopic removal of tissue from the abdominal cavity' was introduced by Steiner in 1993 [71]. Similar instruments according to the Steiner principle have been commercialised since.

Despite the well-established advantages of power morcellation during laparoscopy, the use of power morcellators is not completely without concern. Milad [72] reviewed the FDA's adverse event database "MAUDE" between 1992 and 2013, where injuries to the small/large bowel (31), large blood vessels (27), the kidney (3), ureter (3), bladder (1) and diaphragm (1) have been reported using power morcellation. In six cases, the accidents were fatal. This underlines that direct morcellation injuries are serious and, though underreported, extremely rare. It is recommended to maintain adequate distension and use morcellators with a nozzle to promote lateral pealing preventing the morcellator from coring the tissue and thereby losing the morcellator's tip out of sight [73].

Parasitic fibroids

Traditionally, parasitic fibroids were thought to be pedunculated subserosal fibroids that were accidentally separated from the uterus and had become attached to another organ in the pelvis for their blood supply (3). The increasing number of case reports of parasitic fibroids after the use of laparoscopic morcellation has contributed to the development of an iatrogenic theory. It is thought that seeding of retained small tissue fragments after morcellation can lead to the development of parasitic fibroids in the peritoneal cavity [74]. Most patients presented with symptoms such as abdominal or pelvic pain, dyspareunia, abdominal distension, urinary frequency and constipation. One of five patients is asymptomatic and the presence of a pelvic mass unexpectedly diagnosed during routine examination or another surgical procedure. Additional published cases indicated that although rare, parasitic fibroids can occur long after laparoscopic morcellation and are often asymptomatic or present with abdominal or pelvic pain. Little is known about the incidence and risk factors of this phenomenon.

To answer questions about the *incidence, risk factors and other characteristics* of parasitic fibroids, one of the authors (HP) conducted a systematic literature search the MEDLINE and Embase databases. The report of this systematic review will be submitted elsewhere.

The overall incidence of parasitic fibroids after laparoscopic surgery with the use of morcellation was reported to be between 0.12 and 0.9 % [75–77]. The reported incidence of parasitic myomas after laparoscopic myomectomy was 0.2–1.2 % [76, 78, 79].

With regards to the *risk factors*, gonadal steroids hormones are known to influence the growth of uterine fibroids. It is hypothesised that prolonged exposure to steroid hormones (e.g. hormonal replacement therapy) during postmenopause could be a risk factor for the development of parasitic fibroids. In case of parasitic fibroids, there is often more than one. Statements on parasitic fibroids are listed in Table 4.

'Upstaging' uterine sarcoma

Although reducing a uterine sarcoma with electromechanical power morcellation within the abdominal cavity is contrary to

Table 4 Statements on parasitic fibroids by previous morcellation

Statements	Grade
The overall incidence of parasitic fibroids after laparoscopic surgery with the use of morcellation is reported to be between 0.12 and 0.9 %	D
The reported incidence of parasitic fibroids after laparoscopic myomectomy is 0.2–1.2 %	D
Premenopausal status and hormonal replacement treatment after primary surgery may be considered as risk factors for the development of parasitic fibroids, however not specific	D

oncologic surgical principles, the question remains if sarcoma cells are more inclined to implant in the peritoneum after power morcellation then after 'en bloc' removal of the uterine specimen with sarcoma embedded and if survival is affected given the bad prognosis that the sarcoma already has. These two questions have been addressed in literature. Two case reports support the concept of upstaging by power morcellation [80, 81]. In the reported patients, reintervention showed seeding of sarcomatous tissue, which was not visible during initial surgery. These findings have been confirmed in larger studies where the percentage upstaging ranged from 15 to 64 % [18, 28, 82, 83].

Not only electromechanical power morcellation is associated with the risk of upstaging but also other 'manipulations' of the sarcomatous tumour, such as myomectomy by laparotomy, subtotal hysterectomy and hysteroscopic resection of submucous fibroids, may affect survival suggesting upstaging [84]. The question as to whether seeding affects survival is also addressed by Seidman et al. [18]. In four of seven patients with LMS who were extracted by power morcellation, seeding was visible during reintervention. Three patients died from the disease and one was alive with metastatic disease. Three patients with morcellated sarcoma without signs of seeding were alive without metastases.

Two studies by Park et al. [85, 86] compared the survival of patients with uterine sarcoma with (n=48) and without morcellation (n=58) during surgery and demonstrated a significant difference of survival in favour of the non-morcellated group (Table 5). Although confounding factors cannot be excluded in these retrospective trials, an effect in favour of the morcellation group would have been expected as clinical suspicion of sarcoma based on size and imaging texture could have resulted in a worse prognosis in the laparotomy group.

Recently, a literature review was published by Pritts et al. [87] where she critically appraised the studies that reported on upstaging of sarcoma by morcellation which she evaluated as 'rather poor'. Although this weakens the alarming statements on upstaging, it does not prove the contrary (the innocence of open morcellation of sarcoma) and underlines the need for further studies. Statements on upstaging of uterine sarcoma by morcellation are listed in Table 6.

Table 5 Studies that compared patients operated for uterine sarcoma with and without morcellation. With permission from Nederlands Tijdschrift voor Obstetrie en Gynaecologie [27]

Park 2011 (LGESS)	No.	Age	FU	Recurrence	5 years DFS	ORmv
Morcellation −	27	45.3	64	3/27	84 %	
Morcellation +	23	43.6	66	8/23	55 %	4.03 (1–15)
Park 2011 (LMS)	n	Age	FU	Recurrence	5 years DFS	OR
Morcellation −	31	47.9	52	7/31	65 %	
Morcellation +	25	46.4	27	13/25	40 %	3.11 (1–9)

LGESS low grade endometrial stromal sarcoma, *LMS* leiomyosarcoma, *FU* follow-up, *DFS* disease free survival, *ORmv* odds rate mortality risk after morcellation in a multivariate analysis

Missing the diagnosis of malignancy because of shredded material

Morcellated specimens are poorly amenable to pathologic examination because the morcellation abolishes many of the anatomic features that allow meaningful gross description, including the notions of orientation, dimension, adjacency, border and margin [88]. This has been described in other uterine malignancies and could lead to delayed diagnosis or suboptimal staging, causing treatment delay [89, 90].

How to prevent morcellation complications

Given the scarcity of direct morcellation injuries, no clinical trials are available and all suggestions to prevent them may be considered as good practice points. With regards to preventing direct morcellation injuries, the options are listed in Table 7; regarding the development of parasitic fibroids, the options are mentioned in Table 8. The options to prevent upstaging of uterine sarcomas by power morcellation will be presented under the final options in Table 10.

Table 6 Statements on the complication of morcellation 'seeding' (upstaging uterine sarcoma)

Statements	Grade
The quality of research regarding upstaging of uterine sarcoma by open morcellation is rather poor	D
Electromechanical power morcellation of an unsuspected uterine sarcoma may cause intraperitoneal dissemination ('seeding')	C
Intraperitoneal dissemination ('seeding') may be associated with lower survival rates	C
'En bloc' resection of a uterine sarcoma may be associated with better survival than other tissue retrieval methods going with tumour injury	D

Table 7 Options to prevent direct morcellation injuries

Options	Grade
For safe entry, enlarge the skin and fascia incision to the diameter of the morcellator to reduce the abdominal wall resistance	Good practice point
Make sure that the morcellator's blade remain locked inside the protecting tube during the morcellator insertion into the abdomen	Good practice point
Keep the tip of the morcellator shaft in midline of the lower abdomen while introducing the device into the abdominal cavity and during morcellation	Good practice point
Morcellate only under continuous vision by applying the lateral pealing technique. Prevent penetrating the mass and losing the tip out of sight	Good practice point
Morcellation close to the intestine or to blood vessels increase risk of injury to these structures	Good practice point

Knowledge gaps

The—on some issues—systematic literature search on which this review is based revealed some serious gaps in available knowledge. Due to the low prevalence of uterine sarcomas, most data on prevalence and risk factors are derived from case histories or retrospective trials with low numbers. Prospective data collection of patients after fibroid surgery on age, imaging and laboratory results and subsequent histology is needed to answer questions on individual risk estimation in order to enable the patient to give a well-considered consent prior to minimal invasive surgery.

The development of safer morcellation techniques in the abdominal cavity by technical innovation, including in-bag morcellation, is in its infancy. No doubt that safe in-bag morcellation of fibroids has the potential to avoid many of the reported morcellation complications, such as direct morcellation injuries, parasitic fibroids and the upstaging of morcellated sarcomas. However, not all risks are addressed such as spillage from the content of the bag in the abdomen especially if the bag is punctured to introduce a laparoscope in the bag for better visualisation of the morcellator's tip. The in vitro results are promising. Cohen and Einarsson [91] demonstrated *in-bag* morcellation in an in vitro study, in which they successfully morcellated beef tongue specimens. In only 1 of the 13 trials did leakage of the bag occur. Washings of the container after retrieval of the specimen bag were negative for muscle cells, except for the open control and the trial with leakage of the retrieval bag. A small series of in-bag morcellation have been published with good results [92, 93]. Vaginal morcellation in a bag has been described also [94]. Possible draw backs are the need for a sufficient vaginal entry and the fact that only hysterectomy specimens are suitable for this technique. Future studies must establish the role of vaginal in-bag morcellation.

Table 8 Statements and options on preventing parasitic fibroids after morcellation

Statements and options	Grade
The small risk of parasitic fibroid with laparoscopic morcellation (<1 %) should be discussed with the patient and balanced against alternative treatment options	Good practice point
Avoid spread of cells and tissue fragments in the abdominal cavity by stabilising the specimen and prevent fast rotation	Good practice point
When morcellation is used, efforts should be made to prevent tissue loss during morcellation and to remove all tissue fragments after morcellation:	Good practice point
Place the patient in reverse Trendelenburg position after morcellation and irrigate the abdomen and pelvis extensively	
After irrigation of the peritoneal cavity the abdomen and pelvis should be inspected to identify any remaining tissue fragments	
The potential increased risk of parasitic fibroids after sex steroid exposure (endogenous/exogenous) after laparoscopic morcellation should be considered before hormonal replacement therapy is prescribed	D

In urology in-bag ('contained') morcellation has been performed in low-grade renal cell carcinoma (RCC). In a retrospective study, Wu et al. [95] evaluated in-bag morcellation in 188 patients with low-stage RCC. After a mean follow-up of 21 months, no difference in survival was demonstrated compared to open nephrectomy, although one port site metastases occurred. The safety and effectiveness in terms of survival was confirmed in another study [96]. In low-grade renal cell carcinoma, laparoscopic approach combined with *in-bag* morcellation of the kidney appears to be safe and effective.

Port site metastases after morcellation are thought to be related to the laparoscopic approach itself and not to the morcellation technique as exteriorising the bag before morcellation is meant to prevent contact of the tumour with

Table 9 Statements on technical innovation

Statements	Grade
Research on technical innovation in tissue retrieval from the abdominal cavity mainly focusses on in-bag ('contained') morcellation	D
In-bag morcellation may prevent morcellation complications such as direct morcellation injuries, parasitic fibroids and upstaging eventual malignancies	Good practice point
Potential reported risks of in-bag morcellation is spillage of tumour cells from the bag	C
In urology in-bag morcellation after laparoscopic removal of early stage and low grade renal cell carcinoma is reported to be safe and effective	C
Vaginal in-bag morcellation has also been described and needs further study	D
Development of bags is needed as well as registration of cases to further establish the potential value of on in-bag morcellation in gynaecologic surgery	Good practice point

Table 10 Options in intended fibroid morcellation

Options and considerations	
Informed consent by the patient is the corner stone of preoperative workup. If fibroid morcellation is intended, include its possible complications in the informed consent procedure before operation.	Good practice point
Standardise the clinical management by using a flowchart to classify patients according to global risk of a sarcoma in a presumed fibroid. Use flowchart in the figure as an option.	Good practice point
Use transvaginal ultrasound, transabdominal ultrasound or in case of poor visualisation on ultrasound MRI with or without contrast (Gadolinium-DTPA)	D
Consider including vascularity parameters (RI and PSV in 2D PowerDoppler ultrasound (PDUS) or vascular indices in 3D PDUS)	D
Consider performing LDH and iso-enzyme 3 assay	D
Perform a preoperative endometrial aspiration in case of abnormal uterine bleeding	D
Support the development of potentially beneficial techniques to prevent morcellation complications by participating in clinical trials	Good practice point
Register patient's data after her consent including pre-surgery images and post-surgery histology	Good practice point

the abdominal wall. In a review on port site metastases, the in-bag morcellation technique is recommended to prevent port site metastases [97].

Two studies report on the techniques of containment. Parekh et al. [98] suggested that specimens should be morcellated in fluid-filled retrieval bags. In an in vitro study, five porcine kidneys were morcellated. No perforation or leakage occurred in the fluid-filled bags compared to one perforation in 'dry' morcellation. Also, morcellation time was shorter, when compared to the dry bags.

Meng et al. [99] suggested that washings of a specimen retrieval bag may help the pathological diagnosis after renal morcellation. In their prospective study, 22 consecutive washings were examined. In 9 of 13 patients with carcinoma, the cytological examination confirmed pathology and in three cases cytology provided additional information. In all nine benign cases, cytology was consistent with pathology.

The potential benefits and risks of in-bag morcellation should be further evaluated by clinical studies before it can be recommended in general practice. Furthermore, although in-bag morcellation appears to be very promising as a tool for the prevention of morcellation-related complications, further research is needed to improve the morcellation mechanism itself [100]. The statements on knowledge gaps and potential technical innovations are listed in Table 9.

Concluding remarks

In the previous sections, the results of a literature search are shown to answer questions about fibroid morcellation in laparoscopy, related complications and what is needed to prevent them. It has not been the aim of this study to address morcellation of other structures such as uteri without presumed fibroids (e.g. some cases of LSH) or morcellation of ovarian masses.

As expected, the level of evidence is not sufficient to give recommendations. Therefore, it was decided to present options (Table 10), which are condensed in a flowchart to offer structure in the clinical management (Fig. 1). The flowchart can at best support the clinician to pursue safe and effective fibroid treatment but 'reassuring' does not exclude sarcoma

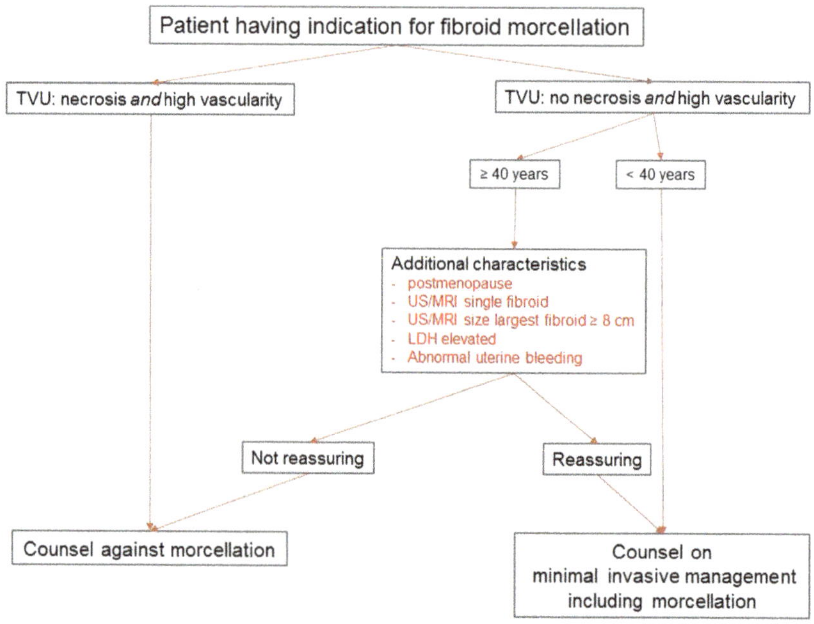

Fig. 1 Flowchart of intended fibroid morcellation

and in 'non-reassuring' cases the diagnosis will likely be benign. Therefore, it cannot have the status of guideline.

The 'additional characteristics' in the flowchart for women over 40 years of age are based on the literature review in the previous sections. These characteristics have been associated with discrimination of sarcomas from fibroids but they lack thorough scientific evaluation. In the case of LDH, the predictive value is based on only one trial [39]. We have to realise we are looking for a needle in a haystack indeed. This means that for each single 'risk factor', we can easily argue that it is of no importance. However, the association of several risk factors is probably more relevant than a single one. If more risk factors are present, it might be wise to be prudent, although the risk of sarcoma remains low.

Fibroid growth has been discussed among the authors at length and it was concluded that 'growth' or 'rapid growth' are not specifically associated with sarcoma but also with fibroids. On the other hand, a stable size during several months without administration of suppressing hormones (GnRH or Ullipristal) does make a sarcoma highly unlikely. Growth of the presumed fibroids during GnRH treatment or in menopause should raise suspicion about the nature of tumour.

The in-bag morcellation of presumed fibroids has the potential to prevent the rare morcellation-related complications typical of 'open' morcellation, such as direct morcellation injuries by distending the morcellation bag, the spread of fibroid chips, sarcoma or other malignant particles and cells in the abdominal cavity. More research is needed to improve the technique and on safety before in-bag morcellation can be recommended as a general tool in laparoscopic surgery.

We have chosen not to list all the literature on the benefits of laparoscopic surgery which are an important argument in the trade-off between laparoscopy with morcellation and laparotomy without. The vast amount of evidence in favour of laparoscopy is elegantly abstracted in the 'second look' article by Pitkin and Parker [101].

Taking needle biopsies before surgery would be an interesting option in case of intended fibroid surgery to rule out sarcoma; however, there are different opinions on the potential harmful effects of tumour manipulation and spread by needle biopsy [45, 69, 70]. Also representativeness of needle biopsies may be a yet unresolved drawback, given the necrotic areas in the sarcoma.

It is clear that there is much research to be done. At first, the issue on sarcoma risk in patients scheduled for fibroid morcellation should be clarified. The preliminary report of Pritts et al. (2014, personal communication) that includes more prospective trials and is based on sound statistics shows much lower prevalences (1:7,400) than previously reported in the meta-analyses based on retrospective trials (1:352) [1].

Secondly, more data must be collected to estimate the risk of sarcoma in individual patients with presumed fibroids, based on epidemiological data from the patient and diagnostic tests such as imaging.

Thirdly, technical innovation, such as in-bag morcellation, should enable safe morcellation of intra-abdominal specimens.

A corner stone in the doctor and patient relationship is the informed consent procedure. This means that the patient needs to be informed as completely as possible and based on the best available evidence in order to let her make the best choice of treatment tailored to her individual situation.

Acknowledgments We are grateful to the members of the ESGE steering committee on fibroid morcellation who are not in the author's list for their critical comments: Andreas Thurkow, Bern Bojahr and Judith Huirne. Also thanks to Rhona O'Flaherty for the administrative support of this initiative.

Author contribution Hans Brölmann-Protocol/manuscript writing/editing
Vasilis Tanos-Manuscript editing
Grigoris Grimbizis-Manuscript editing
Thomas Ind-Data collection and analysis, manuscript writing
Kevin Philips-Manuscript editing
Thierry van den Bosch-Data collection and analysis, manuscript writing
Samir Sawalhe-Data collection and analysis, manuscript writing
Lucas van den Haak-Data collection and analysis, manuscript writing
Frank-Willem Jansen-Data collection and analysis, manuscript writing
Johanna Pijnenburg-Data collection and analysis, manuscript writing
Florin-Andrei Taran-Data collection and analysis, manuscript writing
Sara Brucker-Data collection and analysis, manuscript writing
Arnaud Wattiez-Manuscript editing
Rudi Campo-Manuscript editing
Peter O'Donovan-Manuscript editing
Rudy-Leon de Wilde-Manuscript editing

Conflict of interest Hans Brölmann, Vasilis Tanos, Grigoris Grimbizis, Thomas Ind, Kevin Philips, Thierry van den Bosch, Lucas van den Haak, Frank-Willem Jansen, Johanna Pijnenborg, Florin-Adrei Taran, Sara Brucker, Arnaud Wattiez, Rudi Campo, Peter O'Donovan and Rudy-Leon de Wilde declare that they have no conflict of interest with regards to the manuscript 'options on fibroid morcellation; a literature review'. Samir Sawalhe is the designer of the Sawalhe II supercut morcellator manufactured by Storz.

Informed consent statement This article does not contain any studies with human or animal subjects performed by the any of the authors.

References

1. FDA (2014) FDA discourages use of laparoscopic power morcellation for removal of uterus or uterine fibroids. Food Drug Adm 17:4, Ref Type: Internet Communication
2. Goff BA (2014) SGO not soft on morcellation: risks and benefits must be weighed. Lancet Oncol 15(4):e148–e2045
3. Ankum WA (2014) Food and drug administration ontraadt gebruik van morcellator (redactioneel commentaar). Ned Tijdschr Obstet Gynaecol 127:216–219
4. Patient safety must be a priority in all aspects of care. Lancet Oncol 2014; 15(2):123–2045
5. WGE (2014) Morcelleren: reactie van Werkgroep Gynaecologische Endoscopie op FDA-advies; FDA ontraadt gebruik van morcellator. Ned Tijdschr Obstet Gynaecol 127:215

6. Knight J, Falcone T (2014) Tissue extraction by morcellation: a clinical dilemma. J Minim Invasive Gynecol 21(3):319–320
7. Kho KA, Nezhat CH (2014) Evaluating the risks of electric uterine morcellation. JAMA 311(19):905–906
8. Leung F, Terzibachian JJ (2012) Re: "The impact of tumor morcellation during surgery on the prognosis of patients with apparently early uterine leiomyosarcoma". Gynecol Oncol 124(1):172–173
9. European Society of Gynaecological Endoscopy (ESGE). Statement on morcellation (of presumed fibroids appearing to be sarcomas). ESGE executive board. 2014. Ref Type: Internet Communication
10. Eccles M, Mason J (2001) How to develop cost-conscious guidelines. Health Technol Assess 5(16):1–69
11. Ryan GL, Syrop CH, Van Voorhis BJ (2005) Role, epidemiology, and natural history of benign uterine mass lesions. Clin Obstet Gynecol 48(2):312–324
12. Wallach EE, Vlahos NF (2004) Uterine myomas: an overview of development, clinical features, and management. Obstet Gynecol 104(2):393–406
13. Harlow BL, Weiss NS, Lofton S (1986) The epidemiology of sarcomas of the uterus. J Natl Cancer Inst 76(3):399–402
14. Lurain JR, Piver MS (1992) Uterine sarcomas: clinical features and management. In: Coppleson X, Monagham J, Morrow P, Tattersall M (eds) Gynecologic oncology. Chruchill Livingstone, London, pp 827–840
15. Ng JS, Han A, Chew SH, Low J (2010) A clinicopathologic study of uterine smooth muscle tumours of uncertain malignant potential (STUMP). Ann Acad Med Singap 39(8):625–628
16. Bojhar B, de Wilde RL, Tchartchian. (2014) Malignancy rate of 10, 731 uteri morcellated during laparoscopic supracervical hysterectomy in 2013. (Personal Communication)
17. Ind TEJ, Rajab R, Manyonda I. (2014) Uterine sarcomas and myomectomy—a single institutions experience. (Unpublished Work)
18. Seidman MA, Oduyebo T, Muto MG, Crum CP, Nucci MR, Quade BJ (2012) Peritoneal dissemination complicating morcellation of uterine mesenchymal neoplasms. PLoS ONE 7(11):e50058
19. Rowland M, Lesnoch J, Edwards R, Richard S, Zom K, Sukumvanich P (2012) Occult uterine cancer in patients undergoing laparoscopic hysterectomy with morcellation. Gynecol Oncol 127(1):S29
20. Kamikabeya TS, Etchebehere RM, Nomelini RS, Murta EF (2010) Gynecological malignant neoplasias diagnosed after hysterectomy performed for leiomyoma in a university hospital. Eur J Gynaecol Oncol 31(6):651–653
21. Takamizawa S, Minakami H, Usui R, Noguchi S, Ohwada M, Suzuki M et al (1999) Risk of complications and uterine malignancies in women undergoing hysterectomy for presumed benign leiomyomas. Gynecol Obstet Investig 48(3):193–196
22. Parker WH, Fu YS, Berek JS (1994) Uterine sarcoma in patients operated on for presumed leiomyoma and rapidly growing leiomyoma. Obstet Gynecol 83:414–418
23. Leibsohn S, D'Ablaing G, Mishell DR Jr, Schlaerth JB (1990) Leiomyosarcoma in a series of hysterectomies performed for presumed uterine leiomyomas. Am J Obstet Gynecol 162:968–974, discus:968–974
24. Wright JD, Tergas AI, Burke WM, Cui RR, Ananth CV, Chen L et al. (2014) Uterine pathology in women undergoing minimally invasive hysterectomy using morcellation. JAMA 312(12):1253–1255
25. Paul GP, Naik SA, Madhu KN, Thomas T (2010) Complications of laparoscopic myomectomy: a single surgeon's series of 1001 cases. Aust N Z J Obstet Gynaecol 50(4):385–390
26. Sizzi O, Rossetti A, Malzoni M, Minelli L, La GF, Soranna L et al (2007) Italian multicenter study on complications of laparoscopic myomectomy. J Minim Invasive Gynecol 14(4):453–462
27. Brolmann H, Hehenkamp WJK, Huirne JAF (2014) Heeft het myoom zijn onschuld verloren? Ned Tijdschr Obstet Gynaecol 127:322–325
28. Oduyebo T, Rauh-Hain AJ, Meserve EE, Seidman MA, Hinchcliff E, George S et al (2014) The value of re-exploration in patients with inadvertently morcellated uterine sarcoma. Gynecol Oncol 132(2): 360–365
29. Amant F, Coosemans A, Debiec-Rychter M, Timmerman D, Vergote I (2009) Clinical management of uterine sarcomas. Lancet Oncol 10(12):1188–1198
30. Aviram R, Ochshorn Y, Markovitch O, Fishman A, Cohen I, Altaras MM et al (2005) Uterine sarcomas versus leiomyomas: gray-scale and Doppler sonographic findings. J Clin Ultrasound 33(1):10–13
31. Bell SW, Kempson RL, Hendrickson MR (1994) Problematic uterine smooth muscle neoplasms. A clinicopathologic study of 213 cases. Am J Surg Pathol 18(6):535–558
32. Cormio G, Loizzi V, Ceci O, Leone L, Selvaggi L, Bettocchi S (2014) Unsuspected diagnosis of uterine leiomyosarcoma after laparoscopic myomectomy. J Obstet Gynaecol. doi: 10.1016/j.jmig.2009.08.181
33. Dizon DS, Birrer MJ (2014) Advances in the diagnosis and treatment of uterine sarcomas. Discov Med 17(96):339–345
34. Evans HL, Chawla SP, Simpson C, Finn KP (1988) Smooth muscle neoplasms of the uterus other than ordinary leiomyoma. A study of 46 cases, with emphasis on diagnostic criteria and prognostic factors. Cancer 62(2239–2247):2239–2247
35. Exacoustos C, Romanini ME, Amadio A, Amoroso C, Szabolcs B, Zupi E et al (2007) Can gray-scale and color Doppler sonography differentiate between uterine leiomyosarcoma and leiomyoma? J Clin Ultrasound 35(8):449–457
36. Fukunishi H, Funaki K, Ikuma K, Kaji Y, Sugimura K, Kitazawa R et al (2007) Unsuspected uterine leiomyosarcoma: magnetic resonance imaging findings before and after focused ultrasound surgery. Int J Gynecol Cancer 17(3):724–728
37. Geyer H (1968) LDH isoenzymes in tumors of the human uterus. Klin Wochenschr 46(7):389–390
38. Giuntoli RL, Gostout BS, DiMarco CS, Metzinger DS, Keeney GL (2007) Diagnostic criteria for uterine smooth muscle tumors: leiomyoma variants associated with malignant behavior. J Reprod Med 52(11):1001–1010
39. Goto A, Takeuchi S, Sugimura K, Maruo T (2002) Usefulness of Gd-DTPA contrast-enhanced dynamic MRI and serum determination of LDH and its isozymes in the differential diagnosis of leiomyosarcoma from degenerated leiomyoma of the uterus. Int J Gynecol Cancer 12(4):354–361
40. Hadoux J, Morice P, Lhomme C, Duvillard P, Balleyguier C, Haie-Meder C et al (2013) Uterine leiomyosarcoma: epidemiology, pathology, biology, diagnosis, prognosis and treatment. Bull Cancer 100(9):903–915
41. Hata K, Hata T, Makihara K, Aoki S, Takamiya O, Kitao M et al (1990) Sonographic findings of uterine leiomyosarcoma. Gynecol Obstet Investig 30(4):242–245
42. Hata K, Hata T, Maruyama R, Hirai M (1997) Uterine sarcoma: can it be differentiated from uterine leiomyoma with Doppler ultrasonography? A preliminary report. Ultrasound Obstet Gynecol 9(2): 101–104
43. Janus C, White M, Dottino P, Brodman M, Goodman H (1989) Uterine leiomyosarcoma–magnetic resonance imaging. Gynecol Oncol 32(1):79–81
44. Juang CM, Yen MS, Horng HC, Twu NF, Yu HC, Hsu WL (2006) Potential role of preoperative serum CA125 for the differential diagnosis between uterine leiomyoma and uterine leiomyosarcoma. Eur J Gynaecol Oncol 27(4):370–374
45. Kawamura N, Ichimura T, Ito F, Shibata S, Takahashi K, Tsujimura A et al (2002) Transcervical needle biopsy for the differential diagnosis between uterine sarcoma and leiomyoma. Cancer 94(6):1713–1720
46. Lusby K, Savannah KB, Demicco EG, Zhang Y, Ghadimi MP, Young ED et al (2013) Uterine leiomyosarcoma management,

outcome, and associated molecular biomarkers: a single institution's experience. Ann Surg Oncol 20(7):2364–2372

47. Melia P, Maestro C, Bruneton JN, Gasperoni A, Peyrottes I, Teissier E et al (1995) MRI of uterine leiomyosarcoma. Apropos of 2 cases. J Radiol 76(1):69–72
48. Milman D, Zalel Y, Biran H, Open M, Caspi B, Hagay Z et al (1998) Unsuspected uterine leiomyosarcoma discovered during treatment with a gonadotropin-releasing hormone analogue: a case report and literature review. Eur J Obstet Gynecol Reprod Biol 76(2):237–240
49. Murase E, Siegelman ES, Outwater EK, Perez-Jaffe LA, Tureck RW (1999) Uterine leiomyomas: histopathologic features, MR imaging findings, differential diagnosis, and treatment. Radiographics 19(5):1179–1197
50. Nappi L, Di Spiezio SA, Indraccolo U, Bettocchi S (2008) Hysteroscopic resection of uterine leiomyosarcoma: a case report and literature review. J Minim Invasive Gynecol 15(3):380–383
51. Pattani SJ, Kier R, Deal R, Luchansky E (1995) MRI of uterine leiomyosarcoma. Magn Reson Imaging 13(2):331–333
52. Posy HE, Elkas JC, Yemelyanova AV, Diaz-Montes TP, Bristow RE, Giuntoli RL (2009) Metastatic leiomyosarcoma diagnosed after uterine artery embolization. Eur J Gynaecol Oncol 30(2):199–202
53. Rauh-Hain JA, Oduyebo T, Diver EJ, Guseh SH, George S, Muto MG et al (2013) Uterine leiomyosarcoma: an updated series. Int J Gynecol Cancer 23(6):1036–1043
54. Takemori M, Nishimura R, Sugimura K (1992) Magnetic resonance imaging of uterine leiomyosarcoma. Arch Gynecol Obstet 251(4): 215–218
55. Tulandi T, Ferenczy A (2014) Biopsy of uterine leiomyomata and frozen sections before laparoscopic morcellation. J Minim Invasive Gynecol 14:10
56. Ueda M, Otsuka M, Hatakenaka M, Torii Y (2000) Uterine endometrial stromal sarcoma located in uterine myometrium: MRI appearance. Eur Radiol 10(5):780–782
57. Ueda H, Togashi K, Konishi I, Kataoka ML, Koyama T, Fujiwara T et al (1999) Unusual appearances of uterine leiomyomas: MR imaging findings and their histopathologic backgrounds. Radiographics 19:S131–S145
58. Umesaki N, Tanaka T, Miyama M, Kawamura N, Ogita S, Kawabe J et al (2001) Positron emission tomography with (18) F-fluorodeoxyglucose of uterine sarcoma: a comparison with magnetic resonance imaging and power Doppler imaging. Gynecol Oncol 80(3):372–377
59. Vellanki VS, Rao M, Sunkavalli CB, Chinamotu RN, Kaja S (2010) A rare case of uterine leiomyosarcoma: a case report. J Med Case Rep 4:222. doi:10.1186/1752-1947-4-222-222-224
60. Widy-Kierska K, Roszkowski I (1969) LDH isoenzymes in patients with uterine tumors. Obstet Gynecol 33(2):173–176
61. Yanai H, Wani Y, Notohara K, Takada S, Yoshino T (2010) Uterine leiomyosarcoma arising in leiomyoma: clinicopathological study of four cases and literature review. Pathol Int 60(7):506–509
62. Zhang HJ, Zhan FH, Li YJ, Sun HR, Bai RJ, Gao S (2011) Fluorodeoxyglucose positron emission tomography/computed tomography and magnetic resonance imaging of uterine leiomyosarcomas: 2 cases report. Chin Med J (Engl) 124(14): 2237–2240
63. Schwartz LB, Diamond MP, Schwartz PE (1993) Leiomyosarcomas: clinical presentation. Am J Obstet Gynecol 168:180–183
64. Schwartz LB, Diamond MP, Schwartz PE (1993) Leiomyosarcomas: clinical presentation. Am J Obstet Gynecol 168(1 Pt 1):180–183
65. Kawamura N, Iwanaga N, Hada S, Maeda K, Sumi T, Ishiko O et al (2001) Transient shrinkage of a uterine leiomyosarcoma treated with GnRH agonist for a presumed uterine leiomyoma: comparison of magnetic resonance imaging finding before and during GnRH agonist treatment. Oncol Rep 8(6):1255–1257
66. Wang PH, Lee WL, Chao HT, Shu LP, Kao HL, Wu CW et al (1999) Relationship between hormone receptor concentration and tumor shrinkage in uterine myoma after treatment with a GnRHa. Zhonghua Yi Xue Za Zhi (Tapei) 62(5):294–299
67. Yoshida Y, Kiyono Y, Tsujikawa T, Kurokawa T, Okazawa H, Kotsuji F (2011) Additional value of 16 alpha-[18F] fluoro-17 beta-oestradiol PET for differential diagnosis between uterine sarcoma and leiomyoma in patients with positive or equivocal findings on [18F] fluorodeoxyglucose PET. Eur J Nucl Med Mol Imaging 38 (10):1824–1831
68. Bansal N, Herzog TJ, Burke W, Cohen CJ, Wright JD (2008) The utility of preoperative endometrial sampling for the detection of uterine sarcomas. Gynecol Oncol 110(1):43–48
69. Hansen NM, Ye X, Grube BJ, Giuliano AE (2004) Manipulation of the primary breast tumor and the incidence of sentinel node metastases from invasive breast cancer. Arch Surg 139(6):634–639
70. Martin RC, Scoggins CR, Ross MI, Reintgen DS, Noyes RD, Edwards MJ et al (2005) Is incisional biopsy of melanoma harmful? Am J Surg 190(6):913–917
71. Steiner RA, Wight E, Tadir Y, Haller U (1993) Electrical cutting device for laparoscopic removal of tissue from the abdominal cavity. Obstet Gynecol 81(3):471–474
72. Milad MP, Milad EA (2014) Laparoscopic morcellator-related complications. J Minim Invasive Gynecol 21(3):486–491
73. Milad MP, Sokol E (2003) Laparoscopic morcellator-related injuries. Am J Assoc Gynecol Laparosc 10(3):383–385
74. Nezhat C, Kho K (2010) Iatrogenic myomas: new class of myomas? J Minim Invasive Gynecol 17(5):544–550
75. Donnez O, Jadoul P, Squifflet J, Donnez J (2009) A series of 3190 laparoscopic hysterectomies for benign disease from 1990 to 2006: evaluation of complications compared with vaginal and abdominal procedures. BJOG 116(4):492–500
76. Cucinella G, Granese R, Calagna G, Somigliana E, Perino A (2011) Parasitic myomas after laparoscopic surgery: an emerging complication in the use of morcellator? Description of four cases. Fertil Steril 96(2):e90–e96
77. Leren V, Langebrekke A, Qvigstad E (2012) Parasitic leiomyomas after laparoscopic surgery with morcellation. Acta Obstet Gynecol Scand 91(10):1233–1236
78. Sinha R, Hegde A, Mahajan C, Dubey N, Sundaram M (2008) Laparoscopic myomectomy: do size, number, and location of the myomas form limiting factors for laparoscopic myomectomy? J Minim Invasive Gynecol 15(3):292–300
79. Ordulu Z, Dal CP, Chong WW, Choy KW, Lee C, Muto MG et al (2010) Disseminated peritoneal leiomyomatosis after laparoscopic supracervical hysterectomy with characteristic molecular cytogenetic findings of uterine leiomyoma. Genes Chromosom Cancer 49 (12):1152–1160
80. Anupama R, Ahmad SZ, Kuriakose S, Vijaykumar DK, Pavithran K, Seethalekshmy NV (2011) Disseminated peritoneal leiomyosarcomas after laparoscopic "myomectomy" and morcellation. J Minim Invasive Gynecol 18(3):386–389
81. Della BC, Karini H (2010) Endometrial stromal sarcoma diagnosed after uterine morcellation in laparoscopic supracervical hysterectomy. J Minim Invasive Gynecol 17(6):791–793
82. Morice P, Rodriguez A, Rey A, Pautier P, Atallah D, Genestie C et al (2003) Prognostic value of initial surgical procedure for patients with uterine sarcoma: analysis of 123 patients. Eur J Gynaecol Oncol 24(3–4):237–240
83. Einstein MH, Barakat RR, Chi DS, Sonoda Y, Alektiar KM, Hensley ML et al (2008) Management of uterine malignancy found incidentally after supracervical hysterectomy or uterine morcellation for presumed benign disease. Int J Gynecol Cancer 18(5):1065–1070
84. Perri T, Korach J, Sadetzki S, Oberman B, Fridman E, Ben-Baruch G (2009) Uterine leiomyosarcoma: does the primary surgical procedure matter? Int J Gynecol Cancer 19(2):257–260

85. Park JY, Kim DY, Kim JH, Kim YM, Kim YT, Nam JH (2011) The impact of tumor morcellation during surgery on the outcomes of patients with apparently early low-grade endometrial stromal sarcoma of the uterus. Ann Surg Oncol 18(12):3453–3461
86. Park JY, Park SK, Kim DY, Kim JH, Kim YM, Kim YT et al (2011) The impact of tumor morcellation during surgery on the prognosis of patients with apparently early uterine leiomyosarcoma. Gynecol Oncol 122(2):255–259
87. Pritts E, Parker WH, Brow J, Olive DL (2014) Outcome of occult uterine leiomyosarcoma after surgery for presumed uterine fibroids: a systematic review. J Min Invasive Gynecol 22(1):26–33
88. Hagemann IS, Hagemann AR, LiVolsi VA, Montone KT, Chu CS (2011) Risk of occult malignancy in morcellated hysterectomy: a case series. Int J Gynecol Pathol 30(5):476–483
89. Rivard C, Salhadar A, Kenton K (2012) New challenges in detecting, grading, and staging endometrial cancer after uterine morcellation. J Minim Invasive Gynecol 19(3):313–316
90. Schneider A (1997) Recurrence of unclassifiable uterine cancer after modified laparoscopic hysterectomy with morcellation. Am J Obstet Gynecol 177(2):478–479
91. Cohen SL, Greenberg JA, Wang KC, Srouji SS, Gargiulo AR, Pozner CN et al (2014) Risk of leakage and tissue dissemination with various contained tissue extraction (CTE) techniques: an in vitro pilot study. J Minim Invasive Gynecol 14:10
92. Cohen SL, Einarsson JI, Wang KC, Brown D, Boruta D, Scheib SA et al (2014) Contained power morcellation within an insufflated isolation bag. Obstet Gynecol 124(3):491–497
93. Einarsson JI, Cohen SL, Fuchs N, Wang KC (2014) In bag morcellation (IBM). J Minim Invasive Gynecol 14:10
94. Favero G (2013) Tips and tricks for successful manual morcellation: a response to "vaginal morcellation: a new strategy for large gynecological malignant tumors extraction. A pilot study". Gynecol Oncol 128(1):151
95. Wu SD, Lesani OA, Zhao LC, Johnston WK, Wolf JS Jr, Clayman RV et al (2009) A multi-institutional study on the safety and efficacy of specimen morcellation after laparoscopic radical nephrectomy for clinical stage T1 or T2 renal cell carcinoma. J Endourol 23(9):1513–1518
96. Barrett PH, Fentie DD, Taranger LA (1998) Laparoscopic radical nephrectomy with morcellation for renal cell carcinoma: the Saskatoon experience. Urology 52(1):23–28
97. Tsivian A, Sidi AA (2003) Port site metastases in urological laparoscopic surgery. J Urol 169(4):1213–1218
98. Parekh AR, Moran ME, Newkirk RE, Desai PJ, Calvano CJ (2000) Tissue removal utilizing steiner morcellator within a lapsac: effects of a fluid-filled environment. J Endourol 14(2):185–189
99. Meng MV, Koppie TM, Stoller ML (2003) Pathologic sampling of laparoscopically morcellated kidneys: a mathematical model. J Endourol 17(4):229–233
100. Arkenbout EA, van den Haak L, Driessen SR, Thurkow A.L., Jansen FW (2014) Assessing basic 'physiology' of the morcellation process and tissue spread: a time action analysis. J Minim Invasive Gynaecol. pii: S1553-4650(14)01448-4. doi: 10.1016/j.jmig.2014.10.009
101. Pitkin RM, Parker WH (2010) Operative laparoscopy: a second look after 18 years. Obstet Gynecol 115(5):890–891

29

Single port access laparoscopic myomectomy with X-Cone

Liliana Mereu · Stefano Angioni · Alessandro Pontis · Giada Carri · Luca Mencaglia

Abstract Single-port access laparoscopy (SPAL) technique is developing in the gynecological field but few experiences on SPAL myomectomy have been reported. A case of an infertile nulliparous woman who has been observed to have an intramural–subserosal myoma of 4 cm and bilateral sactosalpinx is reported. The patient underwent a SPAL to remove the myoma and bilateral sactosalpinx. No intraoperative and postoperative complications occurred. Total operative time was 94 min. We describe the technique with strategies to perform surgical treatment of the myoma with a single-access laparoscopic approach.

Keywords Myomectomy · Laparoendoscopic single-site surgery · Single-port access · Minimal access surgery

Background

Leiomyomas represent the most common pelvic tumors, affecting 25% to 45% of women of reproductive age and occurring three times more frequently in African American than white women. They are almost always benign and frequently asymptomatic. When symptomatic, however, uterine leiomyomas may cause heavy menstrual bleeding, pelvic pressure or pain, dyspaurenia, urinary frequency, incontinence, and urgency or constipation. Women with submucosal fibroids may also experience reproductive problems such as infertility, miscarriages, premature labor, or peripartum hemorrhage. After myomectomy, successful pregnancy rates occur in 53% to 70% for submucous fibroids and 58% to 65% for intramural and subserosal fibroids [1, 2].

The mechanisms by which myomas adversely affect fertility are several: displacement of the cervix which may reduce exposure to sperm; enlargement or deformity of the uterine cavity which may interfere with sperm migration and transport; obstruction of the proximal fallopian tube; altered tubo-ovarian anatomy, interfering with ovum capture; increased or disordered uterine contractility that may hinder sperm or embryo transfer or nidation; distortion or disruption of the endometrium; and impaired endometrial blood flow [3].

The removal of leiomyomas with preservation of the uterus is indicated in symptomatic women who wish to preserve their reproductive function and anatomic integrity. Once the decision is made to proceed with the myomectomy, the surgeon must decide whether the patient would be better suited to the laparoscopic or the laparotomic approach. This decision depends on several factors, including the size, the number, the location of the fibroids on the uterus, and the experience of the surgeon. The latter is perhaps the most important determinant as the completeness of the myomectomy and the adequacy of the reconstruction of the uterus after myomectomy will determine the subsequent function of the organ in relieving the symptoms and restoring reproductive potential.

Some investigators have found that uterine myoma have no effect on in vitro fertilization (IVF) outcomes unless they

L. Mereu (✉) · A. Pontis · G. Carri · L. Mencaglia
Division of Gynecology, Centro Oncologico Fiorentino,
Via Ragionieri 101, Sesto Fiorentino,
Florence, Italy
e-mail: Liliana.mereu@lacittadellasalute.it

S. Angioni · A. Pontis
Division of Gynecology, Obstetrics and Pathophysiology of Human Reproduction, University of Cagliari,
Cagliari, Italy

G. Carri
Department of Obstetrics and Gynecology,
Università Cattolica del Sacro Cuore,
Roma, Italy

distort or displace the uterine cavity; other investigators suggest that IVF success rates are also lower in women with intramural myomas, particularly when larger than 5 cm in diameter. Recent findings suggest that the size of the fibroids is positively related to implantation failure, especially when the diameter of the lesion exceeds 4 cm [4] and 5 cm [5].

The size, the number, and the location of fibroids that can be removed by a minimally invasive approach depend largely on the endoscopic skills and experience of the surgeons [6]. The latest advancements in terms of technical expertise and surgical instrumentation have allowed minimal-access surgery to become even more minimal with the development of single-access laparoscopic surgery (SALS). Reducing the number of working ports decreases the risk of bleeding, infection, concomitant iatrogenic visceral injury, hernia formation with better pain control, and cosmetic outcome. After initial applications on animal models, the subsequent development of specialized purpose-built instrumentation coupled with advances in skills led to the successful application of single-port access laparoscopy (SPAL) in human patients and this minilaparoscopic procedure has emerged as one of the viable, feasible, and widely applicable minimally invasive procedures. Preliminary advances in SPAL were applied to urologic and gastrointestinal surgery, and only recently papers have been published about the application of SPAL also in gynaecology [7, 8]. These preliminary experiences have shown good results in terms of feasibility, operative time, and complications particularly in the treatment of adnexal pathologies. At the moment, few experiences on SPAL myomectomy have been reported [8]. We present our technique to perform SPAL myomectomy using a new re-usable trocar (X-Cone).

Method

A 38-year-old infertile woman affected by bilateral sactosalpinx and uterine myoma underwent myomectomy and bilateral salpingectomy by single-access transumbilical laparoscopy.

The patient had previously undergone appendicectomy surgery. She had a regular menstrual cycle with a normal hormonal profile. Abdomino-pelvic examination was negative while transvaginal ultrasound found an anterior intramural myoma of 4 cm in diameter which distorted the endometrium and bilateral hydrosalpinx.

Laparoscopy was performed using a reusable single-site trocar with five integrated access ports (S-Portal X-Cone, Karl Storz, Tuttlingen, Germany). This new device consists of two symmetrical metal half-shells that are connected and sealed by one large silicon cap containing the access port. Once in the peritoneal cavity, the two half-shells fit together to form an X shape and the final access portal. The silicon cap comprising three 5-mm and one 12-mm port is connected on top of the X-Cone, which forms an airtight seal. A clamp integrated into the rubber sealing prevents the X-Cone from opening unintentionally. The external and internal diameters at the level of the X-Cone's waistline are 25 and 20 mm, respectively. Under general anesthesia, each patient was positioned in the dorsal lithotomic position with both legs supported in Allen stirrups and the arms resting alongside the body. An intrauterine device was used to mobilise the uterus. A 2.0-cm intraumbilical vertical skin incision and a 2–2.5-cm rectus fasciotomy were performed to enter the peritoneal cavity. The single-port trocar was inserted into the abdominal cavity and the abdomen was insufflated to 12 mmHg. The patient was then put in a Trendelemburg position. Following placement of the X-Cone, the surgeon stood behind the patient's left shoulder at the level of the patient's right shoulder, and the monitor was positioned between the patient's legs. We routinely used a rigid 30°, 5-mm-diameter, 50-cm-length Hopkins high definition laparoscope in combination with a high definition three-chip video camera (Karl Storz) [8, 9].

For the bilateral salpingectomy, rigid single curved forceps or *scissors* (S Portal, Karl Storz) and a standard straight bipolar dissector or device with grasping, coagulating, and transecting functions (En Seal; Ethicon) were used simultaneously. A 10-mm endobag through the 12-mm X-Cone access was used to remove the specimens.

The myometrium overlying the fibroid is injected with a 1:20 diluted solution of vasopressin using a laparoscopic needle. After the injection of 40 to 60 mL of solution, the uterus pales, indicating diminished blood flow. The myometrial incision was made with a flexible monopolar hook (Karl Storz) and was deep enough to the dissection plane between the myoma and the myometrium. Enucleation of the myoma was performed with a 10-mm myoma drill (Fig. 1).

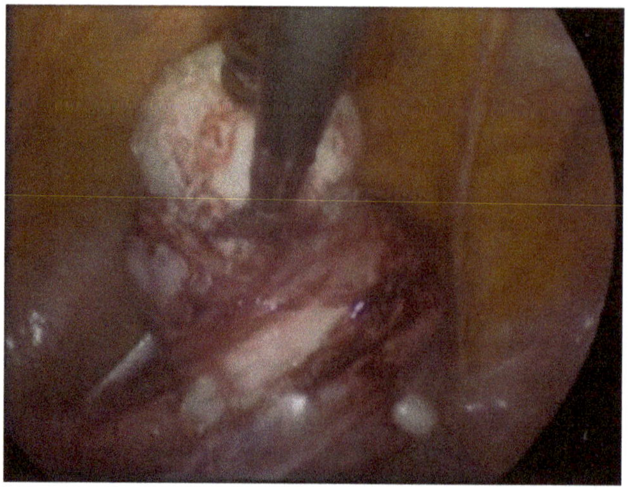

Fig. 1 Enucleation of the myoma performed with a 10-mm myoma drill

An intracorporeal double-layer suture of myometrium was performed by 2-0 absorbable barbed monofilament (V-Loc 180, Covidien). For stitching, a straight needleholder and a curved Kelly forcep as a contra-needleholder were used. Removal of the specimen was obtained under a vision with a 10-mm morcellator (Rotocut, Karl Storz) through the X-Cone 12 mm port.

No intraoperative and postoperative complications were detected. The estimated blood loss was less than 20 ml and the total operative time (skin to skin) was 94 min.

The patient was discharged after 1 day of hospitalization with a complete satisfaction in terms of pain and cosmetic outcome. The postoperative control after 1 month revealed a complete recovery of the umbilical scar at clinical exploration and of the uterus at ultrasound.

Findings—discussion

We describe a new surgical approach for transumbilical single-port access surgery in infertile patient with uterine leiomyoma and bilateral sactosalpinx. The surgical strategy planned for this patient has been bilateral salpingectomy and myomectomy to improve the IVF pregnancy rate. In our experience, we believe that the removal of the myoma in infertile patients which are 4 cm or more in diameter, which distort the endometrium causing defects in embryo implantation, is effective. SALS provides an opportunity to further enhance the cosmetic benefits of minimally invasive surgery while minimising the potential morbidity associated with multiple incisions but it has to be taken in consideration that SPAL approach has intrinsic limits such as absence of triangulation, inline vision, and instruments crowding. Therefore, to improve the performance and the application of this surgery, some suggestions and techniques should be taken into account. To facilitate the correct ergonomy, the monitor should be placed between the patient's legs and the first surgeon should stand by the left shoulder (lateral to the head of the patient) to recreate the correct axis for eyes–hands–monitor; the assistant should stand at the level of the patient's right shoulder. Since a third assistant's hand is not required in single-port procedures, an intrauterine device should be placed to aid in the manipulation of the uterus and exposition of the surgical field. The use of a 5-mm, 30° telescope is mandatory for both avoiding inline view and a constant clashing between instruments and a video camera and a 50-cm extended-length scope is useful since it allows the assistant to move the scope without hindering the surgeon's movements outside of the abdominal cavity.

During laparoscopic surgery, instrument triangulation allows proper tissue retraction which is essential for proper dissection along anatomical tissue planes and helps to avoid crossing between the instruments and the camera. The use of at least one flexible or curved instrument moves the shaft's axis out of the center sufficiently, thus allowing the surgeon to operate with some degree of triangulation. The use of curved instruments (single or double curve) consents the mobilization and traction of the organs using rotating, forward, and backward movements.

To reduce crowding instruments, the profile should be as slim as possible. If one camera and two instruments occupy the multichannel port, varying lengths prevent the bulkiest portion of each instrument (the external handle) from overlapping extracorporeally. A straight rotating handle is preferable.

In addition, multifunctional devices capable of grasping, dissecting, coagulating, and cutting overcome the limitation imposed by the reduced numbers of ports.

Stitching and suturing remain one of the most difficult skills in laparoscopy and more so in the single-port approach [9–12]. Standard rules have to be followed in order to simplify the technique as much as possible. To overcome the difficulty of the intracorporeal knot, we decided to use a barbed monofilament capable of safely fixing the tissue with a constant tension along the wound. A double-layer suture was needed to correctly close the myometrium, and to reduce adhesions an intraflexion suture at the level of the perimetrium was performed. Continuous suturing technique and absence of tying knots permit a considerable reduction in operating time. A good rule to keep in mind in performing laparoscopic stitching is that the suture axe should be parallel to the needleholder and perpendicular to the needle axe and in the single-port approach this means that the uterine incision, at the level of the anterior or posterior wall, should always be longitudinal. Even if the cosmetic advantage of the SPAL is realistic and more patients start to request this particular approach, it is important to define correct indications and to standardize techniques. With this report, we describe the technique used to perform SPAL myomectomy but we will need further experience and studies to correctly define the best reproducible technique.

Conclusion

Single-port laparoscopic myomectomy with X-Cone is feasible; however, further reports are needed to better define patients selection, to standardize the technique, and to develop specific instruments.

Declaration of interest The authors report no conflicts of interest. The authors alone are responsible for the content and writing of the paper.

References

1. Luciano AA (2009) Myomectomy. Clin Obstet Gynecol 52 (3):362–371
2. Baird DD, Dunson DB, Hill MC et al (2003) High cumulative incidence of uterine leiomyoma in black and white woman. Am J Obstet Gynecol 188:100–107
3. (2008) The Practice Committee of the American Society for Reproductive Medicine in collaboration with the Society of Reproductive Surgeons. Myomas and reproductive function. Fertil Steril 90(Suppl 3): S125–130
4. Oliveira FG, Abdelmassih VG, Diamond MP, Dozortsev D, Melo NR, Abdelmassih R (2004) Impact of subserosal and intramural uterine fibroids that do not distort the endometrial cavity on the outcome of in vitro fertilization—intracytoplasmic sperm injection. Fertil Steril 81(3):582–587
5. Bulletti C, DE Ziegler D, Levi Setti P, Cicinelli E, Polli V, Stefanetti M (2004) Myomas, pregnancy outcome, and in vitro fertilization. Ann NY Acad Sci 1034:84–92
6. William H, Parker MD (2007) Uterine myomas: management. Fertil Steril 88(2):255–271
7. Kim T-J, Lee Y-Y, Kim KMJ, CJ KH, Choi CH, Lee J-W, Kim B-G, Bae D-S (2009) Single port access laparoscopic adnexal surgery. J Minim Invasive Gynecol 16:612–615
8. Lee JH, Choi JS, Jeon SW, Son CE, Lee SJ, Lee YS (2010) Eur J Obstet Gynecol Reprod Biol 153:81–84
9. Kaouk JH, Haber GP, Goel RK, Desai MM, Aron M, Rackley RR et al (2008) Single port laparoscopic surgery in urology: initial experience. Urology 71(1):3–6
10. Fader AN, Escobar PF (2009) Laparoendoscopic single-site surgery (LESS) in gynecology oncology: technique and initial report. Gynecol Oncol 114(2):157–161
11. Mereu L, Angioni S, Melis GB, Mencaglia L (2010) Single access laparoscopy for adnexal pathologies using a novel reusable port and curved instruments. Int J Gynecol Obstet 109(1):78–80
12. Fagotti A, Fanfani F, Marocco F, Rossito C, Gallotta V, Scambia G (2009) Laparoendoscopic single-site surgery (LESS) for ovarian cyst nucleation: report of first 3 cases. Fertil Steril 92(3):1168: 13–16

30

Uterine manipulation in operative laparoscopy by suction disposable uterine device

S. Tamburro · E. Nouhz · F. Calonaci · A. Wattiez ·
M. Canis · G. Mage

Abstract The uterine mobilization is important to expose correctly the vesico-uterine plane, the adnexae, and the posterior cul-de-sac. Several studies compared different types of uterine manipulator and their maneuvrability, underlining the limitations or advantages related to the head and shaft when they are fixed together, limiting exposition or in the other, once there is dye injection capability. A new model of uterine manipulator by suction of endometrial cavity has been studied. Patients were not selected by uterine dimension or by gynecological disease; only the cases of endometrial cancer were excluded. In ten patients, we performed an hysteroscopic study associated to an endometrial specimen before installing the uterine device. No endometrial modification was found between normal endometrial specimen before surgery and after surgical treatment. The Vectec uterine manipulator has been demonstrated to be easy and safe to use.

S. Tamburro (✉) · E. Nouhz · F. Calonaci
Department of Obstetrics & Gynecology, CH Thiers,
Route du Fau,
63300 Thiers, France
e-mail: s.tamburro@cice.fr

A. Wattiez
CHU Hôpital Hautepierre, Chirurgie gynécologique,
1 Avenue Molière,
67098 Strasbourg Cedex 2, France

S. Tamburro · E. Nouhz · M. Canis · G. Mage
Department Obstetrics and Gynecology, CHU Clermont Ferrand,
CHU Estaing,
1 Place Lucie Aubrac,
63003 Clermont-Ferrand CEDEX 1, France

Keywords Laparoscopy · Uterine manipulator · Suction · New device

Introduction

Our aim and objective is to evaluate the efficacy and ergonomy of a new uterine manipulator and of the consequences of a suction system on endometrial tissue.

Laparoscopic surgery is currently accepted worldwide as an excellent diagnostic and treatment tool for many gynecologic problems. The uterine manipulator is essential, assisting the control of the uterus during a laparoscopic operation.

The uterine mobilization is important to expose correctly the vesico-uterine plane, the adnexae, and the posterior cul-de-sac. Otherwise, peritoneal lesions or defect of anterior and posterior space may not be evidenced and treated. In addiction pushing and lateralizing the uterus, more anatomical structures and spaces are visualized, such as paravesical and pararectal spaces. They could be accessible to dissection if necessary. Several studies compared different types of uterine manipulator and their maneuvrability, underlining the limitations or advantages related to the head and shaft when they are fixed together, limiting exposition or in the other once there is dye injection capability [2]. The uterine manipulator play the major role during operative laparoscopy approach showing uterine ligaments, parametrial spaces, uterine vessels, and to make colpotomy and hysterectomy; however, also during laparoscopy for adnexal pathology, it is revealed important to expose pelvic space [1–3, 5, 6].

More recently, in 2006, Banerjee, for the first time, suggested a suction cannula as uterine manipulator [4]. According to this idea, we developed a new model of uterine manipulator by suction of endometrial cavity, easy to install with the possibility to make a dye test. As part of a gynecologic procedure, dye is injected into the uterine cavity to observe its passage through the fimbria for evaluation of the fallopian tube patency in infertile patient [7–9].

Materials & methods

The design of the study has been reported here. Ten patients, between 25 and 50 years old, were included in the study independently of uteri dimensions or previous surgery. Before the cannulation, an endometrial biopsy with a Cornier pipelle and a diagnostic hysteroscopy were performed in all patients to assess the endometrium. The Pipelle endometrial sampler obtains a small sample of endometrium for histological assessment without dilatation of the cervix, and as there is usually minimal discomfort associated with the procedure, it may be conducted in the outpatient setting. Tissue samples obtained were collected into 10% neutral buffered formalin, routinely processed in the pathology laboratory and embedded in paraffin. About 5-mm tissue sections were cut, mounted, dewaxed, and stained with haematoxylin and eosin. No uterine cervical forceps or cervical dilatation was necessary to install the uterine vacuum manipulator (Fig. 1).

Uteri dimension study by Vectec, hysterometer is made to adapt the manipulator to endometrial cavity with or without the use of a reducer device. The blunt upper extremity of the manipulator with holes is inserted in the uteri and connected to the vacuum by a tube with a luer lock link. Particular attention is necessary to push closely in contact the extremity of Vectec manipulator with the cervix to obtain the good vacuum and to solidarize it with uteri. The dye test was made, blocking the tap on manipulator and linking a syringe to inject methylene blue inside.

After surgical laparoscopic procedure, at the end of the surgery, the uterine manipulator has been removed, and a second endometrial study by Cornier device and diagnostic hysteroscopy were performed, as previously described above.

Adequacy of both preparations was assessed as satisfactory when sufficient cellular material was present to make a pathological diagnosis, or to exclude a pathological process with confidence.

After the use of a manipulator, we have focused the attention to compare the endometrial glands and stromal cells characteristics, cytoplasm, and basal lamina; in the vessels' endothelial structure and integrity, in luminal gland secretion, and inflammatory infiltration cells.

Specimens described as "barely adequate" contained scanty endometrial material that was adequate for assessment, but suboptimal for exclusion of pathology.

In contrast, a specimen was assessed as "inadequate" if there was insufficient cellular material in both the cytological slide and the cell block to exclude a pathological diagnosis. The stromal cells, the endometrial glands, vessels, and inflammatory cells infiltration were compared between the two specimens to study the modification caused by manipulator application.

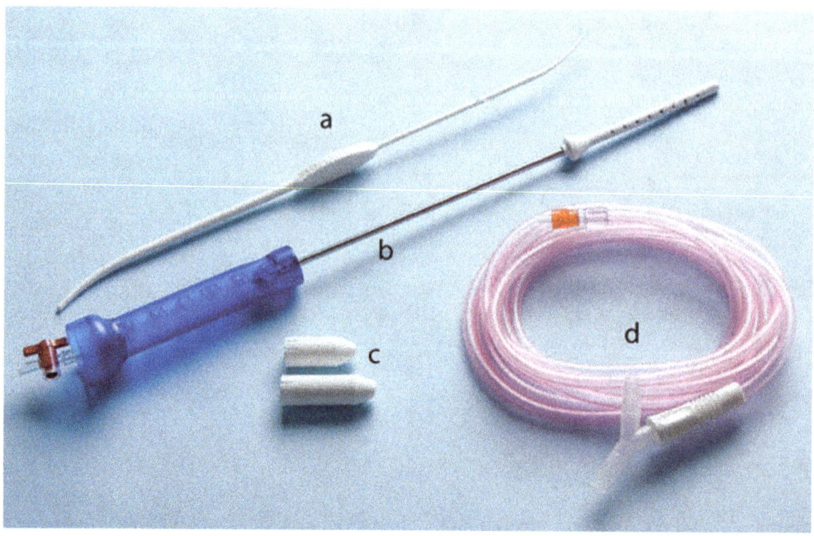

Fig. 1 The Vectec manipulator: **a** hysterometer, **b** manipulator, **c** reducer device, **d** vacuum tube

Results

No difficulties were found to insert the uterine manipulator, and the suction system allowed the surgeon to obtain a good exposition and mobility of uteri during surgery, independently of the uterine size. The Vectec manipulator has the advantage to be adaptable to each endometrial cavity; light and easy to mobilize. Using the manipulator, a blue dye test easily showed the bilateral tubal permeability, despite a fluid blue reflux which occurred around the cannula in three cases. In these cases, we checked that in a no right position of manipulator, which was not in contact with the uterine external orifice consequently, a non-optimal aspiration was obtained.

In the two groups of biopsies obtained before (Fig. 2, 3) and after manipulating, no differences were evidenced in specimens. Endometrial glands conserved their structure in multiple organization around the lumen, with the mucinous cell layers correctly represented. Glandular cells appeared normal, characterized with mucinous drops in cytoplasm and morphologically regular nuclei. The negative pressure induced by vacuum showed no modified basal cells layer and basal lamina of glands; however, in some lumen of glands, the gliar secretion induced by the suction action was visible. Among glands and stromal cells, mononuclear and other inflammatory cells were sometimes present to testify the consequences of suction induced by the manipulator, but no important distortions of tissue structure were found. (Fig. 4)

In all cases, no difference was found between two biopsies before and after uterine Vectec manipulator application. Tissue structures were well preserved, permitting an adequate analysis of tissue.

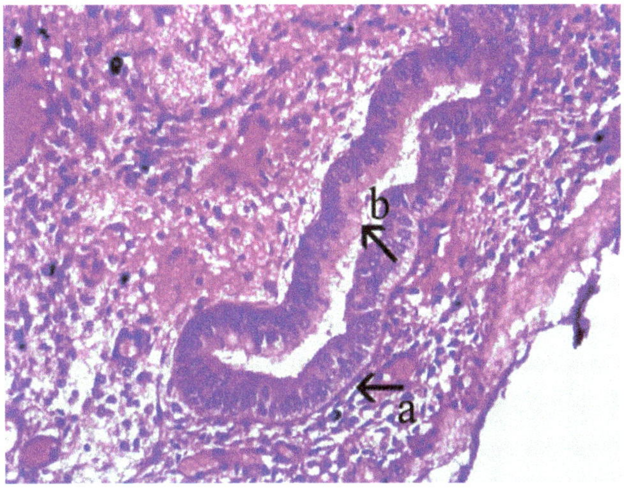

Fig. 3 Normal endometrial gland and stromal tissue. Basal layer (**a**) and mucinous fluid cells (**b**) are clearly evident (*arrows*)

Conclusions

The Vectec suction manipulator has demonstrated to be easy to install, cheap, and safe. The respect of hystological structure by suction is an important concept, because it could open other possibilities for others pathologies as application in oncology, where the integrity of tissue structures and cells is necessary to distinguish normal cells from atypical cells or neoplasia. In addition, the vacuum action in oncology could limit the neoplastic endometrial cells diffusion in peritoneal cavity during laparoscopic surgery. To evaluate this potential role, several studies are necessary which the results will be next published.

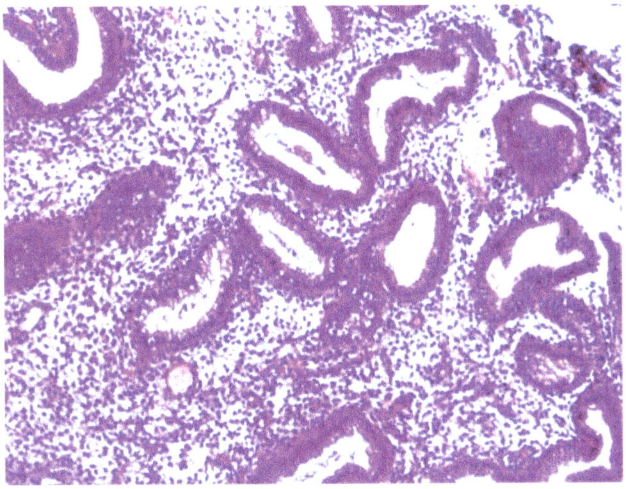

Fig. 2 Normal endometrial tissue before the use of the uterine manipulator

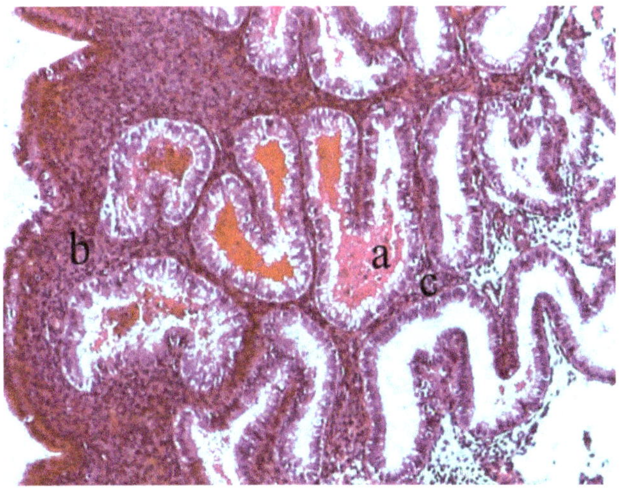

Fig. 4 Endometrium after manipulator use. Glands are intact with an important mucinous fluid in gland cavity (**a**); inflammatory cells are present among stromal cells (**b**). Basal layer is preserved and presented in normal structure (**c**)

Declaration of interest The authors report no conflicts of interest. The authors alone are responsible for the content and writing of the paper.

References

1. Ramirez PT, Frumovitz M, Dos Reis R, Milam MR, Bevers MW, Levenback CF et al (2008) Modified uterine manipulator and vaginal rings for total laparoscopic radical hysterectomy. Int J Gynecol Cancer 18:571–575
2. Choksuchat C, Getpook C, Watthanagamthornkul S, Choobun T, Dhanaworavibul K, Tintara H (2008) Comparison of the TINTARA uterine manipulator with the Cohen cannula in gynecologic laparoscopy. J Med Assoc Thai 91:439–444
3. Agdi M, Tulandi T (2008) The benefits of intrauterine balloon: an intrauterine manipulator and balloon proved useful in myomectomy. A J Obstet Gynecol 199:581
4. Banerjee AK, Emembolu JO (2006) Plastic suction curette as uterine manipulator at combined laparoscopic sterilization: a prospective study of 531 cases. Eur J Contracept Reprod Health Care 11:310–313
5. Wu HH, Yeh GP, Hsieh TC (2005) Iatrogenic uterine rupture caused by overinflation of RUMI manipulator balloon. J Minim Invasive Gynecol 12:174–176
6. Bernstein P (1995) A new uterine manipulator for operative laparoscopic hysterectomy. J Am Assoc Gynecol Laparosc 2:331–333
7. Gregersen E (1994) The U-elevator. A new manipulator for gynecologic laparoscopy. Acta Obstet Gynecol Scand 73:508–510
8. Letterie GS (1991) Simple modification of an intrauterine manipulator. Int J Fertil 36:358–359
9. Scott JW (1983) A new uterine manipulator for use at laparoscopy. Am J Obstet Gynecol 147:458–459

The effect of patient body mass index on surgical difficulty in gynaecological laparoscopy

Kate McIlwaine • M. Cameron • E. Readman • J. Manwaring • P. Maher

Abstract The objective of this pilot study was to evaluate the extent to which laparoscopic gynaecological surgery could be completed as planned in overweight and obese patients versus patients of normal weight. A prospective surgical audit was conducted of 64 women undergoing laparoscopy for benign gynaecological conditions. Patients were grouped according to their body mass index (BMI). The number of attempts required for successful laparoscopic entry, the ability to identify key surgical landmarks, the ability to complete the planned surgery, the rate of conversion to laparotomy and the complication rates were recorded. Surgery was completed as planned in 95.31% of participants. Completion rates declined with increasing BMI. Increased entry attempts and an inability to identify key surgical landmarks were associated with increased BMI, although the sample size was insufficient to provide any statistically significant conclusions. The overall complication rate was 6.25%. There was a higher mean BMI in patients with a complication; however, there was insufficient data to show a significant difference. This study suggests an association between increasing BMI and increased entry attempts for laparoscopy, increased difficulty in surgical landmark identification and an overall reduction in completion of gynaecological laparoscopy as planned.

Keywords Laparoscopic surgery · Body mass index · Obesity · Surgical outcomes · Complications

K. McIlwaine (✉) · M. Cameron · E. Readman · J. Manwaring · P. Maher
Department of Endosurgery, Mercy Hospital for Women, 163 Studley Rd., Heidelberg, VIC 3084, Australia
e-mail: KMcilwaine@mercy.com.au

Introduction

Overweight and obesity are measured using the body mass index (BMI)—the ratio of weight (measured in kilogrammes) over the square of height (measured in metres). A normal BMI is between 18.5 and 24.99. A BMI of 25 kg/m^2 or greater indicates overweight, and 30 kg/m^2 or greater indicates obesity [1]. Obesity has reached epidemic proportions in the Western World with more than one billion adults overweight and at least 300 million clinically obese [2]. In Australia, obesity has almost tripled over the past 20 years [3] and costs the country $21 billion annually [4]. According to the 2007–2008 National Health Survey, 55% of Australian women are either overweight or obese [5].

Obesity is associated with numerous chronic health issues such as respiratory difficulties, musculoskeletal problems and infertility. It is also a major risk factor for cardiovascular disease, type 2 diabetes, hypertension and stroke and some forms of cancer such as cancers of the endometrium, breast and colon [2].

Obesity has been well studied in obstetrics and is linked to a number of adverse obstetric outcomes, as well as increased maternal and neonatal morbidity and mortality [6]. These complications include gestational hypertension, pre-eclampsia, gestational diabetes, caesarean section, postpartum haemorrhage, foetal macrosomia, congenital abnormalities and antepartum stillbirth [6–10]. In contrast to the plethora of research on obesity in the obstetric population, there is comparatively little data to guide the pre-operative counselling process in overweight and obese patients presenting to their gynaecologists requiring laparoscopic surgery.

An Ovid Literature Search, using the search terms 'laparoscopic surgery and obesity', yielded 758 results. The papers reviewed, however, mostly assessed surgical difficulties and outcomes in bariatric surgery and robot-assisted laparoscopic radical prostatectomy, specifically in older male patients with medical comorbidities. Few of the papers reviewed were relevant to our younger female population undergoing elective laparoscopic gynaecological procedures. The currently available literature supports laparoscopic surgery in favour of open surgery in the obese population given the reduction in post-operative hospital stay, post-operative pain and wound infection rates, as well as reduced post-operative ileus and fever, compared with obese patients undergoing laparotomy [11].

Most of the data regarding the effect of obesity on surgical outcomes in gynaecological laparoscopy comes from retrospective reviews in the gynaecology oncology population [12–14]. The available evidence suggests that laparoscopic surgery is feasible in most obese patients; however, there is an increased risk of conversion to laparotomy compared with non-obese patients.

Whilst the available literature shows that laparoscopic surgery is a safe alternative to laparotomy in patients with an increased BMI, there is a definite paucity of good quality prospective data assessing the limitations and risks of surgery in this clinically important group of patients. In particular, there is a lack of data regarding the risks associated with increased BMI in laparoscopies for benign conditions where the level of risk acceptable to patients may be less than what would be accepted by those undergoing emergency or life-saving surgery for malignant disease.

Gynaecologists are therefore somewhat limited in the information they can provide for overweight and obese women regarding the increased risks (if any) that their weight adds to having a laparoscopic procedure and whether their BMI is likely to impact on the ability to complete the surgery as planned. This pilot study aims to address some of the gaps in the currently available data and help answer these important clinical questions.

Methods

The study group included women undergoing diagnostic or operative laparoscopy for benign gynaecological conditions. Women aged over 18 years attending for laparoscopy from January to October 2009 at our centre were invited to participate in the study after an interview with one of the authors (KM). Women included in the study were required to have an adequate grasp of the English language and be able to give informed consent. Ethical approval for this study was obtained from The Mercy Hospital for Women Human Research Ethics Committee.

Baseline demographic data were recorded including patient age, height, weight, waist and hip circumference and any prior abdominal or pelvic surgery (Table 1). Each patient was measured and weighed without shoes and wearing a hospital gown or light street clothing using the same height measuring device and scales. Waist circumference was measured with the patient in the standing position around the narrowest point between the ribs and hips when viewed from the front after exhaling. Hip circumference was measured at the point where the buttocks extend the maximum, when viewed from the side. Measurements were taken to the nearest centimetre without compression of the skin.

After obtaining written informed consent, women recruited to the study had their laparoscopic procedures performed in the usual manner as determined by the treating surgeon. Details of the operation, including

Table 1 Patient demographics

BMI	<25	25–29.9	≥30	>35	Overall
Age (mean)	30.43	39.27	36.62	39.33	35.50
Waist, Hip (mean)	0.77	0.85	0.82	0.85	0.81
Prior surgery	61.90%	50.00%	90.48%	77.78%	67.19%
Laparoscopy	47.62%	27.27%	42.86%	11.11%	40.63%
Laparotomy	14.29%	22.73%	47.62%	66.67%	26.56%
Procedure					
Diagnostic	19.00%	13.64%	33.33%	44.44%	21.88%
Simple Op	52.38%	40.91%	33.33%	33.33%	42.19%
Complex Op	19.00%	22.73%	0.00%	0.00%	14.06%
Advanced Op	9.52%	22.73%	33.33%	22.22%	21.88%
Adhesions					
Nil	33.33%	31.82%	28.57%	33.33%	31.25%
Mild	38.10%	27.27%	19.05%	11.11%	28.13%
Moderate	28.57%	18.18%	28.57%	33.33%	25.00%
Severe	0.00%	22.73%	23.81%	22.22%	15.63%

indications for the procedure, complexity of the procedure, degree of pelvic adhesions, primary operator, surgical outcomes, entry technique and any difficulties encountered, surgical landmark identification, any surgical or anaesthetic complications, and whether conversion to laparotomy was required, were documented by the operating surgeon at the conclusion of the procedure on a data collection sheet. Simple operative procedures included ovarian cystectomies, bilateral salpingo-oophorectomy (BSO), management of ectopic pregnancies and excision of stages I–II endometriosis. Complex operative procedures included excision of stage III endometriosis, and advanced procedures included total laparoscopic hysterectomy (TLH) and management of stage IV endometriosis. The degree of pelvic adhesions was scored qualitatively from nil to severe.

A further data collection sheet was completed by the gynaecologist reviewing the patient at their 6-week post-operative visit in order to detect any complications encountered following the patient's discharge from hospital.

The primary outcome of this study was whether the planned surgery could be completed in overweight and obese patients undergoing laparoscopy. Secondary outcomes were the number of attempts required for successful laparoscopic entry, the ability to identify key surgical landmarks, the conversion rate to laparotomy and the rate of surgical and anaesthetic complications.

All data were analysed using Minitab® Release 14 statistical package. Power and sample size calculations were completed using a Power=0.80 and α=0.05. The two-sample t test and the two-sample p test were used for calculations involving means and proportions respectively.

Results

A total of 64 women were recruited to the study with an even distribution across the various BMI categories of normal (BMI <25), overweight (BMI 25–29.99) and obese (BMI ≥30). Patients with a BMI exceeding 35 were analysed as a subgroup of the obese category. Nine women (14% of the study sample) had a BMI over 35.

There was no significant difference across the various BMI categories with regards to mean age, waist-to-hip ratio or the complexity of the laparoscopic procedure performed (Table 1). There was, however, a higher prior laparotomy rate in obese patients, particularly in the morbidly obese group, which may have translated to a larger proportion of patients with moderate to severe adhesions in this BMI category.

The overall completion rate of the planned surgery was 95.31% (61 patients). The completion rate of surgery declined with increasing BMI from 100% completion in the normal BMI category—95.45% in the overweight group, 90.48% in the obese group to 77.78% in the subgroup of patients with a BMI over 35 (Fig. 1).

There was a trend towards an increased number of attempts at laparoscopic entry in the subgroup of patients with a BMI exceeding 35 (Fig. 2). The majority of entries (92%) were made using the Veress needle. The Endopath® Xcel Bladeless Trocar (Ethicon Endo-Surgery, LLC Guaynabo, Puerto Rico 00969, USA) and the open technique were also used for primary entry at the discretion of the operating surgeon.

There was a trend towards a reduced ability to identify key surgical landmarks with increasing patient BMI (Table 2). The inferior epigastric vessels and ureters were recorded as being identified if they were either partially or completely visible.

One patient (1.56%) required conversion of their procedure to laparotomy. This postmenopausal patient had a BMI of 29.64 and was undergoing a laparoscopic BSO for a persistent ovarian cyst. Laparoscopic access to the pelvis was poor due to fat and adhesions.

The overall complication rate in the study group was 6.25%. There were two major and two minor complications. The major complications were a right ureterovaginal fistula following a complex TLH for severe endometriosis in a patient with a BMI of 27.24 and an episode of asystole on Veress insufflation of CO2 in a patient with a BMI of 28.58, which required atropine and cardiac compressions for correction. There were two patients with minor cases of wound cellulitis requiring oral antibiotic therapy. There was a higher mean BMI in the patients who had a complication (29.80) compared with the patients who did not have a complication (28.04); however, the sample size was insufficient to show a significant difference.

Based on the data of this pilot study, it was calculated that 299 patients would be required to demonstrate whether there is a statistically significant relationship between patient BMI and the ability to complete the surgery as planned.

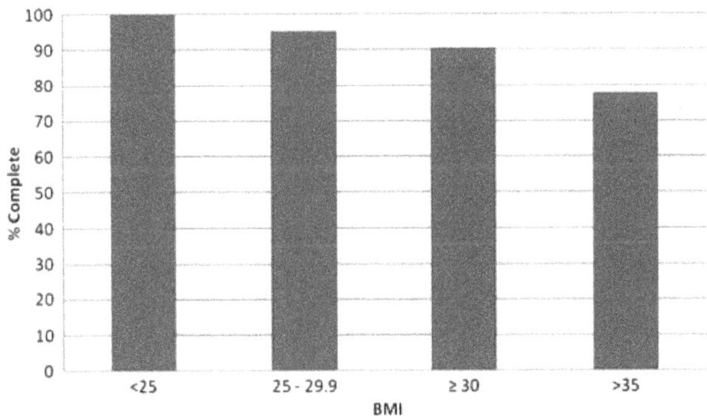

Fig. 1 Surgery completed as planned

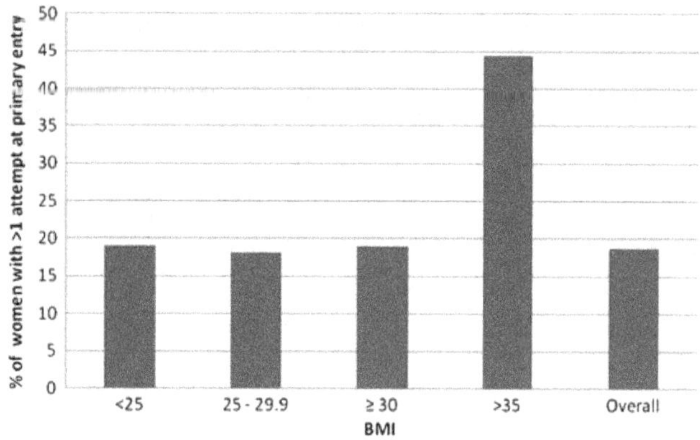

Fig. 2 Attempts at laparoscopic entry

Discussion

Obesity is fast becoming a global epidemic, and we are increasingly presented with overweight and obese patients requiring laparoscopic gynaecological surgery for a host of benign gynaecological conditions. Whilst the ideal approach for these individuals is pre-operative weight loss, this is often difficult to attain [15]. Obesity was once considered a contraindication to laparoscopic surgery; however, the laparoscopic approach is well suited to obese patients given their increased susceptibility to thromboembolic events and poor wound healing following laparotomy [15].

Most of the studies examining the effects of obesity on outcomes in laparoscopic surgery to date are non-gynaecologic in nature. The available research supports the laparoscopic approach for the treatment of endometrial cancer in obese patients although most of these studies are retrospective reviews with their attendant limitations [13, 14]. A further retrospective cohort study in 270 general gynaecology patients demonstrated that TLH could be performed successfully in most obese patients with similar complication rates to those for non-obese patients although operating times and intra-operative blood loss were increased in the obese group [16]. The observational nature of this study again makes it difficult to draw absolute conclusions. There remains little, therefore, to guide the pre-operative counselling process in patients requiring laparoscopic gynaecological surgery for benign conditions.

Table 2 Surgical landmark identification

Surgical landmark	Identified	Mean BMI
Left inferior epigastric artery	Y	27.44
	N	33.92
Right inferior epigastric artery	Y	27.44
	N	32.53
Left ureter	Y	26.96
	N	32.84
Right ureter	Y	26.99
	N	35.21

It is of critical importance to the process of obtaining informed consent to be able to advise the patient on the risks and benefits associated with the proposed surgery and to provide a realistic expectation of the likely surgical outcome. Our study aims to address the gaps in the currently available data in order to help answer these important clinical questions.

With regards to the primary outcome of this study, our results suggest a reduced ability to complete the planned surgery with increasing BMI. This was most pronounced in the subgroup of patients with a BMI over 35 where the ability to complete the surgery as planned was 77.78% compared with a completion rate of 100% in patients of normal BMI. Where surgery was unable to be completed as planned, this was attributed to poor access due to fat and/or adhesions precluding safe access to the pelvis.

Obtaining a pneumoperitoneum in obese patients can be particularly challenging due to increased abdominal wall thickness and preperitoneal fat. The percentage of women requiring more than one attempt at laparoscopic entry was highest in the morbidly obese group when compared with women in all other weight ranges. This is likely due to the Veress needle dissecting into the preperitoneum more frequently in the morbidly obese patients despite attempting insertion through the base of the umbilicus. Direct entry under vision using the Endopath® Xcel Bladeless Trocar was a useful way of obtaining primary entry in the morbidly obese and was selected more frequently in this subgroup of patients.

Technical obstacles, associated with open pelvic surgery in the obese, are primarily those related to operative exposure and access to deep pelvic structures. These obstacles present similar challenges when laparoscopy is attempted [16]. In the patient whose procedure was converted to laparotomy, fat and adhesions precluded safe access to the pelvis, and the decision was made to open through a Pfannenstiel incision. The surgery was completed uneventfully, and the patient had an unremarkable post-operative course.

Of the two major complications occurring in this series, one was a right-sided ureterovaginal fistula occurring in an overweight patient undergoing a TLH for severe endometriosis and adenomyosis. A cystoscopy that demonstrated bilateral ureteric jets was performed at the conclusion of the procedure. Post-procedure cystoscopy with intravenous injection of indigo carmine is increasingly used to demonstrate ureteric patency following gynaecologic surgery [17] and is routinely performed in our unit following TLH. This method, however, can still provide a false negative result in cases of urological injury secondary to thermal damage or where there is partial obstruction [17, 18]. The fistula in this case was thought to have formed post-operatively from a diathermy injury to the ureter whilst obtaining haemostasis at the vaginal vault. The patient underwent further surgery for reimplantation of the right ureter, and subsequently, made a full recovery. There was a higher mean BMI in patients with a complication (29.8) compared to the group with no complications (28.04); however, there was insufficient data to show a significant difference.

Conclusion

The results of this pilot study suggest an association between increasing BMI and reduced completion of planned gynaecological laparoscopy, an increased number of attempts at laparoscopic entry and increased difficulty in surgical landmark identification. A larger study is currently underway with the aim of recruiting 300 women in order to answer the question, 'Can the planned surgery be completed in overweight and obese women undergoing gynaecological laparoscopy and what are the excess risks associated with an increased BMI?'

Disclosure The authors of this paper have no commercial, proprietary or financial interest in any aspect of the work pertaining to this article.

References

1. www.naaso.org—North American Association for the Study of Obesity. Accessed 26 March 2010
2. WHO (2010) Obesity and overweight. www.who.int/dietphysical activity/publications/facts/obesity/en/print.html. Accessed 26 March 2010
3. OECD (2009) Health at a glance 2009: OECD indicators. OECD Publishing. doi:10.1781_glance-2009-en.
4. Colagiuri S, Lee CM, Colagiuri R et al (2010) The cost of overweight and obesity in Australia. MJA 192(5):260–264
5. Australian Bureau of Statistics 2009 National Health Survey Summary of Results. 43640.0 2007–2008 viewed 26 March 2010.
6. Jarvie E, Ramsay JE (2010) Obstetric management of obesity in pregnancy. Semin Fetal Neonatal Med 15:83–88
7. Rowlands I, Graves N, de Jersey S et al (2010) Obesity in pregnancy: outcomes and economics. Semin Fetal Neonatal Med 15:94–99
8. Usha Kiran TS, Hemmadi J, Bethel J et al (2005) Outcome of pregnancy in a woman with an increased body mass index. BJOG 112:768–772
9. Weiss JL, Malone FD, Emig D et al (2004) Obesity, obstetric complications and caesarean delivery rate—a population-based screening study. Am J Obstet Gynecol 190:1091–1097
10. Magriples U, Kershaw TS, Schindler Rising S et al (2009) The effects of obesity and weight gain in young women on obstetric outcomes. Am J Perinatol 26(5):365–371
11. Lamvu G, Zolnoun D, Boggess J et al (2004) Obesity: physiologic changes and challenges during laparoscopy. Am J Obstet Gynecol 191(2):669–674
12. Eltabbakh GH, Piver MS, Hempling RE et al (1999) Laparoscopic surgery in obese women. Obstet Gynecol 94(5):704–708
13. O'Hanlan KA, Lopez L, Dibble S et al (2003) Total laparoscopic hysterectomy: body mass index and outcomes. Obstet Gynecol 102(6):1384–1392
14. Obermair A, Manolitsas TP, Laung Y et al (2005) Total laparoscopic hysterectomy versus total abdominal hysterectomy for obese women with endometrial cancer. Int J Gynecol Cancer 15:319–324
15. Matory WE Jr, O'Sullivan J, Fudem G et al (1994) Abdominal surgery in patients with severe morbid obesity. Plast Reconstr Surg 94(7):976–987
16. Heinberg EM, Crawford BL, Weitzen SH et al (2004) Total laparoscopic hysterectomy in obese versus non-obese patients. Obstet Gynecol 103(4):674–680
17. Dandolu V, Mathai E, Chatwant A et al (2003) Accuracy of cystoscopy in the diagnosis of ureteral injury in benign gynaecologic surgery. Int Urogynecol J Pelvic Floor Dysfunct 14:427–431
18. Siow A, Nikam YA, Ng C et al (2007) Urological complications of laparoscopic hysterectomy: a four-year review at KK Women's and Children's Hospital. Singapore Med J 48(3):217–221

The efficacy of laparoscopic uterosacral nerve ablation (LUNA) in the treatment of unexplained chronic pelvic pain

Hossam El-Din Shawki

Abstract The aim of this work is to explore the efficacy , safety, and patients' satisfaction of laparoscopic uterosacral nerve ablation (LUNA) in relief of pain in women with chronic pelvic pain in whom diagnostic laparoscopy reveals either no pathology or mild endometriosis (AFS score ≤5). The study was a prospective, single-blind, randomized trial with 12 months follow-up. It was conducted at the endoscopy unit of the Gynecology Department of El Minia University Hospital, Egypt. One hundred ninety Egyptian women consented to participate in the study. These eligible patients were randomized using computer-generated tables and were divided into two equal groups, including the control group (diagnostic laparoscopy with no pelvic denervation) and the study group (diagnostic laparoscopy plus LUNA). Diagnostic laparoscopy with or without laparoscopic uterosacral nerve ablation was done. There were no statistically significant difference between both groups regarding the efficacy and the overall success rate (between group I and group II, it was 77.64%, 76.47%, and 74.11% versus 79.06%, 75.58%, and 73.25% at 3, 6, and 12 months, respectively) and the cumulative patients' satisfaction rate (it was 74.11%, 74.11%, and 71.76% versus 75.58%, 75.58%, and 72.09% at 3, 6, and 12 months between group I and group II, respectively; $P \leq 0.05$). There was no statistically significant difference between both groups as regards the effectiveness of LUNA in the treatment of primary (spasmodic) and secondary (congestive) dysmenorrhea ($P \leq 0.05$), while there was a statistically significant difference between both groups in the treatment of dyspareunia ($P \geq 0.05$). LUNA can be a last alternative option in well-selected patients for control of chronic pelvic pain without endometriosis; however, its effectiveness may not extend to other indications. Also, preliminary experience in the treatment of primary deep dyspareunia presents a promising perspective on the management of deep dyspareunia, especially if it will involve a team of social, psychological, and gynecological specialists.

Keywords Chronic pelvic pain · LUNA · Dysmenorrhea · Laparoscopy · Dyspareunia

Background

Chronic pelvic pain (CPP) can be defined as intermittent or constant pain in the lower abdomen or pelvis of at least 6 months' duration, not occurring exclusively with menstruation or intercourse, and not associated with pregnancy; it is a symptom, not a diagnosis and dysmenorrhea, deep dyspareunia, and intermenstrual pain constitute its main symptom complex [1]. CPP is one of the commonest symptomatology in gynecological outpatient clinics. It accounts for 10% of office visits to gynecologists, general clinics, and about a quarter of outpatient consultations in general gynecological practice and for 40–60% of all diagnostic laparoscopies [2]. In our department, it varies from 40–46% of all diagnostic laparoscopy annually. CPP has a profound impact on a woman's personal health and quality of life, including an economic impact through loss of working hours [1].

Laparoscopy is a valuable tool in the evaluation of undiagnosed CPP, as it can establish a definite diagnosis and modify the treatment without resorting to exploratory laparotomy [3]. In the absence of pathology, there is no

H. El-Din Shawki (✉)
Obstetrics and Gynecology Department, Faculty of Medicine, El Minia University,
El Minia, Egypt
e-mail: Hossam20002003@yahoo.com

established treatment, therefore, treatment is sometimes unsuccessful, and hysterectomy often becomes the final resort. Therefore, a conservative surgery, if shown to be effective, would represent a major improvement in its management [1]. Recent developments in minimal access surgery using laparoscopy make ablation of the nerve plexuses and ganglions in the uterosacral ligaments (laparoscopic uterosacral nerve ablation (LUNA)) a practicable treatment option [4].

Some recent reports of randomized controlled studies have clarified some roles of LUNA in the control of pelvic pain [5, 6] ,but systematic review and recent Cochrane reviews [7, 8] have shown that the currently available research evidence on LUNA is inconclusive, and therefore, further research is required among patients in different communities with different demographic and clinical characteristics to generate effectiveness evidence in the form of a high-quality, randomized, controlled trial to assess the principal hypothesis that, in women with chronic pelvic pain in whom diagnostic laparoscopy reveals either no pathology or mild endometriosis (American Fertility Society (AFS) score ≤5), LUNA alleviates pain and improves life quality [4].

Aim of the work

The primary aim of this work is to explore the efficacy and the safety of LUNA in the relief of pain in women with CPP in whom diagnostic laparoscopy reveals either no pathology or mild endometriosis (AFS score ≤5). The secondary aim was to evaluate the patients' satisfaction from the procedure during 3, 6, and 12 months follow-up, and to test the hypothesis that response to LUNA differs according to type of the pain by two secondary analyses: (1) women with primary or secondary dysmenorrhea, and (2) women with deep dyspareunia.

Patients and methods

This prospective, randomized, controlled trial was conducted at the endoscopy unit of the Gynecology Department at El Minia University Hospital, Egypt between the period of June 2004 to December 2008 with single-blind assessment of outcomes in eligible consenting patients randomized at diagnostic laparoscopy to LUNA (study group) or to no pelvic denervation (control group).

Eligibility

All new patients (280 women) who presented to the Gynecology outpatient clinic with pelvic pain (cyclical or noncyclical) and/or dyspareunia and who required diagnostic laparoscopy for evaluation of these conditions were invited to participate. When they consented to participate, they were registered prior to randomization (registered patients). Only 190 patients were eligible to randomization into one of the study groups according to strict inclusions criteria, and the study protocol was in concordance with the protocol guidelines of the LUNA Trial Collaboration [3] (Fig. 1).

1. Inclusion criteria

Patients with pelvic pain of longer than 6 months in duration, that was located within the true pelvis or between and below the anterior iliac crests, associated with functional disability, did not respond to medical treatment, and planned diagnostic laparoscopy revealed no pelvic pathology were considered as eligible patients for the study.

2. Exclusion criteria

Patients with previous LUNA, moderate and severe endometriosis (AFS score >5), previous surgery for endometriosis or for pelvic inflammatory disease, previous hysterectomy, and adnexal pathology were excluded from the study.

Eligible patients were thoroughly counseled, and informed consent was taken from all the patients. Complete history was taken, including the patients' present symptoms, past medical history, medication used, known allergies, and previous similar attack(s), and method(s) of treatment. Detailed, general, abdominal, and pelvic examinations were performed, including a vaginal examination using sterile speculum. Cervical cytology, pelvic and vaginal ultrasound was done for all patients. At this point, the women were randomly assigned to diagnostic laparoscopy to start therapy according to protocol that has been approved by the medical ethical committee of the department.

Randomization

Consenting patients (280 patients) were subjected to diagnostic laparoscopy first, and in the same sitting, consenting eligible patients (190 patients) were randomized using computer-generated tables into two equal groups, including the control group (diagnostic laparoscopy with no pelvic denervation) and the study group (diagnostic laparoscopy plus uterosacral nerve ablation).

The patients were allocated to groups using a chance procedure, blocking, and stratification. Stratified block randomization was employed to ensure that there was nearly equal numbers of patients in the two groups within the prognostic subgroups, even if the study ends prematurely so that a chance imbalance in the stratification variable does not have an effect on the outcome.

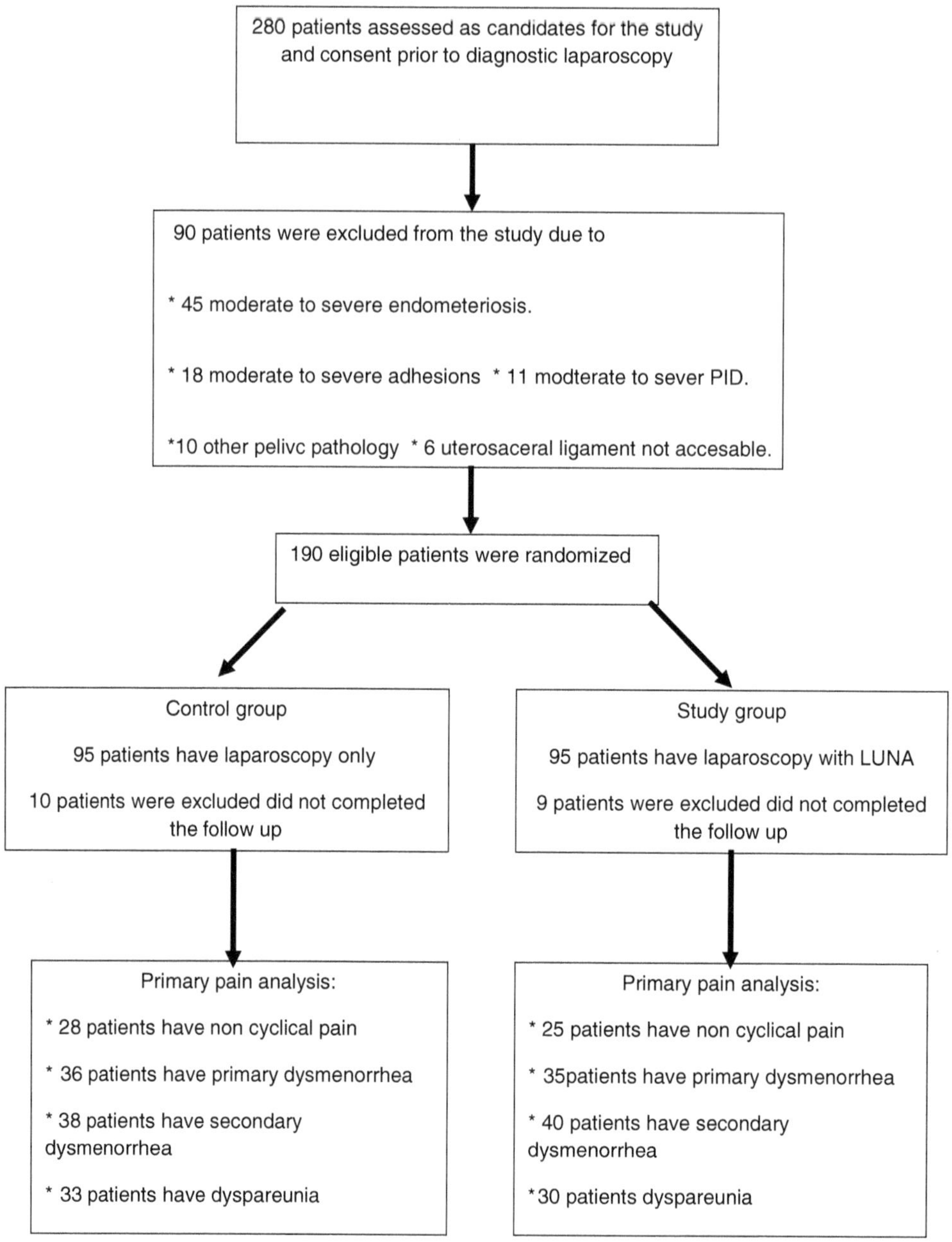

Fig. 1 Flow chart of the study protocol

Blinding

In this study, patients were kept blind to their treatment allocation until the follow-up in the trial was completed to avoid the placebo effect that may occur if they know they have received the active treatment. Unfortunately, single-blind approach was used, as it was difficult to keep the surgeon blind to the procedure.

Interventions

Routine preparation was made for a diagnostic laparoscopy with the patient under general anesthesia. Following pneumoperitoneum, a laparoscope was used to visualize the pelvis. Before embarking on operative laparoscopy, an anatomical pelvic assessment was performed to identify pelvic structures and pathology. At this stage, patients with pathology outlined in the exclusion criteria were excluded. It is expected that around 30% to 50% of women will be unsuitable for LUNA at operation and were "registered only" cases. Eligible patients were randomized into one of the study groups: first group, the control group, laparoscopy without pelvic denervation, and the second group, the study group, laparoscopy with uterosacral nerve ablation.

The posterior leaf of the broad ligament was carefully inspected to identify the course of the ureters, which, on rare occasions, could be particularly close to the uterosacral ligaments. Care was also taken to note thin-walled pelvic veins, which often lie lateral to the uterosacral ligaments. If accidentally punctured, they may cause troublesome bleeding, requiring further endoscopic endocoagulation. The uterosacral ligaments were identified by manipulation of the uterus in the right and left lateral planes. Clear identification of the uterosacral ligaments was a prerequisite for treatment, and ablation of the ligament was carried out using 5-mm bipolar electrodiathermy using bipolar Meyerland forceps (the main unit of the diathermy is adjusted at 30 W, and energy is applied for 5 s in order to deliver a dose power of coagulation 150 J to every uterosacral ligament), and then complete transaction of the uterosacral ligaments was done using a 5-mm curved scissors supplied with the ability to use monopolar electrodiathermy if needed. The ablation was started as close to the posterior aspect of the cervix as possible and continued for a minimum of 1 cm posterolaterally on either side. The aim of the procedure was to destroy the sensory nerve fibers and the secondary ganglia as they leave the uterus and come to lie within the uterosacral ligaments [3]. Patients with moderate pelvic adhesion obliterating the douglas pouch or making access to either uterosacral ligament difficult were excluded from the study.

Following surgery, the surgeon filled the operation details on a post-surgery form, including the laparoscopic finding, technique, the operative time, intraoperative blood loss, and intraoperative and postoperative complications.

Follow-up protocol and statistical analysis

All patients were followed up after 3, 6, and 12 months after the ablation. Follow-up visits included: history taking, clinical examination, and ultrasound (abdominal and vaginal) examination. The effectiveness of the procedure was estimated using a 10-cm visual analog scale (VAS), anchored at one end as no pain at all, and at the other as the worst imaginable pain. Also, the VAS ratings were obtained at 3, 6, and 12 months for each of the types of pain: noncyclical pain (pain at any other time other than during periods or during intercourse), primary (spasmodic) dysmenorrhea, secondary (congestive) dysmenorrhea, and dyspareunia (pain during intercourse). The success rate was defined as the percentage of women who reported no, minimal, or tolerable pain during the period of follow-up and without hysterectomy or repeated LUNA, and this PAS was calculated as percentage to simplify the results (*excellent =10–9, **good =6–8 PAS , ***tolerable =3–5, ****minimal =0–2 PAS). The patients' satisfaction was estimated by asking the patients a direct question (did the procedure improve your health status?, regarding the need for additional treatments, resource usage, days off work, and complications of surgery), and the patients' answers determine the degree of satisfaction (if it is excellent [4], good [3], average [2], or no improvement [1]). Also, the option if the pain was "worse than before" was evaluated and was only restricted to complications of the procedure that worsen the patients' condition. All patients were followed up for long-term complication and the need for additional treatment (medical or surgical), which was considered as treatment failure. Statistical analysis was performed on an IBM personal computer using SPSS statistical package for windows (SOSS, Inc, USA). Results were expressed as mean±SD for quantitative characteristics, and number and percentage for qualitative characteristics. Among different groups, statistical comparison was made using chi-square X2 test or Fisher exact test for qualitative characteristics and one-way ANOVA for numerical results among different groups. P values of ≤0.05 were considered as the level of significance.

Findings

There was no statistically significant difference between both groups regarding demographic and clinical characteristics of patients (Tables 1 and 2). The efficacy was comparable between group I and group II at 3, 6, and 12 months of follow-up ($P\leq0.05$). Also, the overall success rate between group I and group II was comparable to each other, as it was 77.64%, 76.47%, and 74.11% versus 79.06%, 75.58%, and 73.25% at 3, 6, and 12 months, respectively($P\leq0.05$; Table 3). Patients' satisfaction rate did not vary significantly between group I and group II at 3, 6, and 12 months follow-up ($P\leq0.05$). The cumulative satisfaction rate was 74.11%, 74.11%, and 71.76% versus 75.58%, 75.58%, and 72.09% at 3, 6, and 12 months between group I and group II, respectively ($P\leq0.05$; Table 4). In evaluating the effectiveness of LUNA (when compared to a control or no treatment) in the treatment of primary (spasmodic) dysmenorrhea and secondary (congestive) dysmenorrhea, there was no statistically significant difference between both groups, ($P\leq0.05$); on the other hand, as regarding the effectiveness of LUNA in the treatment of dyspareunia, there was a statistically significant difference between both groups, ($P\geq0.05$; Fig. 2). There were no statistically significant difference between group I and group II regarding the intraoperative and postoperative complications ($P\leq0.05$; Table 2).

Discussion

Definitive diagnosis of CPP is usually by laparoscopy or laparotomy. Treatment for CPP depends on the underlying cause. In some patients, a cause cannot be identified, so conservative treatments will be tried. If these medical treatments fail, conservative surgical treatment options which include vaginal uterosacral ligament resection, uterine nerve ablation, and presacral neurectomy may be beneficial [1–4].

Table 1 Clinical characteristics of patients in both study groups

		Group I (control) N=85	Group II (study) N=86	P value
Age (years)	Range (Mean±SD)	25–45 31.90±2.44	24–43 30.25±2.55	NS
Weight (kg)	Range (Mean±SD)	48–75 66–11±5.31	50–72 67.18±4.34	NS
Height (cm)	Range (Mean±SD)	153–170 163±1.17	152–173 161±2.10	NS
BMI (kg/m^2)	Range (Mean±SD)	24.40–29.55 24.80±1.46	23.66–28.41 25.23±1.25	NS
Parity (N)	Range (Mean±SD)	1–8 4.78±1.65	1–7 5.43±1.61	NS
Clinical presentation(s), N (%)				
Acyclic lower abdominal pain		28 (32.9%)	25 (29%)	NS
Congestive dysmenorrhea		38 (44.7%)	40 (46.5%)	NS
Spasmodic dysmenorrhea		36 (42.3%)	35 (40.6%)	NS
Deep dyspareunia		33 (38.8%)	30 (34.8%)	NS
Pervaginal findings, N (%)				
Pelvic tenderness		18/85 (21.1%)	19/86 (22.9%)	NS
Localized to one fornix		6/18 (33.3%)	7/19 (36.8%)	NS
Bilateral		3/18 (16.6%)	3/19 (15.7%)	NS
Diffuse		9/18 (50%)	12/19 (63.3%)	NS
Fornical fullness		14/85 (16.4%)	12/86 (13.9%)	NS
Unilateral		5/14 (35.7%)	5/12 (41.6%)	NS
Bilateral		9/14 (64.2%)	7/12 (85.3%)	NS
Cul-de-sac nodularity		3/85 (3.5%)	2/86 (2.3)	NS
Fixed retroverted uterus		1/85 (1.1%)	1/86 (1.1%)	NS
No significant finding		16/85 (18.8%)	18/86 (20.9%)	NS

NS not significant

Table 2 Operative and postoperative data for both study groups

		Group I (N=85)	Group II (N=86)	P value
Operative time	Range (min) (Mean±SD)	25–35 27.50±4.51	30–48 36.33±7.68	S
Intraoperative complications (N %)				
Bleeding		4/85 (4.70%)	5/86 (5.8%)	NS
Visceral injuries		0	0	NS
Vascular injuries		0	0	NS
Conversion to open surgery		0	0	NS
Discharge time	Range (days) (Mean ± SD)	1–2 1.33±0.22	1–2 1.33±0.22	NS
[a]Postoperative complications, N (%)				
Fever		5/85 (5.88%)	6/86 (6.9%)	NS
Postoperative bleeding		0	0	NS
Constipation		0	3 (3.48%)	NS
Urinary urgency		0	4 (4.65%)	NS
Uterine prolapse		0	2 (2.32%)	NS
Painless labor		0	0	NS
Time to return to normal lifestyle	Range (days) (Mean ± SD)	4–10 6.78±1.55	5–10 6.34±1.22	NS

[a] Including immediate and remote complications during the period of follow-up

S significant, *NS* not significant

Table 3 The summation of success rate according to the mean PAS after treatment at 3, 6, 12 month follow-up in both study groups

	Group I (*N*=85)			Group II (*N*=86)			*P* value
	3MS	6MS	12MS	3MS	6MS	12MS	
[a]No pain, *N* (%)	20 (23.52%)	18 (21.17%)	18 (21.17%)	21 (24.41%)	19 (22.09%)	18 (20.93%)	NS
[b]Minimal pain, *N* (%)	19 (22.35%)	19 (22.35%)	17 (20%)	20 (23.25%)	19 (22.09%)	18 (20.93%)	NS
[c]Tolerable pain, *N* (%)	27 (31.76%)	28 (32.94%)	28 (32.94%)	27 (31.39%)	28 (32.55%)	27 (31.39%)	NS
[d]Severe pain, *N* (%)	19 (22.35%)	20 (23.52%)	22 (25.88%)	18 (20.93%)	21 (24.41%)	22 (25.58%)	NS
Overall success rate	(66/85) (77.64%)	(65/85) (76.47%)	(63/85) 74.11%	(68/86) 79.06%	(65/86) 75.58 %	(63/86) 73.25%	NS

NS not significant

[a] excellent=10–9

[b] good=6–8 PAS

[c] tolerable=3–5

[d] minimal=0–2 PAS

In the present study, There was no statistically significant difference as regards the efficacy and the overall success rate between group I and group II at 3, 6, and 12 months of follow-up ($P \leq 0.05$). This is in agreement with the results of other studies, in which LUNA was used to treat patients with CPP in whom laparoscopy revealed no pathology as the systematic review (Cochrane) and meta-analysis including six randomized, controlled trials (RCTs) [9], reported that there were no significant differences overall in pain relief between women treated with LUNA and controls (women treated with diagnostic laparoscopy or conservative surgery alone) as pain relief up to 6 months (five studies, *N*=258): odds ratio (OR) 1.15, 95% confidence interval (CI) 0.66 to 1.99, pain relief up to 12 months (four studies, *N*=285): OR 1.20, 95% CI 0.72 to 1.99 and pain relief up to 36 months (one study, *N*=116): OR 0.84, 95% CI 0.39 to 1.80). The review states that the effect of treatment may overlap with the placebo effect of laparoscopy, reducing differences in short-term efficacy between groups, and the lack of power to detect a clinically important difference was an issue of concern in the trials with null results, and they stated that lack of sustained long-term benefit could be due to regrowth of nerves or pain signals being transferred via alternative routes and consequently, because of this last speculation, in the present study, uterosacral nerve cauterization using bipolar electrosurgical current and then nerve transaction was used rather than any procedure alone. In a recent randomized, controlled trial [10], 80 women were studied with CPP treated with LUNA or vaginal uterosacral nerve resection with a follow-up till 12 months, there were no significant differences between the two study groups with regard to pain relief. The same results were obtained from recent meta-analysis [11] used by collecting individual patient data from the existing trials to provide a comprehensive assessment of the effectiveness of LUNA that will be generalizable in various clinical contexts. Also, in the most recent multicentric, randomized, controlled trial [12] including 487 women with CPP lasting longer than 6 months without or with minimal endometriosis, adhesions, or pelvic inflammatory disease, recruited to the study by consultant gynecological surgeons from 18 UK hospitals, with follow-up conducted by questionnaires mailed at 3 and 6 months and at 1, 2, 3, and 5 years, it concluded that after a median follow-up of 69 months, there were no significant differences reported on the visual analog pain scales for the

Table 4 Patients' satisfaction rate of the treatment during 3, 6, and 12 months follow-up in both study groups

	Group I (*N*=85)			Group II (*N*=86)			*P* value
	3MS	6MS	12MS	3MS	6MS	12MS	
Excellent	19/85 (22.35%)	17/85 (20%)	17/85 (20%)	20/86 (23.25%)	19/86 (22.09%)	19/86 (22.09%)	NS
Good	26/85 (30.58 %)	24/85 (28.23%)	22/85 (25.88%)	25/86 (29.06%)	23/86 (26.74 %)	22/86 (23.25 %)	NS
Moderate	18/85 (21.17%)	22/85 (25.88%)	22/85 (25.88%)	20/86 (23.86 %)	23/86 (26.74%)	21/86 (24.41%)	NS
No improvement	22/85 (25.88%)	22/85 (25.88%)	24/85 (28.23%)	21/86 (24.41%)	21/86 (24.41%)	24/86 (27.90%)	NS
[a]Cumulative satisfaction rate	63/85 (74.11%)	63/85 (74.11%)	61/85 (71.76%)	65/86 (75.58%)	65/86 (75.58%)	62/86 (72.09%)	NS

[a] Cumulative satisfaction rate = Excellent + Good + Moderate.

Worse than before = restricted only to patients with surgery complications, and it was 0%

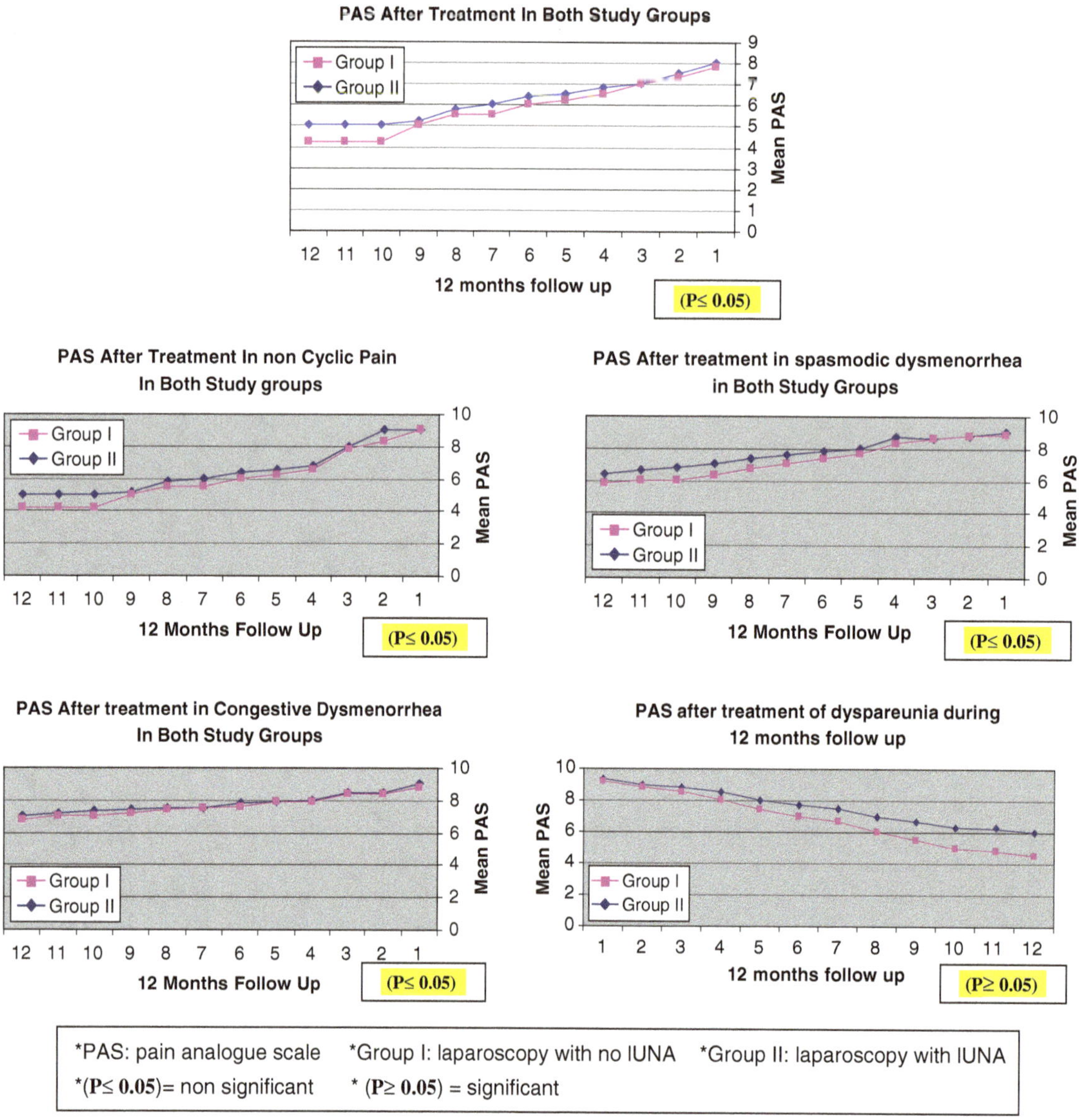

Fig. 2 Effect of LUNA at 12 months follow-up in both study groups

worst pain between the LUNA group and the no LUNA group for quality of life.

The cumulative satisfaction rate was 74.11%, 74.11%, and 71.76% versus 75.58%, 75.58%, and 72.09% at 3, 6, 12 months between group I and group II, respectively ($P \leq 0.05$). This results go hand in hand with the overall satisfaction rate in the meta-analysis study [9] and other studies [13, 14], as it stated that there is no significant difference at the satisfaction rate, or the need of additional treatment between the study and the control group among six RCTs they evaluated.

As regarding the effectiveness of LUNA (when compared to a control or no treatment) in treatment of primary (spasmodic) dysmenorrhea and secondary (congestive) dysmenorrhea, there was no statistically significant difference between both groups, ($P \leq 0.05$); on the other hand, as regarding the effectiveness of LUNA in the treatment of dyspareunia, there was a statistically significant difference between both groups, ($P \geq 0.05$). The previous results were in agreement with that of the report of Proctor et al. [9], as in his systematic review of six RCTs, he reported that, for women with primary dysmenorrhea, the OR for pain relief at 6 and 12 months was 0.67 (95% CI 0.17 to 2.61) and 0.10 (95% CI 0.03 to 0.03), respectively, in favor of LUNA. For women with secondary dysmenorrhea, the OR for pain relief at 6 and 12 months was 1.03 (95% CI 0.52 to 2.02) and 0.77 (95% CI 0.43 to 1.39), respectively. In *Cochrane Database of Systematic Reviews* [15], regarding the treatment of primary dysmenorrhea, there was some evidence of the effectiveness of LUNA when compared to a control or no treatment.

In the present study, endometriosis with an AFS score of >5 was excluded from the study, as in the majority of women who had endometriosis that was treated with conservative laparoscopic procedure alone or with conservative medical therapy, as well as with LUNA, it will be difficult to attribute their response to the LUNA alone or to the adjuvant therapy of endometriosis, and this is in agreement with the conclusion of different studies as that of Guyer et al. [13] and Davis et al. [14]. Also, in a randomized trial of 180 patients with symptomatic endometriosis, the addition of LUNA to conservative laparoscopic surgery for endometriosis did not reduce the medium- or long-term frequency and severity of recurrent dysmenorrheal [6]. Another randomized study of 67 patients with CPP and laparoscopic evidence of endometriosis found no significant difference in the pain outcome [5].

In the present study, the effectiveness of the LUNA in relief or improvement of deep dyspareunia was taken with great interest and discussion because to my knowledge, there has been few similar reports specifically on the treatment of primary deep dyspareunia by the LUNA procedure, as Jung et al. [16] found that of his 12-month follow-up study of LUNA for treating primary deep dyspareunia, the satisfactory rates at 3 and 12 months were 66.7% and 50%, respectively, while on the other hand, Vercellini et al. [6] found no significant advantage on sexual satisfaction by the LUNA procedure. In a multicentric, randomized, controlled trial (*JAMA* trial) [12], after a median follow-up of 69 months, there were no significant differences reported on the visual analog pain scales for the worst pain (mean difference between the LUNA group and the no LUNA group, −0.04 cm (95% CI −0.33 to 0.25 cm; $P = 0.80$), noncyclical pain (−0.11 cm, 95% CI, −0.50 to 0.29 cm]; $P = 0.60$), dysmenorrhea (−0.09 cm, 95% CI, −0.49 to 0.30 cm; $P = 0.60$), or dyspareunia (0.18 cm, 95% CI, −0.22 to 0.62 cm; $P = 0.40$), and they concluded that in women with CPP, LUNA did not result in improvements in pain, dysmenorrhea, dyspareunia, or quality of life compared with laparoscopy without pelvic denervation. However, in our opinion, deep dyspareunia is very complicated in its pathogenesis, which includes both physical and psychiatric/psychologic aspects; hence, a verified system comprising of clarified definitions and criteria in the assessment of satisfaction or improvement is mandatory, and will be very difficult to be practiced in our community and with our patients with the lack of group evaluators, including social personnel who are qualified for appraising a sexologic and psychiatric/psychologic questionnaire to give more informed insight, and so these results need to be evaluated carefully in a large, randomized trial before it will be generalized.

In the present study, there was no statistically significant difference between group I and group II regarding intraoperative and postoperative complications ($P \leq 0.05$); only urge incontinence was significantly observed among patients with LUNA. All of these complications were minimal and treated conservatively with no additional measures. This was in agreement with that of Yuan [1] who stated that the adverse events of LUNA were less common. Also, a meta-analysis [9] found that few complications were reported, while two case reports described a total of five women with uterine prolapse after having LUNA; three women were young nulliparous, and the other two women had a history of vaginal childbirth [14, 16]. In *Cochrane Database of Systematic Reviews* [15], adverse events were significantly more common for presacral neurectomy; however, the majority had complications such as constipation, which may spontaneously improve.

The National Institute for Health and Clinical Excellence [17] examined LUNA for CPP and will publish guidance on its safety and efficacy to the NHS in England, Wales, Scotland, and Northern Ireland. This overview is based on one Cochrane systematic review and meta-analysis [9–14]. They concluded that there was some evidence for the effectiveness of LUNA when compared with controls or no treatment in women with primary dysmenorrhea, and there were no significant differences in short-term pain relief between LUNA and LPSN. On the other hand, The European Society for Human Reproduction and Embryology published a guideline for the diagnosis and treatment of endometriosis in 2005 [18]. This guideline states that "ablation of endometriotic lesions reduces endometriosis-associated pain and the smallest effect is seen in patients with minimal disease; there is no evidence that also performing LUNA is necessary". A guideline published by the Royal College of Obstetricians and Gynecologists states that "There is no evidence that laparoscopic uterine nerve ablation is necessary when ablating endometriotic lesions and laparoscopic uterine nerve ablation by itself has no effect on dysmenorrhea associated with endometriosis" [19]. So, both uncontrolled or controlled randomized studies and the present study had proven that LUNA showed no statistically significant difference in complete relief of CPP, but it has a role in substantial reduction in CPP level in well-selected patients, and this may be due the complicated anatomical and physiological picture of CPP as anatomically, at least five pathways transmit signals from noxious stimuli in the pelvis, and these nerve trunks vary in location and can intersect, with the potential for neuronal crosstalk so LUNA may obliterate some of the nerve fibers, but others are interwoven with the pelvic arteries and ureters [12]. This explanation that LUNA has no role in reducing CPP was an objective one, not subjective, and if we generalized this opinion, at the same step, it will be of no value to ligate the uterine arteries or the internal iliac arteries to stop severe postpartum hemorrhage, as the uterus has many other blood sources, but the philosophy of the LUNA is that it has a short-term effect in complete or incomplete relief of CPP that will give the patients the chance to return to their normal lifestyle, and then accommodation and less pain habituation will take place making their PAS fall to its minimal level, especially when the patients know that their diagnostic laparoscopy was free, and these results, if obtained from the LUNA, will be considered as a relative success event, not an absolute one. So, after this controversial explanations, LUNA, in well-selected patients, can be added as an adjuvant last treatment in patients with CPP when other options of treatment failed, and laparoscopy was recommended for diagnosis, but it is not recommended as an indication for LUNA in patients with CPP.

Conclusion

In conclusion, LUNA can be a last alternative option in well-selected patients for control of CPP without endometriosis; however, its effectiveness may not extend to other indications. Also, preliminary experience in the treatment of primary deep dyspareunia presents a promising perspective on the management of deep dyspareunia, especially if it will involve a team of social, psychological, and gynecological specialists.

Acknowledgments To all my colleges in the endoscopy unit , El-Minia university hospital, and all of my patients for their cooperation. Also with great appreciation to my colleges in the statistical section of the public health department about their cooperation in performing these results.

Declaration of interest The authors report no conflicts of interest. The authors alone are responsible for the content and writing of the paper.

References

1. Yuan Ch-Ch (2006) Laparoscopic uterosacral nerve ablation and chronic pelvic pain. J Chin Med Assoc 69(3):101–103
2. Hebbar S, Chawla C (2005) Role of laparoscopy in evaluation of chronic pelvic pain. J Min Access Surg 1(issue 3):116–120
3. The LUNA Trial Collaboration: a randomized controlled trial to assess the efficacy of laparoscopic uterosacral nerve ablation (LUNA) in the treatment of chronic pelvic pain: the trial protocol. BMC Womens Health. 2003 3:6. Published online 2003 December 8. doi:10.1186/1472-6874-3-6
4. Hammoud A, Gago LA, Diamond MP (2004) Adhesions in patients with chronic pelvic pain: a role for adhesiolysis? Fertil Steril 82:1483–1491
5. Johnson NP, Farquhar CM, Crossley S, Yu Y, Van Peperstraten AM, Sprecher M, Suckling J (2004) A double-blind randomized controlled trial of laparoscopic uterine nerve ablation for women with chronic pelvic pain. BJOG 111:950–959
6. Vercellini P, Aimi G, Busacca M, Apolone G, Uglietti A, Crosignani PG (2003) Laparoscopic uterosacral ligament resection for dysmenorrhea associated with endometriosis: results of a randomized, controlled trial. Fertil Steril 80:310–319
7. Proctor ML, Latthe PM, Farquhar CM (2005) Surgical interruption of pelvic nerve pathways for primary and secondary dysmenorrhea. Cochrane Database of Systematic Reviews Issue 4: CD001896
8. Stones, RW, Mountfield, J (2000) Interventions for treating chronic pelvic pain in women. [update of Cochrane Database Syst Rev. ;(2): CD000387 ; 10796713.]. [Review] [15 refs]. Cochrane Database Syst Rev. p. CD000387
9. Wilson ML, Farquhar CM, Sinclair OJ, Johnson NP (2000) Surgical interruption of pelvic nerve pathways for primary and secondary dysmenorrhea. [Review] [6 refs]. Cochrane Database Syst Rev.: (2000) CD001896
10. Palomba S, Russo T, Falbo A (2006) Laparoscopic uterine nerve ablation versus vaginal uterosacral ligament resection in postmenopausal women with intractable midline chronic pelvic pain: a randomized study. Eur J Obstet Gynaecol 129:84–91
11. Xiong T, Daniels J, Middleton L, Champaneria R, Khan KS, Gray R, Johnson N, Lichten EM, Sutton C, Jones KD, Chen FP, Vercellini P, Aimi G, Lui WM (2007) International LUNA IPD Meta-analysis Collaborative Group: meta-analysis using individual patient data from randomised trials to assess the effectiveness of laparoscopic uterosacral nerve ablation in the treatment of chronic pelvic pain: a proposed protocol. BJOG. Dec;114(12):1580, e1-7
12. Daniels J, Gray R, Hills RK, Latthe P, Buckley L, Gupta J, Selman T, Adey E, Xiong T, Champaneria R, Lilford R, Khan KS, LUNA Trial Collaboration (2009) Laparoscopic uterosacral nerve ablation for alleviating chronic pelvic pain: a randomized controlled trial. JAMA 302(9):955–961
13. Guyer C, Moors A, Louden K (2000) An audit of conservative surgery for endometriosis in a district general hospital 1995–1998. J Obstet Gynaecol 20(5):514–516
14. Davis GD (1996) Uterine prolapse after laparoscopic uterosacral transection in nulliparous airborne trainees. J Reprod Med 41:279–282
15. Proctor ML, Latthe PM, Farquhar CM, Khan KS, and Johnson NP: Surgical interruption of pelvic nerve pathways for primary and secondary dysmenorrhea Cochrane Database of Systematic Reviews 2007 Issue 3 Copyright © 2007 The Cochrane Collaboration. Published by Wiley
16. Juang CM, Yen MS, Horng HC, Cheng CY, Yu HC, Chang CM (2006) Treatment of primary deep dyspareunia with laproscopic uterosacral nerve ablation procedure: a pilot study. J Chin Med Assoc 69:110–114
17. National institute for health and clinical excellence: interventional procedure overview of laparoscopic uterine nerve ablation (LUNA) for chronic pelvic pain. February 2007. Available from www.nice.org.uk/ip376overview
18. Kennedy S, Bergqvist A, Chapron C (2005) ESHRE guideline for the diagnosis and treatment of endometriosis. Hum Reprod 20 (10):2698–2704
19. Royal College of Obstetricians and Gynaecologists (2006) The investigation and management of endometriosis. Green-top guideline no. 24. London

33

Laparoscopic management of urachal remnants in women affected of pelvic pain

Juan Gilabert-Estelles · Juan Gilabert-Aguilar

Abstract Symptomatic urachal cysts are very infrequently encountered in women affected of pelvic pain and uterine myomas. We report on two female patients aged 40 and 49 years, who underwent complete transperitoneal laparoscopic excision of urachal cysts at our unit. The first patient suffered from infertility and presented a uterine myoma, which was treated with laparoscopic myomectomy. The second case referred was menorrhagia and chronic pelvic pain, and she was treated with a total laparoscopic hysterectomy with complete excision of urachal cyst. All two operations had no serious immediate complications and minimal blood loss. Cysts were located at the lower third of the urachus, and no communication was detected between the cyst and the bladder. The bladder apex was reinforced using suturing in both cases, and a postoperative cystoscopy confirmed the integrity of the bladder wall. Patients were discharged uneventfully on the second postoperative day. In conclusion, complete excision of urachal remnants in women affected of pelvic pain is advisable in order to treat the symptoms and can be safely performed by a laparoscopic approach.

J. Gilabert-Estelles (✉) · J. Gilabert-Aguilar
Unit of Gynecological Endoscopy, Hospital Casa de Salud,
Av. Manuel Candela 41,
46010, 46009 Valencia, Spain
e-mail: juangilaeste@yahoo.es

J. Gilabert-Estelles
Department of Gynecology, University Hospital La Fe,
Valencia, Spain

J. Gilabert-Aguilar
Department of Gynecology, Hospital Arnau de Vilanova,
Valencia, Spain

Keywords Urachus · Laparoscopy · Cyst · Abnormalities · Pelvic pain

Introduction

The urachus is the embryological remnant of the allantois, which communicates the apex of the bladder with the umbilicus and usually becomes obliterated shortly after birth. Urachal cysts account for one third of urachal obliteration defects with an observed incidence of 1/5,000 live borns [1, 2]. Even though males are affected three times more than females [3], gynecologists should be aware of this rare condition, which may be encountered while managing women affected of pelvic pain and midline cysts. Cysts of the urachus rarely become symptomatic and may be encountered often during a surgical endoscopy exploration. Complications of these abnormalities have been described, including infection [4], formation of urachal calculi [5], and the potential risk for a malignant change of the, otherwise, benign urachal remnant [6, 7]. Symptoms of urachal cysts at adult age may be unspecific and include lower abdominal pain, irritative voiding symptoms, periumbilical pain, or palpable abdominal masses [2]. A number of gynecological pathologies, such as ovarian cysts or uterine myomas, may cause these symptoms and might, therefore, hamper an early diagnosis of urachal cysts in menstruating women

A surgical approach is not always necessary in small uncomplicated urachal cysts as symptoms are often related to complications. In women referring pelvic pain, any abdominal abnormalities found during surgery should be corrected, taking into account the fertility status. Therefore, the recommended management of the incidental finding of these embryologic defects, in this type of patients, is surgical excision.

Considering the potential complications and the risk of recurrence, excision of the urachal cyst is recommended over drainage [1]. Traditional approach includes the resection of the urachus by open surgery, but an increasing number of cases have been reported detailing minimally invasive approaches to urachal cysts [8–12].

Our experience in the management of urachal cysts in two women affected of pelvic pain and uterine myomas supports that laparoscopy offers a safe and effective management of both gynecological and urachal pathology.

Case 1

A 49-year-old Caucasian multigravid woman was referred to our endoscopy unit with a 2-year history of hypermenorrea and lower abdominal pain that increased during menstruation. The patient had a good physical status and did not have any previous surgery. Gynecological examination revealed a tenth week myomatous uterus. Vaginal ultrasound showed multiple intramural myomas with normal adnexa and a 6-cm midline unilocular simple cyst that was located next to the uterine fundus. A computed tomography revealed a 61×48 mm low density image located at midline cranial to the bladder apex, suggesting the diagnosis of urachal cyst. The preoperative laboratory tests were normal. An informed consent was obtained, and risks and benefits of removing the urachal remnant were discussed. A total laparoscopic hysterectomy with bilateral salpingo-oophorectomy (BSO), and transperitoneal excision of the urachal cyst was planned.

Laparoscopy was performed under general endotracheal anesthesia with the patient in a dorsal lithotomy position. After induction of pneumoperitoneum with a veress needle, an 11-mm trocar was inserted 3 cm over the umbilicus under direct vision for the 0° laparoscope (Ternamian endotip, Karl Storz, Germany). A 6-cm preperitoneal cystic mass consistent with a cyst of the lower urachus was detected (Fig. 1). Three accessory 5-mm trocars were placed, one at midline 3 cm infraumbilically and the other two, laterally to it. First, a standard total laparoscopic hysterectomy with BSO was performed; otherwise, a possible bleeding of the anterior peritoneum while performing the excision of the urachal cyst could have impaired the operative field. The cystoscopy performed discarded the patency of any communication between the cyst and the bladder apex. Then, 200 cm^3 of saline serum with methylene blue were left in the bladder in order to facilitate further dissection. Peritoneum was sectioned cranially to the cyst and blunt dissection proceeded laterally. Bipolar courant was used for sealing and cold scissors allowed a complete enucleation of the cyst, including the urachal tract located cephalad. A wall defect comprising the muscular and serosa layers of the bladder was observed but without any leakage. The bladder was sutured transversally with an interrupted intracorporeal polyglactine 3–0 suture (Fig. 2). The specimen was removed vaginally and extracorporeal polyglactine 0 sutures were used to close the vaginal cuff.

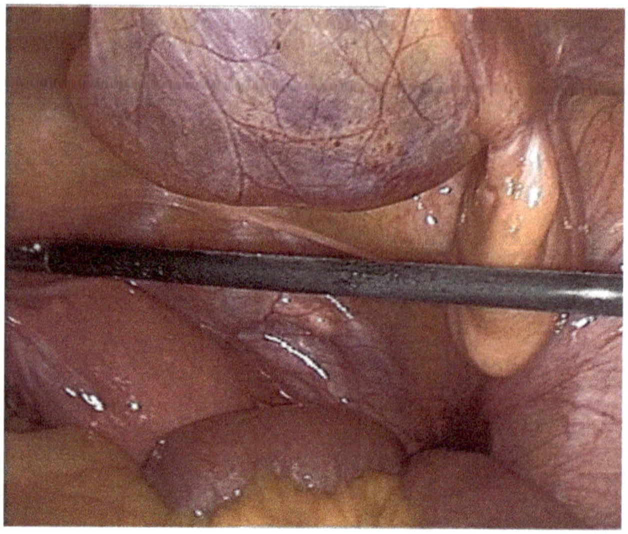

Fig. 1 Laparoscopic view of urachal cyst (Case 1)

Case 2

A 40-year-old nulligravid Hispanic woman consulted with the diagnosis of uterine leiomyoma. This patient referred a 2-year history of infertility with no other known additional etiologic factors. She had no medical pathological con-

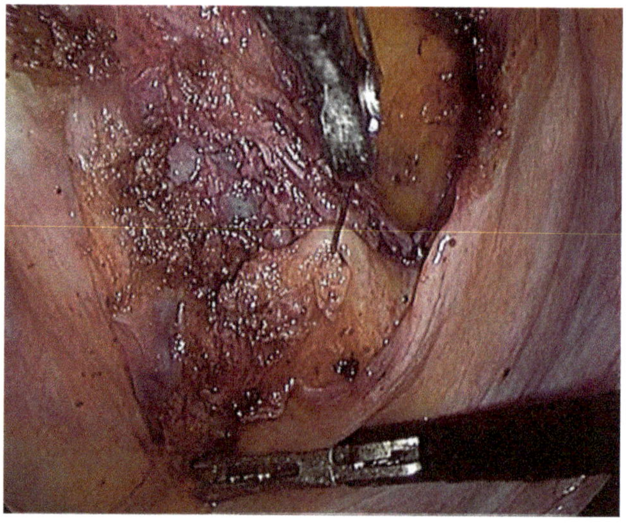

Fig. 2 Reinforcement of the bladder wall with extracorporeal suturing (Case 1)

ditions except from a mild obesity. Gynecological ultrasound detected a posterior 60×58 mm intramural myoma, which did not distort the endometrial cavity and ovaries appeared to be normal. A laparoscopic approach to perform a myomectomy and assess tubal patency was planned. Laparoscopic access was performed using an umbilical visual port insertion with a ternamian trocar. The diagnosis of a posterior 6-cm intramural myoma was confirmed. In addition, the examination of the abdominal cavity showed a 3×2 cm cystic mass subperitoneally located at midline in the anterior abdominal wall (Fig. 3) and an intraoperative cystoscopy ruled out the presence of intraluminal alterations of the bladder. At this point, a small uncomplicated urachal cyst was highly suspected. Given the fact that myomectomy requires the placement of a 12-mm suprapubic trocar for morcellation, we decided to excise the cystic lesion previously. Two lateral 5 mm trocars were used in order to remove the lesion with a similar procedure to the previous case, after having distended the bladder with 200 ml of saline serum. A polydioxanone endoloop was used in order to seal the urachus cranially to the bladder dome. Once lower resection was completed, urachus was removed cranially to the cyst, including the parietal peritoneum. At the end of the procedure, the bladder was once again distended to check for leaks. Myomectomy was performed uneventfully, and the specimen was extracted after drainage inside an endoscopic bag through the suprapubic trocar.

The total operating time was 120 min in case 1 and 100 min in case 2. Neither intraoperative nor postoperative complications occurred. A bladder catheter was maintained for 24 h in order to avoid bladder distension. Both patients were discharged uneventfully within 2 days after surgery. The excised specimens were sent for histopathological assessment, and the diagnosis of benign urachal remnants was confirmed.

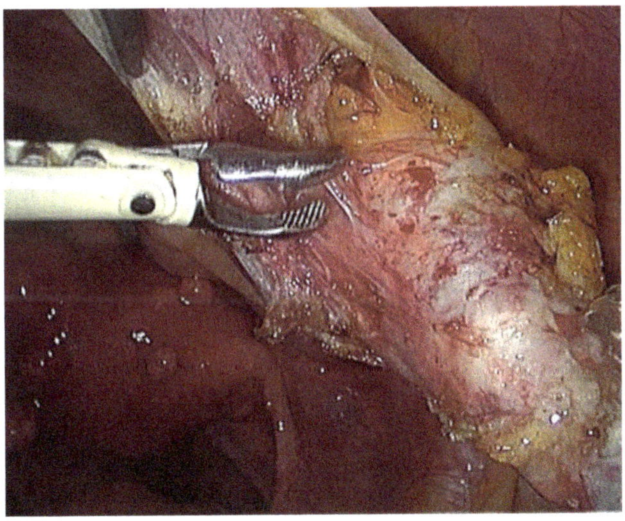

Fig. 3 Opening of the Retzius space cranially to the urachal cyst (Case 2)

Currently, both patients remain dry and have not experienced recurrent symptoms with a follow-up period of 8 and 27 months, respectively.

Discussion

Urachal congenital anomalies are secondary to an abnormal involution of the allantois. Bauer and Retik [13] described four types of anomalies according to the portion of this embryonic structure that remains patent. If the urachus remains patent from the bladder to the umbilicus, it forms a urachal fistula. However, when a patent urachus communicates with the umbilicus but not the bladder, this is called urachal-umbilical sinus. On the contrary, a vesicourachal diverticulum defines a communication between the patent urachus and the dome of the bladder. Finally, the fourth and most common type of urachal remnant is a urachal cyst, which results from the accumulation of mucinous and serous secretions in a cavity suspended at any level of the urachus without communication to either the bladder or to the umbilicus. The most relevant complications of urachal cysts include infection with possible rupture in the peritoneal cavity leading to peritonitis [4] and the risk of malignant degeneration. The most accepted treatment for congenital patent urachus is the excision of the urachal tract, including the parietal peritoneum, from the umbilicus to the bladder. Partial resections of patent urachus may recur up to 30% [14]. Several authors perform a partial colpectomy, including the dome of the bladder to prevent malignant degeneration. However, we did not consider necessary this practice as the estimated risk of malignancy is lower than 0.1% [15] and other authors have reported favorable outcomes without resection of the bladder cuff in all the cases [16].

Women at their reproductive age present frequently ovarian cysts, most of them functional and which do not require surgery. The urachal cysts are frequently located at the lower portion of the urachus, and differential diagnosis is mandatory with other adnexal pathology. Gynecological ultrasound is usually performed vaginally with previous voiding of the bladder. Therefore, low urachal cysts are encountered at midline near to the uterine fundus, quite similar to ovarian cysts, and might lead to misdiagnosis of the urachal abnormality. A useful tip consists in filling the bladder, a maneuver which cranially displaces the cyst and facilitates its correct diagnosis [17].

Symptomatic urachal remnants have been traditionally managed by midline infraumbilical incision. Open approach is usually associated with long recovery periods and negative cosmetic results. Neufang et al. reported the first laparoscopic excision of a urachal fistula in 1992 [18]. In 1993, Trondsen described a laparoscopic approach in a patient affected of urachal sinus [12], being the first laparoscopic excisions of a urachal cyst reported by Siegel et al. [19] and Jorion [20] in 1994. Since then, several case reports have described successful laparoscopic managements of urachal cysts in different clinical conditions [9, 21, 22]. There have also been short series describing the laparoscopic management of urachal remnants with a complete excision and a reduced morbidity [6, 8, 23, 24]. Cutting et al. reported one recurrence in five patients treated by laparoscopy due to a lack of resection of the subcutaneous part of the urachus below the umbilicus in an obese patient [11]. Based on their comparative study between the laparoscopic and the open approach to urachal remnants, Okegawa et al. stressed the clinical advantages of minimal invasive surgery [25].

Different techniques have been described for the surgical management of urachal remnants. Transperitoneal technique allows the examination of the abdominal cavity both to rule out other entities and to treat concomitant findings. This approach was mandatory in our cases, as treatment of uterine leiomyomas was the main indication for surgery and was also preferred by Takeda et al., who excised an ovarian dermoid cyst and a urachal cyst found at preoperative examination [26]. LePicard et al. exploited the unique preperitoneal localization of the urachal cyst at the Retzius space to describe an extraperitoneal approach, with an easy blunt dissection and a very selective use of electrocoagulation, which remains a feasible option in cases of isolated urachal pathology [27]. Umbilical access offers good cosmetic results but may reduce the operative field and impair a proper instrument triangulation. In keeping with other authors, we have found the supraumbilical port to be very useful [11, 23] and unhampered of limitations to perform a concomitant hysterectomy.

In conclusion, the present report underlines that the laparoscopic excision of urachal remnants in women affected of benign gynecological pathology is a safe and reliable technique. A urachal cyst in the presence of pelvic pain should be removed as soon as an accurate diagnosis has been achieved, even though etiologic relationship is not confirmed.

Conflict of interest There is no actual or potential conflict of interest in relation to this article.

References

1. Blichert-Toft M, Nielsen OV (1971) Diseases of the urachus simulating intra abdominal disorders. Am J Surg 122:123–128
2. Goldman IL, Caldamone AA, Gauderer M et al (1988) Infected urachal cyst: a review of 10 cases. J Urol 140:375–378
3. Bunch PT, Kline-Fath BM, ImhoV SC, Calvo-Garcia MA, Crombleholme TM, Donnelly LF (2006) Allantoic cyst: a prenatal clue to patent urachus. Pediatr Radiol 36:1090–1095
4. Macneily AE, Koleilat N, Kiriuluta HG et al (1992) Urachal abscesses: protean manifestations, their recognition and management. Urology 40:530
5. Seo IY, Han DY, Oh SJ, Rim JS (2008) Laparoscopic excision of a urachal cyst containing large stones in an adult. Yonsei Med J 49:869–871
6. Cadeddu J, Boyle K, Fabrizio M et al (2000) Laparoscopic management of urachal cysts in adulthood. J Urol 164:1536–1539
7. Navarrete S, Sanchez-Ismayel A, Sanchez-Salas RE et al (2005) Treatment of urachal anomalies: a minimally invasive surgery technique. JSLS 9:422–425
8. Fahlenkamp D, Schonberger B, Lindeke A, Loening S (1995) Laparoscopic excision of the sinusoidal remnants of the urachus in a 3-year-old boy. Br J Urol 76:135–137
9. Stone NN, Garden R, Weber H (1995) Laparoscopic excision of a urachal cyst. Urology 45:161–164
10. Linos D, Mitropolus F, Patoulis J, Psomas M, Parasyris V (1997) Laparoscopic removal of urachal sinus. J Laparoendosc Adv Surg Tech 7:135–138
11. Cutting CW, Hindley RG, Poulsen J (2005) Laparoscopic management of complicated urachal remnants. BJU Int 966:1417–1421
12. Trondsen E, Reiertsen O, Rosseland AR (1993) Laparoscopic excision of a urachal sinus. Eur J Surg 159:127–128
13. Bauer SB, Retik AB (1978) Urachal abnormalities and related umbilical disorders. Urol Clin North Am 5:195–211
14. Nix J, Menville J, Albert M, Wendt D (1958) Congenital patent urachus. J Urol 79:264–273
15. Pantuck A, Vates T, Javidian P, Weiss R (1997) Urachal adenocarcinoma. Can J Urol 4:450–452
16. Mesrobian HG, Zacharias A, Balcom AH, Cohen RD (1997) Ten years of experience with isolated urachal anomalies in children. J Urol 158:1316–1318
17. Robert Y, Hennquin C, Chaillet D (1996) Urachal remnants: sonographic assessment. J Clin Ultrasound 24:339
18. Neufang T, Ludtke FE, Lepsien G (1992) Laparoscopic excision of a urachal fistula-new therapy for a rare disorder. Minim Invasive Ther 1:245–249
19. Siegel JF, Winfield H, Valderrama E, Smith A (1994) Laparoscopic excision of urachal cyst. J Urol 151:1631–1633
20. Jorion JL (1994) Laparoscopic removal of urachal cyst. J Urol 151:1006
21. Yamada T, Okamoto Y, Kasamatsu H, Mori H (2001) Laparoscopic assisted removal of a large urachal cyst. J Am Assoc Gynecol Laparosc 8:159–160
22. Turial S, Hueckstaedt T, Schier F, Fahlenkamp D (2007) Laparoscopic treatment of urachal remnants in children. J Urol 177:1864–1866
23. Khurana S, Borzi PA (2002) Laparoscopic management of complicated urachal disease in children. J Urol 168:1526–1528
24. Nakagawa K (2002) Laparoscopic excision of urachal remnant. JJCS 27:884–888
25. Okegawa T, Odagane A, Nutahara K, Higashihara E (2006) Laparoscopic management of urachal remnants in adulthood. Int J Urol 13:1466–1469
26. Takeda A, Manabe S, Mitsui T, Nakamura H (2005) Laparoscopic excision of urachal cyst found at preoperative examination for ovarian dermoid cyst. Gynecol Surg 3:1
27. LePicard P, Carion G (2002) Extraperitoneal laparoscopic treatment of urachal cyst. J Chir 139:286–287

Laparoscopic management of cornual heterotopic pregnancy with the use of Harmonic ACE®

Sonia Chachan • N. Waters • A. Kent

Abstract Heterotopic pregnancy is the simultaneous coexistence of both intrauterine and extrauterine pregnancies. Cornual heterotopic pregnancies can cause catastrophic haemorrhage because of their location. Available evidence suggests that they have usually been managed surgically by laparotomy and cornual resection, few were managed medically and two expectantly. Of the surgical group, only three underwent laparoscopic management. We report the first case of successful management of cornual heterotpic pregnancy by Harmonic ACE® and a favourable outcome of the intrauterine pregnancy.

Keywords Cornual · Heterotopic · Laparoscopy · Ultracision®

Introduction

Heterotopic pregnancy is the simultaneous coexistence of both intrauterine and extrauterine pregnancies. The universal quotation of incidence of heterotopic pregnancy of one in 30,000 comes from Devoe and Pratt (1948) [1]. Since then, a rise in incidence has been documented due to the increase in use of artificial reproductive technologies (ART) and also increased incidence of pelvic inflammatory diseases.

S. Chachan (✉)
Department of Gynaecology, Royal Surrey County Hospital, Guildford, Surrey GU2 7XX, UK
e-mail: soniac@doctors.org.uk

N. Waters · A. Kent
Department of Gynaecology,
Institution: Minimal Access Therapy Training Unit, Post Graduate Medical School, University of Surrey, Manor Park, Guildford, Surrey GU2 7WG, UK

The incidence of heterotopic pregnancy after ART seems to be as high as one in 100 to one in 500 [2–5]. The incidence of cornual heterotopic pregnancy has been estimated as one in 3,600 IVF pregnancies [6]. There is no known incidence of cornual heterotopic pregnancy following ovulation induction with clomiphene citrate but an incidence of one in 900 [7] has been reported for heterotopic pregnancy in general with this drug. Alongside intrauterine pregnancy, the location of heterotopic pregnancies may be abdominal [8], bilateral tubal [9], twin gestation in the tube [3], bilateral simultaneous tubal sextuplet [10] and cornual [11].

The term cornual pregnancy is sometimes used synonymously with interstitial pregnancy. Cornual pregnancy implants in the muscular interstitial part of the fallopian tube. This allows the pregnancy to grow and distend and usually develop into the second trimester. Rupture of this pregnancy can result in catastrophic haemorrhage in up to 2% cases requiring laparotomy and even hysterectomy [11–13].

An early diagnosis and management has become possible due to advances in ultrasound resolution. The ultrasound picture of cornual heterotopic pregnancy shows two gestational sacs separated by a thick bridge of myometrium. The specific feature of cornual pregnancy is that the position of chorionic sac is separate and is more than 1 cm from the most lateral edge of the uterine cavity [14]. The management of cornual heterotopic pregnancy poses clinical and ethical dilemma because of coexisting intrauterine pregnancy and the history of infertility. Traditionally cornual pregnancies have been managed by laparotomy by either cornual resection or hysterectomy for uncontrollable haemorrhage. However, cornual pregnancies have been successfully managed laparoscopically.

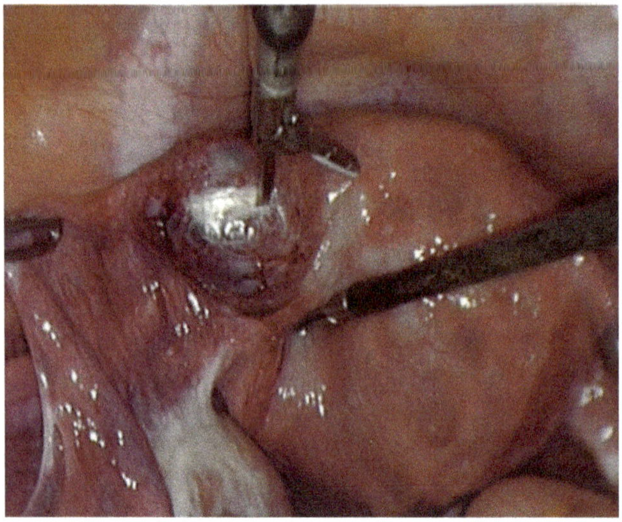

Fig. 1 Left cornual ectopic being shelled out by Harmonic ACE®

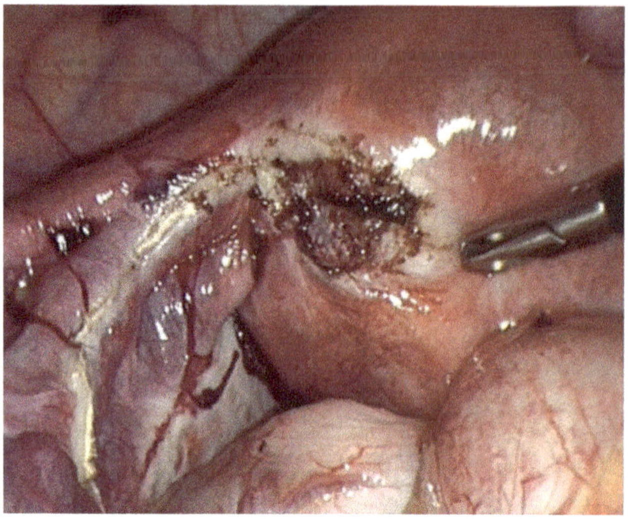

Fig. 3 Cornual pregnancy along with the left tube removed

There are 48 published cases of cornual heterotopic pregnancy [6, 15–25]. Only seven were from spontaneous conception, all others were from some form of assisted reproduction techniques. They were managed mainly surgically by laparotomy and cornual resection, few were managed medically and two expectantly. Of the surgical group, only three underwent laparoscopic management [15, 24, 25].

Case report

In this case report, we present a case of cornual heterotopic pregnancy managed laparoscopically by Harmonic ACE® with excellent outcome. Our patient was a 36-year-old woman, gravida 3. She had one previous full term spontaneous vaginal delivery and one early miscarriage. She also had a history of secondary infertility for 2 years prior to this pregnancy. She had regular periods with ovulatory cycles and patent fallopian tubes confirmed on hysterosalphingogram. She was prescribed clomiphene citrate for unexplained infertility and conceived in the third cycle. She had no known risk factors for ectopic pregnancy. She was seen in the early pregnancy clinic for pain in the left iliac fossa with a positive pregnancy test. Transvaginal ultrasound scan (TVS) revealed a viable intrauterine pregnancy with crown rump length (CRL) of 9.8 mm corresponding to 7 weeks of gestation. A second gestational sac was seen in the left cornual region of the uterus. It also had a yolk sac with foetal echoes with heart action with a CRL of 8.2 mm, corresponding to 6 weeks and 5 days. A diagnosis of intrauterine pregnancy with coexisting cornual pregnancy was made. We decided to resect the cornual

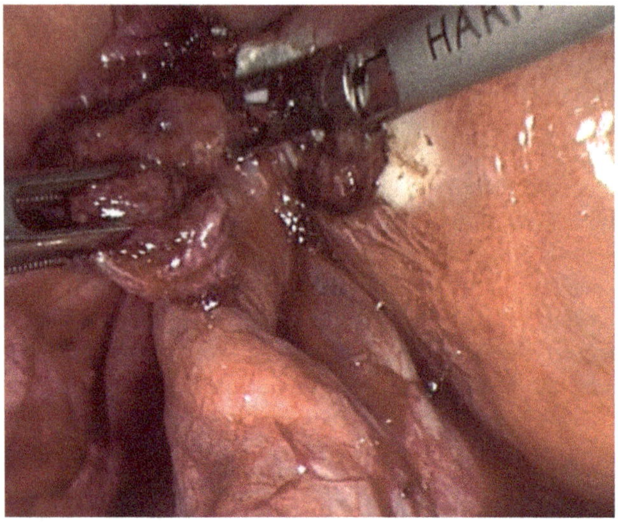

Fig. 2 Dissection continued

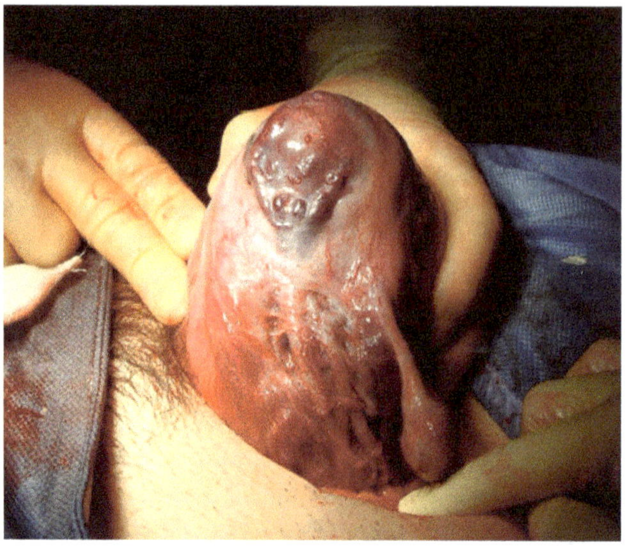

Fig. 4 Left cornu at caesarean section

pregnancy laparoscopically and allow the intrauterine pregnancy to continue after counselling the patient about the risks involved.

At laparoscopy, a 4×4 cm left cornual ectopic pregnancy was identified. The other tube looked normal. There were filmy adhesions surrounding the liver suggesting Fitz-Hugh-Curtis syndrome. Using Harmonic ACE® shears, the left cornual ectopic including the entire left fallopian tube was excised with minimal blood loss (see Figs. 1, 2 and 3). The uterine cavity was not breached. Peritoneal washout was carried out with heparinised saline. The patient had a short postoperative recovery and was discharged the next day. The intrauterine pregnancy was closely monitored with regular ultrasound scans for foetal wellbeing. An elective caesarean section was performed at 38 weeks and a live male baby weighing 3,821 g was delivered. The operation was uncomplicated. The site of the previous cornual ectopic pregnancy was very vascular but intact (see Fig. 4). The patient made an uneventful recovery and discharged home on day 3.

Discussion

Cornual heterotopic pregnancies are not as rare as previously thought. Advancement in TVS and colour flow Doppler and MRI and establishment of early pregnancy assessment units have made immense contribution to diagnosing this condition before catastrophic haemorrhage in many cases. Early diagnosis, available surgical expertise and patient choice remain the mainstay of management of heterotopic pregnancies.

Medical management of heterotopic pregnancy has certain disadvantages as the available agents used i.e. methotrexate and prostaglandins are contraindicated in viable intrauterine pregnancies and result in high miscarriage rate. It is also difficult to monitor the resolution of the cornual pregnancy after medical management because of the increased βhCG of the ongoing intrauterine pregnancy. However, there is a possibility of selective feticide by injection of 0.5 mL of 15% potassium chloride into the foetal heart [23]. This treatment does not have the disadvantages mentioned above.

Review of current literature suggests a better outcome with surgical techniques especially with laparoscopy if expertise is available. Sherer et al. [24] reported a ruptured right interstitial pregnancy which was managed by resection with endo-GIA staples. The intrauterine pregnancy went on to deliver at 33 weeks by emergency lower segment caesarean section. Vilos et al. [25] reported cornual heterotopic pregnancy which was managed laparoscopically after ligation with endoloop and resection with CO2 laser. The patient delivered vaginally at term. Pasic et al. [15] described laparoscopic management using unipolar scissors to incise the cornual pregnancy, evacuating it and controlling the haemostasis with combination of unipolar and bipolar energy. The patient had an elective caesarean section at 38 weeks. Our patient was also delivered by elective caesarean section because we could not establish the integrity of the cornu and if it would withstand labour. Vaginal delivery however has been reported in the literature in similar situation [25].

To date in our unit, we have treated three cases of cornual ectopic with Harmonic ACE® but only this one was a heterotopic pregnancy. One of them had simultaneous sterilisation of the other tube and was uneventful. The other patient fell pregnant just 3 months after surgery and had perforation of the affected cornua at 12 weeks of pregnancy with miscarriage and needed evacuation of the uterus under laparoscopic control. The cornua was repaired simultaneously.

The harmonic scalpel is becoming increasingly popular in gynaecological surgery in recent times. It uses ultrasound energy which operates at lower temperatures compared with electrosurgery, and has simultaneous cutting and coagulating properties with minimum lateral spread and no production of smoke, only a fine mist of water or fat droplets. Harmonic ACE® therefore allows a minimally invasive surgical management in complicated cases such as this. It is a multifunctional tool combining dissection, coagulation and cutting with minimum need for change of equipment. It causes little lateral thermal spread and eliminates the danger of electrical injuries and would appear to be safe to use in cases with concurrent intrauterine pregnancy.

References

1. De VR, Pratt JH (1948) Simultaneous intrauterine and extrauterine pregnancy. Am J Obstet Gynecol 56(6):1119–1126
2. In vitro fertilization-embryo transfer (IVF-ET) (1992) in the United States: 1990 results from the IVF-ET Registry. Medical Research International. Society for Assisted Reproductive Technology (SART), The American Fertility Society. Fertil Steril 57(1):15–24
3. Goldman GA, Fisch B, Ovadia J, Tadir Y (1992) Heterotopic pregnancy after assisted reproductive technologies. Obstet Gynecol Surv 47(4):217–221
4. Lund PR, Sielaff GW, Aiman EJ (1989) In vitro fertilization patient presenting in hemorrhagic shock caused by unsuspected heterotopic pregnancy. Am J Emerg Med 7(1):49–53
5. Molloy D, Deambrosis W, Keeping D, Hynes J, Harrison K, Hennessey J (1990) Multiple-sited (heterotopic) pregnancy after in vitro fertilization and gamete intrafallopian transfer. Fertil Steril 53(6):1068–1071
6. Habana A, Dokras A, Giraldo JL, Jones EE (2000) Cornual heterotopic pregnancy: contemporary management options. Am J Obstet Gynecol 182(5):1264–1270
7. Honarbakhsh A, Khoori E, Mousavi S (2008) Heterotopic pregnancy following ovulation induction by Clomiphene and a healthy live birth: a case report. J Med Case Reports 2:390

8. Abdalla HI, Ahuja KK, Morris N, Lynn J (1986) Combined intra-abdominal and intrauterine pregnancies after gamete intrafallopian transfer. Lancet 2(8516):1153–1154
9. Olive DL, Taylor N, Cothran GE, Schenken RS (1988) Gamete intrafallopian transfer (GIFT) complicated by bilateral ectopic pregnancy. Fertil Steril 49(4):719–720
10. Chang CC, Wu TH, Tsai HD, Lo HY (1998) Bilateral simultaneous tubal sextuplets: pregnancy after in-vitro fertilization–embryo transfer following salpingectomy. Hum Reprod 13(3):762–765
11. Bisca BV, Felder ME (1960) Coexistent interstitial and intrauterine pregnancy following homolateral salpingo-oophorectomy: report of a case. Am J Obstet Gynecol 79:263–265
12. Lau S, Tulandi T (1999) Conservative medical and surgical management of interstitial ectopic pregnancy. Fertil Steril 72 (2):207–215
13. Rock J, Thompson J (2003) Telinde's Operative Gynecology. Lippincott-Raven, Philadelphia
14. Timor-Tritsch IE, Monteagudo A, Matera C, Veit CR (1992) Sonographic evolution of cornual pregnancies treated without surgery. Obstet Gynecol 79(6):1044–1049
15. Pasic RP, Hammons G, Gardner JS, Hainer M (2002) Laparoscopic treatment of cornual heterotopic pregnancy. J Am Assoc Gynecol Laparosc 9(3):372–375
16. Divry V, Hadj S, Bordes A, Genod A, Salle B (2007) Case of progressive intrauterine twin pregnancy after surgical treatment of cornual pregnancy. Fertil Steril 87(1):190
17. van der Weiden RM, Karsdorp VH (2005) Recurrent cornual pregnancy after heterotopic cornual pregnancy successfully treated with systemic methotrexate. Arch Gynecol Obstet 273(3):180–181
18. Lam PM, Lok IH, Yip SK (2004) Two cases of heterotopic cornual pregnancy with initially missed diagnosis. Aust NZ J Obstet Gynaecol 44(3):256–259
19. Ozgur K, Isikoglu M (2005) Cornual heterotopic pregnancy: conservative treatment with transvaginal embryo reduction. Arch Gynecol Obstet 271(1):73–75
20. Oyawoye S, Chander B, Pavlovic B, Hunter J, Gadir AA (2003) Heterotopic pregnancy: successful management with aspiration of cornual/interstitial gestational sac and instillation of small dose of methotrexate. Fetal Diagn Ther 18(1):1–4
21. Ghazeeri GS, Phillips OP, Emerson DS, Kutteh WH, Ke RW (2002) Live birth after treatment of a heterotopic cornual pregnancy with fetal intrathoracic KCI. A case report. J Reprod Med 47(12):1038–1040
22. Sills ES, Perloe M, Kaplan CR, Sweitzer CL, Morton PC, Tucker MJ (2002) Uncomplicated pregnancy and normal singleton delivery after surgical excision of heterotopic (cornual) pregnancy following in vitro fertilization/embryo transfer. Arch Gynecol Obstet 266(3):181–184
23. van der Weiden RM, Brandenburg H (2001) Cornual heterotopic pregnancy: contemporary management options. Am J Obstet Gynecol 185(2):522
24. Sherer DM, Scibetta JJ, Sanko SR (1995) Heterotopic quadruplet gestation with laparoscopic resection of ruptured interstitial pregnancy and subsequent successful outcome of triplets. Am J Obstet Gynecol 172(1 Pt 1):216–217
25. Vilos GA (1995) Laparoscopic resection of a heterotopic cornual pregnancy followed by term vaginal delivery. J Am Assoc Gynecol Laparosc 2(4):471–473

35

Laparoscopic management of a pelvic retroperitoneal leiomyoma

William Kondo · Revaz Botchorishvili · Fanny Desvignes · Gérard Mage

Abstract Leiomyomas are benign tumors frequently found in the fourth and fifth decades of life. Although the uterus is the most common site of origin of leiomyomas, they can develop at any site where there is smooth muscle cell. Extrauterine leiomyomas are not common and usually their diagnostic are more challenging. In this paper, we report one case of pelvic retroperitoneal leiomyoma associated to vulvar/perineal leiomyomas. A 47-year-old female patient presented with a 6-month history of deep dyspareunia, abdominal pain, dysuria, and pain during defecation. She had a previous history of two open myomectomies, a supracervical hysterectomy associated to the exeresis of a vulvar leiomyoma, and a left salpingo-oophorectomy. On vaginal examination, there was a tender and firm mass at the vaginal vault and along the posterior vaginal wall. There was another tumor at the left vulvar/perineal region measuring around 6 cm. Magnetic resonance imaging demonstrated the presence of a mass at the Douglas pouch measuring 14×10×10 cm suggestive of uterine leiomyomatosis. She underwent a successful laparoscopic resection of the pelvic tumor with an operative time of 210 min. The vulvar/perineal lesions were resected by vaginal approach. She presented an uneventful postoperative course and was discharged home 3 days after surgery. Histopathology confirmed the diagnosis of leiomyomas. Laparoscopic approach for pelvic retroperitoneal leiomyoma is feasible. It is important to keep in mind the possibility of this entity as a differential diagnosis of retroperitoneal masses in women.

W. Kondo · R. Botchorishvili · F. Desvignes · G. Mage
C.H.U. Clermont-Ferrand,
Department of Gynecology and Obstetrics,
Polyclinique de l'Hôtel Dieu,
Clermont Ferrand, France

W. Kondo (✉)
Boulevard Leon Malfreyt,
63058 Clermont-Ferrand CEDEX 1, France
e-mail: williamkondo@yahoo.com
URL: drwilliamkondo.site.med.br

Keywords Retroperitoneal leiomyomatosis · Leiomyoma · Retroperitoneal mass · Laparoscopy

Introduction

Leiomyomas are benign tumors, which are mainly composed of smooth muscle and some fibrous connective tissue elements [1]. They represent the most common gynecologic and uterine neoplasms [2], and 20% to 30% of women older than 35 years have uterine leiomyomas that are manifested clinically [3, 4].

Occasionally, leiomyomas can develop with uncommon growth patterns or in unusual locations, making their identification more challenging both clinically and radiologically. Diffuse peritoneal leiomyomatosis, intravenous leiomyomatosis, benign metastasizing leiomyomas, retroperitoneal leiomyomas, and parasitic leiomyomas are examples of leiomyomas with unusual growth patterns. Unusual sites of origin include the vulva, ovaries, urinary bladder, and urethra [2]. In this paper, we report one case of pelvic retroperitoneal leiomyoma associated to vulvar/perineal leiomyomas.

Case report

A 47-year-old female patient was referred to our service due to a pelvic mass. She had a previous history of two open myomectomies (in 1995 and 1996), a cesarean section (in 1997), and a supracervical hysterectomy associated to the exeresis of a vulvar leiomyoma (in 2004). There was no evidence of disseminated intraperitoneal leiomyomatosis or myomas at any extrauterine location at the time of the last surgery. One year ago, she underwent a left salpingo-oophorectomy for a 9.2-cm pelvic mass with the pathological finding of follicular ovarian cyst and tubal endometriosis.

She presented a 6-month history of deep dyspareunia, abdominal pain, dysuria, and pain during defecation. Her body mass index was 44.4 kg/m^2. On vaginal examination, there was a tender and firm mass at the vaginal vault and along the posterior vaginal wall. There was another tumor at the left vulvar/perineal region measuring around 6 cm.

Transvaginal ultrasound showed a heterogeneous mass at the Douglas pouch measuring 11×10×9 cm, with no atypical vascularization, and a heterogeneous, multilobulated, and well-delimited left perineal/vulvar mass measuring 6.3×6.7 cm with no continuity to the pelvic mass. Magnetic resonance imaging demonstrated a multilobulated pelvic mass measuring 14×10×10 cm with large areas of fibrous remnants suggestive of uterine leiomyomatosis (Fig. 1). Based on these findings on imaging studies suggestive of benign leiomyoma, we decided to perform a laparoscopy with intraoperative frozen section.

Under general anesthesia, she underwent a laparoscopic surgery with the intraoperative finding of a retroperitoneal mass bulging the Douglas pouch and displacing the rectum to the right. All adhesions from the previous surgeries were released. The cervix was anteriorly retracted using a transparietal suspension to improve exposition. There was no direct communication between the residual uterine cervix and the mass. The retroperitoneum was opened over the mass (Figs. 2a and b) and a biopsy was performed for intraoperative frozen section which confirmed the preoperative diagnosis of leiomyoma. Careful dissection was conducted to free the tumor from adjacent structures (Fig. 2c), including posterior vaginal wall, pararectal fossa and levator ani muscules, rectum, and pevic sidewalls (Fig. 2d). After releasing the mass, it was morcellated to allow extraction from the abdominal cavity (Fig. 3). Right salpingo-oophorectomy completed the laparoscopic procedure. The second step of the surgery was the exeresis of the left vulvar/perineal tumor by vaginal approach. There were three leiomyomas measuring 0.5×0.4, 4×2.5×1, and 4×2.5×2 cm. Total weight of the pelvic mass retrieved after morcellation was 405 g. Operative time was 210 min. The difference between pre- and postoperative hemoglobin levels was 1.9 g/dl.

She presented an uneventful postoperative course and was discharged home 3 days after surgery.

Histopathology confirmed all masses to be leiomyomas. The retroperitoneal mass presented no areas of nuclear atypia or mitosis. There was extensive hyalinization and the residual smooth muscle fibers showed fibrinoid necrosis. The vulvar/perineal leiomyomas were well encapsulated and benign, and contained large areas of collagen deposits. Immunohistochemistry demonstrated the absence of hormonal receptors in all lesions. On postoperative day 30, she was asymptomatic.

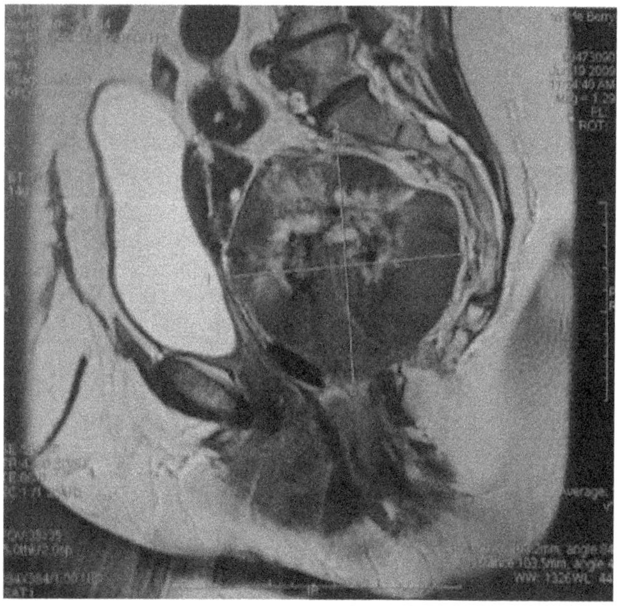

Fig. 1 Preoperative IRM demonstrating the presence of a pelvic tumor measuring 14×10×10 cm

Discussion

Leiomyoma is more frequently found in the fourth and fifth decades of life [1]. Although the uterus is the most common site of origin of leiomyomas, the lesions arise as proliferations of smooth muscle cells, and they may develop at any site where such cells are found [2]. Rarely, extrauterine leiomyomas may be seen in the retroperitoneum [1, 2, 5–11] and along the labia majora [2, 12–14].

The etiology and pathogenesis of retroperitoneal leiomyomas are unclear. Leiomyomatous masses can be seen in the pelvic retroperitoneum in women with a concurrent uterine leiomyoma or a history of uterine leiomyoma. Rarely, the extrauterine masses may extend to the upper retroperitoneum, as high as the level of the renal hilum [2]. Several mechanisms of spread have been theorized on the basis of a spectrum of pathologic processes. There are some cases reported in patients previously submitted to hysterectomy [5, 6], and it might be speculated that retroperitoneal leiomyomas may be unrelated to uterine leiomyomas. Stutterecker et al. [5] proposed that retroperitoneal lesions could originate from embryonal remnants of müllerian or

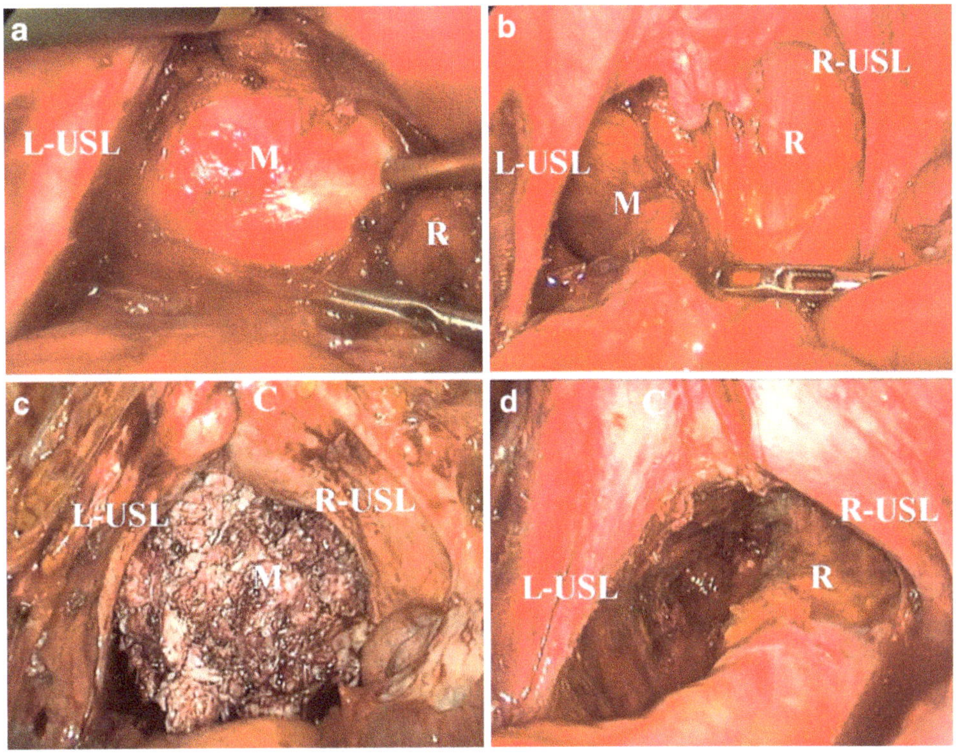

Fig. 2 **a** Opening the Douglas pouch retroperitoneum and visualization of the leiomyoma (*M*) between the left uterosacral ligament (*L-USL*) and the rectum (*R*). **b** Presence of a leiomyoma (*M*) at the Douglas pouch between the left uterosacral ligament (*L-USL*) and the rectum (*R*); the rectum is displaced to the right, next to the right uterosacral ligament (*R-USL*). **c** Dissection of the leiomyoma (*M*) from the adjacent structures. *L-USL* left uterosacral ligament, *R-USL* right uterosacral ligament, *C* uterine cervix. **d** Final view after resection of the mass. *C* uterine cervix, *L-USL* left uterosacral ligament, *R-USL* right uterosacral ligament, *R* rectum

wolffian ducts. It also has been suggested that leiomyomas that are adherent to the broad ligament originate from hormonally sensitive smooth muscle elements of that ligament [15, 16]. Occasionally, leiomyomas become adherent to surrounding structures (e.g., the broad ligament, omentum, or retroperitoneal connective tissue), develop an auxiliary blood supply, and lose their original attachment to the uterus, thus becoming "parasitic" [17, 18]. Classically, parasitic myomas occur spontaneously; however, part of the myometrium (or a small residual fibroid) can be left after vaginal [19] or abdominal hysterectomy and can receive blood supply, growing under stimulation by ovarian estrogen (residual parasitic theory) [9]. Alternatively, the recent prevalence of minimally invasive endoscopic procedures [20, 21] may promote a new type of parasitic myoma that can be called an iatrogenic parasitic myoma [22, 23]. In this situation, the electric tissue morcellator produces minute fragments of myoma tissue and there is a possibility that these fragments will implant onto peritoneal or omental tissue [24] and grow. In addition, these retroperitoneal tumors can represent metastatic or synchronous primary lesions. Several hypotheses have been proposed to explain the metastasizing theory (the lungs are the most common site of metastatic involvement): (1) it could be a benign uterine tumor that spreads via a hematogenous route to the lungs or other organs [25], (2) it could be a surgically induced hematogenous spread, and the tumor would gain venous access from surgical trauma during hysterectomy [26], and (3) it could be a low-grade metastatic leiomyosarcoma [27]. Retroperitoneal tumors are sometimes seen on autopsy or are detected incidentally on routine checkup; so, they could also represent primary extrauterine leiomyomatosis unrelated to but coexisting with uterine leiomyomata [28]. In our patient, it is difficult to believe in the iatrogenic or the residual parasitic theories because the previous hysterectomy was supracervical. Therefore, the retroperitoneal space was not opened during the procedure. It is difficult to imagine that a piece of the myometrium left after morcellation infiltrated the retroperitoneum and developed there without any intraperitoneal lesion. Also, the metastasizing theory is not justified in our patient because neither pelvic lymph nodes nor blood vessels were involved in the retroperitoneal leiomyoma.

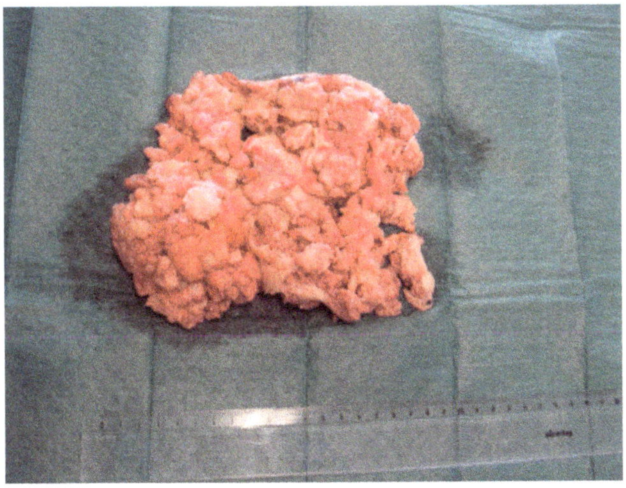

Fig. 3 Surgical specimen

We are not sure about the actual pathogenesis of this case, but maybe it could be a spontaneous parasitic leiomyoma arising from the residual cervix or a primary leiomyoma arising from embryonal remnants of müllerian or wolffian ducts.

More than 40% of patients affected by retroperitoneal leiomyomas have a concurrent uterine leiomyoma or a remote history of hysterectomy for treatment of a uterine leiomyoma. These tumors may enlarge considerably yet remain asymptomatic. Common symptoms include abdominal discomfort, fatigue, urinary symptoms, weight loss, and pelvic pain [11]. Rarely, they grow to become clinically apparent [1].

Although preoperative imaging and gross appearance are frequently typical for uterine leiomyomas, retroperitoneal leiomyomas are frequently misdiagnosed as malignant tumors [1]—tumors due to its unusual localization. Even though magnetic resonance imaging is the most reliable technique for evaluating retroperitoneal masses [2], the differential diagnosis between leiomyomas and leiomyosarcomas based on radiologic findings is difficult [29, 30]. Therefore, definitive diagnosis of a leiomyoma requires pathologic examination. US-guided percutaneous biopsy of the mass is helpful for determining its histologic composition preoperatively [2]. In some instances, determination of the exact nature of the retroperitoneal mass in a small histologic specimen might be difficult, and the true nature of the retroperitoneal mass can be only determined by complete histologic examination of the resected specimen [1].

Despite the difficulties of approaching a pelvic retroperitoneal mass by laparoscopy, the performance of a minimally invasive surgery provides many advantages for the patient and is feasible and safe even for overweight/obese women [31]. Compared with laparotomy, obese patients who undergo laparoscopy have reduced intraoperative bleeding, shorter hospitalization, less postoperative pain [32], and lower rates of postoperative wound infection [33]. Although most of previous reported cases of retroperitoneal leiomyomata were operated by laparotomy [1, 6–9], the laparoscopic approach is also feasible [34]. In our patient, the procedure was successfully performed by laparoscopy. The intraoperative frozen section was compatible with leiomyoma and the entire tumor could be dissected from the surrounding structures and removed. Reviewing 37 cases of retroperitoneal leiomyomata, Poliquin et al. [11] found that surgery was mostly curative with five reported cases of recurrence, three of which were then considered sarcomatous. In this setting, they recommend heightened surveillance after surgical treatment.

Differential diagnosis of retroperitoneal pelvic masses includes common benign and malignant neoplasms of neurogenic origin (schwannoma, paraganglioma, ganglioneuroma, and extraadrenal pheochromocytoma) as well as teratoma, desmoid tumor, hemangioma, extraadrenal angiomyelolipoma, sarcoma, lymphoma, and metastatic tumors [35].

Our patient presented also vulvar/perineal leiomyomas which were resected by vaginal approach, because there was no sign of continuity with the retroperitoneal leiomyoma on preoperative pelvic magnetic resonance imaging (MRI). Fewer than 120 cases of smooth muscle tumors of the vulva have been reported in the literature [2]. They are thought to arise from smooth muscle cells within erectile tissue, blood vessel walls, or the round ligament [36]. The average tumor size varies from 0.5 to 15 cm [37], and findings at preoperative MRI may be suggestive of the benign nature of these tumors. The differential diagnosis includes benign and malignant entities such as Bartholin cysts, fibromas, lymphangiomas, soft-tissue sarcomas, and neurogenic tumors [2].

Conclusions

Pelvic retroperitoneal and vulvar leiomyomas are rare occurrences. In this paper, we reported one patient with concomitant retroperitoneal and vulvar lesions. Preoperative diagnosis based on MRI was suggestive of benign leiomyoma and laparoscopic approach for the retroperitoneal tumor was successfully performed. It is important to keep in mind the possibility of a retroperitoneal leiomyoma as a differential diagnosis of retroperitoneal masses in premenopausal women with previous history of hysterectomy for leiomyomas.

Conflict of interest There is no actual or potential conflict of interest in relation to this article.

References

1. Dursun P, Salman MC, Taskiran C, Yüce K, Ayhan A (2005) Retroperitoneal leiomyomatosis: a case report. Int J Gynecol Cancer 15:1222–1225
2. Fasih N, Prasad Shanbhogue AK, Macdonald DB, Fraser-Hill MA, Papadatos D, Kielar AZ et al (2008) Leiomyomas beyond the uterus: unusual locations, rare manifestations. Radiographics 28:1931–1948
3. Szklaruk J, Tamm EP, Choi H, Varavithya V (2003) MR imaging of common and uncommon large pelvic masses. Radiographics 23:403–424
4. Buttram VC Jr, Reiter RC (1981) Uterine leiomyomata: etiology, symptomatology, and management. Fertil Steril 36:433–445
5. Stutterecker D, Umek W, Tunn R, Sulzbacher I, Kainz C (2001) Leiomyoma in the space of Retzius: a report of 2 cases. Am J Obstet Gynecol 185:248–249
6. Maskery PJ (1970) Retroperitoneal leiomyomatosis following hysterectomy. Proc R Soc Med 63:55–56

7. Sayer RA, Amundsen CL (2003) Giant pelvic retroperitoneal leiomyoma arising from the rectal wall. Obstet Gynecol 101:1132–1134
8. Kang WD, Kim SM, Kim YH, Choi HS (2009) Three isolated, large retroperitoneal leiomyomas. Arch Gynecol Obstet 280 (3):499-501
9. Fukamachi N, Togami S, Iwamoto I, Tsuji T, Nomoto M, Goto M et al (2007) Retroperitoneal uterine leiomyoma occurring 5 years after hysterectomy for fibroids. J Obstet Gynaecol Res 33:878–881
10. Paal E, Miettinen M (2001) Retroperitoneal leiomyomas: a clinicopathologic and immunohistochemical study of 56 cases with a comparison to retroperitoneal leiomyosarcomas. Am J Surg Pathol 25:1355–1363
11. Poliquin V, Victory R, Vilos GA (2008) Epidemiology, presentation, and management of retroperitoneal leiomyomata: systematic literature review and case report. J Minim Invasive Gynecol 15:152–160
12. Reyad MM, Gazvani MR, Khine MM (2006) A rare case of primary leiomyoma of the vulva. J Obstet Gynaecol 26:73–74
13. Guven S, Esinler D, Salman MC, Gultekin M, Ayhan A (2005) Recurrent vulval leiomyoma in a postmenopausal patient mimicking vulval carcinoma. J Obstet Gynaecol 25:732–733
14. Pitukkijronnakorn S, Leelachaikul P, Chittacharoen A (2005) Labial leiomyoma: a case report. J Med Assoc Thai 88:118–119
15. Billings SD, Folpe AL, Weiss SW (2001) Do leiomyomas of deep soft tissue exist? An analysis of highly differentiated smooth muscle tumors of deep soft tissue supporting two distinct subtypes. Am J Surg Pathol 25:1134–1142
16. Rader JS, Binette SP, Brandt TD, Sreekanth S, Chhablani A (1990) Ileal hemorrhage caused by a parasitic uterine leiomyoma. Obstet Gynecol 76:531–534
17. Hendrickson MR, Kempson RL (1994) The uterine corpus. In: Hendrickson MR (ed) Diagnostic surgical pathology, 2nd edn. Raven Press, New York, pp 2091–2193
18. Brody S (1953) Parasitic fibroid. Am J Obstet Gynecol 65:1354–1356
19. Shukunami K, Nishijima K, Kurokawa T, Orisaka M, Yoshida Y, Kotsuji F (2006) A benign solitary uterine leiomyoma on the pelvic peritoneum detected long after the hysterectomy for fibroids. J Obstet Gynaecol 26:589
20. Istre O, Langebrekke A, Qvigstad E (2007) Changing hysterectomy technique from open abdominal to laparoscopic: new trend in Oslo, Norway. J Minim Invasive Gynecol 14:74–77
21. Hurst BS, Matthews ML, Marshburn PB (2005) Laparoscopic myomectomy for symptomatic uterine myomas. Fertil Steril 83:1–23
22. Paul PG, Koshy AK (2006) Multiple peritoneal parasitic myomas after laparoscopic myomectomy and morcellation. Fertil Steril 85:492–493
23. Sinha R, Sundaram M, Mahajan C, Sambhus A (2007) Multiple leiomyomas after laparoscopic hysterectomy: report of two cases. J Minim Invasive Gynecol 14:123–127
24. Takeda A, Mori M, Sakai K, Mitsui T, Nakamura H (2007) Parasitic peritoneal leiomyomatosis diagnosed 6 years after laparoscopic myomectomy with electric tissue morcellation: report of a case and review of the literature. J Minim Invasive Gynecol 14:770–775
25. Harper RS, Scully RE (1961) Intravenous leiomyomatosis of the uterus. A report of four cases. Obstet Gynecol 18:519–529
26. Wolff M, Silva F, Kaye G (1979) Pulmonary metastases (with admixed epithelial elements) from smooth muscle neoplasms. Report of nine cases, including three males. Am J Surg Pathol 3:325–342
27. Cho KR, Woodruff JD, Epstein JI (1989) Leiomyoma of the uterus with multiple extrauterine smooth muscle tumors: a case report suggesting multifocal origin. Hum Pathol 20:80–83
28. Goyle KK, Moore DF Jr, Garrett C, Goyle V (2003) Benign metastasizing leiomyomatosis: case report and review. Am J Clin Oncol 26:473–476
29. Schwartz LB, Zawin M, Carcangiu ML, Lange R, McCarthy S (1998) Does pelvic magnetic resonance imaging differentiate among the histologic subtypes of uterine leiomyomata? Fertil Steril 70:580–587
30. Arakawa A, Yasunaga T, Yano S, Morishita K, Nakashima K, Sato R et al (1993) Radiological findings of retroperitoneal leiomyoma and leiomyosarcoma: report of two cases. Comput Med Imaging Graph 17:125–131
31. O'Hanlan KA, Dibble SL, Fisher DT (2006) Total laparoscopic hysterectomy for uterine pathology: impact of body mass index on outcomes. Gynecol Oncol 103:938–941
32. Eltabbakh GH, Shamonki MI, Moody JM, Garafano LL (2000) Hysterectomy for obese women with endometrial cancer: laparoscopy or laparotomy? Gynecol Oncol 78:329–335
33. Obermair A, Manolitsas TP, Leung Y, Hammond IG, McCartney AJ (2005) Total laparoscopic hysterectomy versus total abdominal hysterectomy for obese women with endometrial cancer. Int J Gynecol Cancer 15:319–324
34. Hilger WS, Magrina JF (2006) Removal of pelvic leiomyomata and endometriosis five years after supracervical hysterectomy. Obstet Gynecol 108:772–774
35. Nishino M, Hayakawa K, Minami M, Yamamoto A, Ueda H, Takasu K (2003) Primary retroperitoneal neoplasms: CT and MR imaging findings with anatomic and pathologic diagnostic clues. Radiographics 23:45–57
36. Kaufman RH, Gardner HL (1965) Tumors of the vulva and vagina. Benign mesodermal tumors. Clin Obstet Gynecol 8:953–981
37. Nielsen GP, Rosenberg AE, Koerner FC, Young RH, Scully RE (1996) Smooth-muscle tumors of the vulva. A clinicopathological study of 25 cases and review of the literature. Am J Surg Pathol 20:779–793

36

A case report of incisional hernia through a 5-mm lateral port site following laparoscopic right ovarian cystectomy

A. Sayasneh • H. Nosib • H. Abdel-Rahman

Abstract We report a case of postoperative bowel obstruction with early onset hernia presenting through a 5-mm port. A 43-year-old woman having undergone laparoscopic ovarian cystectomy 2 days before presented with features of intestinal obstruction in the form of persistent abdominal pain, vomiting, and inability to pass stool or flatus. Computed tomography scan of her abdomen showed collapsed large bowel and a loop of small bowel protruding through the lateral 5-mm sheath defect. A secondary laparoscopic procedure allowed both confirming diagnosis and surgical repair of the hernia. Our case describes this rare complication through a 5-mm lateral port, with complete bowel obstruction, in the absence of any of the recognized risk factors following a straightforward short surgical procedure, performed as an open laparoscopy with the sample retrieved through the 10-mm trocar. Body mass index was normal, with no significant health problems preoperatively.

Keywords Port site hernia · Laparoscopic ovarian cystectomy · Small bowel obstruction

Abbreviations

USS	ultrasound scan
CA125	cancer antigen 125
CO_2	carbon dioxide
A&E	Accident and Emergency Department
FBC	full blood count
Us and Es	urea and electrolytes
LFTs	lever function tests
CRP	C-reactive protein
CXR	chest X-ray
AXR	abdominal X-ray
CT	computed tomography
°C	degree Celsius
mmHg	millimeters of mercury
mm	millimeters
cm	centimeters
BMI	body mass index

A. Sayasneh (✉) · H. Nosib · H. Abdel-Rahman
Department of Obstetrics and Gynaecology,
Hinchingbrooke Hospital,
Huntingdon, UK
e-mail: sayasneh@gmail.com

Introduction

Trocar site hernia is a rare cause of major morbidity after laparoscopic surgery. It is a common practice to close 10 mm rectal sheath defect to prevent this serious complication. However, there is not enough evidence to suggest closing 5-mm laparoscopic incisions. In our case, we report a 5-mm lateral port hernia, and we discussed the incidence, etiology, and prevention of this very rare laparoscopic surgery complication.

Case report

A 43-year-old nulliparous woman was admitted for an elective laparoscopic right ovarian cystectomy. Her body mass index was 26, she had no known medical problems, and had never undergone abdominal surgery. She had a simple-looking ovarian cyst on USS measuring 5 cm diameter, and CA125 was 11.

Three ports were used for carrying out the procedure, of which one was 10 mm and two were 5 mm. The 10-mm

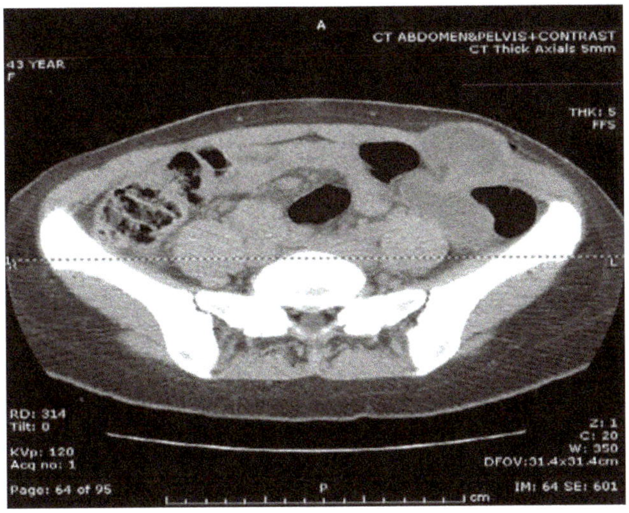

Fig. 1 Small bowel hernia through left 5-mm port site on CT scan

port was an umbilical camera port, and the two 5 mm were working ports. A Hasson entry was performed, and a 10-mm umbilical port was introduced. Carbon dioxide was insufflated to a pressure of 20 mmHg and then lowered to 15 mmHg when all trocars were in the abdominal cavity. Two 5-mm lateral pyramidal-tipped trocars were inserted on each lower abdominal quadrant outside the rectus sheath under direct vision. Insertion of all ports was obtained at first attempt, with one trocar pass for each port, and no stretching of port sites took place during the procedure. The cyst was dissected using a laparoscopic grasper and retrieved in an endobag via the 10-mm umbilical port under direct vision from the right lateral port. The procedure was uncomplicated; hemostasis was achieved with bipolar diathermy. The lateral ports were removed under direct vision, and the CO_2 was expelled through the ports. The umbilical port was removed after complete evacuation of CO_2. The umbilical rectus sheath was closed with vicryl 1. The skin was closed with interrupted monocryl in the umbilical and lateral ports.

On the third postoperation day, she presented to A&E with features of intestinal obstruction in the form of persistent abdominal pain, vomiting, and inability to pass stool or flatus. Her general condition was average, and she was conscious. Her temperature was 37.4°C, blood pressure was 123/67 mmHg, and pulse was 70/min. Her abdomen was non-distended and soft. A 4-×5-cm hard lump was palpated under the left 5-mm port site and was tender and non-reducible. There were no erythematic changes, local temperature fluctuation, or any other sign of infection at any of the trocars' sites. Bowel sounds were negative. Blood tests including FBC, Us and Es, LFTs, amylase, and CRP were normal. CXR was normal and showed no signs of perforation. Erect AXR showed multiple fluid levels in the small bowel with no gas in the rectum. Surgical opinion was sought, and an urgent CT scan of her abdomen on the same day showed collapsed large bowel and an ovoid area of fluid within the abdominal wall musculature immediately lateral to the left rectus measuring 2.5×4.5 cm with an internal structure resembling bowel. This confirmed the diagnosis of incisional hernia (Fig. 1).

Management

She was immediately taken to the theater for laparoscopy/laparotomy for exploration and reduction of the hernia with possible bowel resection depending on the viability of the herniated bowel. She was maintained on intravenous fluids only, and a nasogastric tube was inserted, which drained 1 l of bilious fluid. A urinary catheter was also inserted.

The operation was performed jointly by the general surgical and the gynecology teams. The previous umbilical incision was reopened bluntly, and a scope was inserted through with CO_2 insufflation. A small bowel loop was found to have herniated through the left lateral port (see Figs. 2, 3, and 4).The right lateral port was reentered under laparoscopic guidance, and the left lateral port site was enlarged to 3 cm externally. The herniated bowel was reduced gently through the fascial defect using a finger, applying downward pressure from the skin incision on the left side. The herniated loop of bowel was dusky after reduction but looked well perfused and viable after irrigation with warm saline and observation for 20 min. The rest of the bowels and pelvis looked normal. Bowel resection was not deemed necessary. All the extra CO_2 was expelled, and all the port sites were closed with prolene to the sheath and monocryl to the skin.

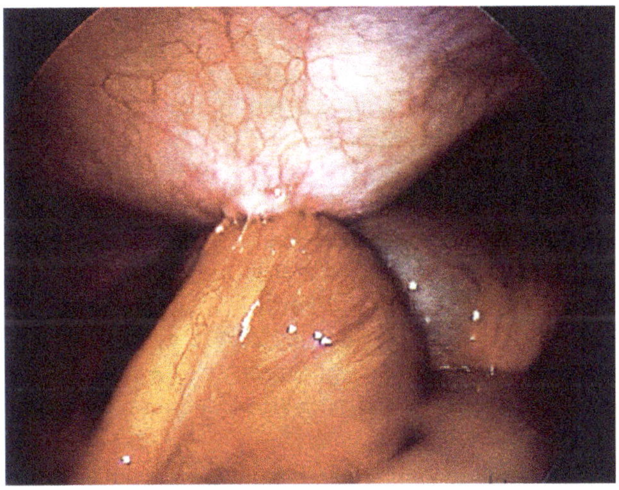

Fig. 2 Small bowel hernia through left 5-mm port site as seen in laparoscopy. Note that part of the mesentery is included in the hernia as well

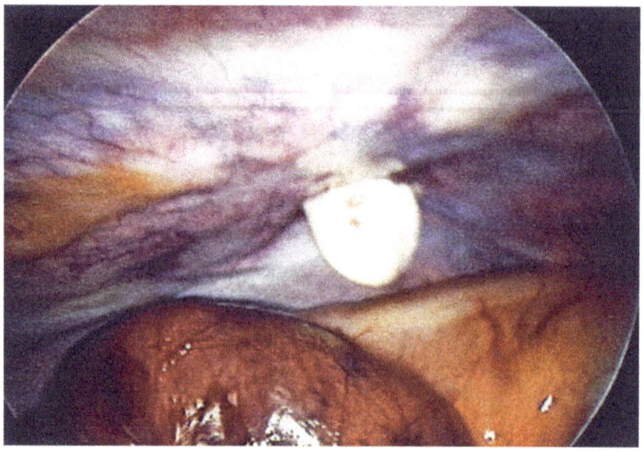

Fig. 3 Small bowels reduced through the old 5-mm port site assisted by the surgeon's index finger, which is seen in the image. Note the dark color, early incarceration changes of the reduced bowel

The patient made a good postoperative recovery. Her initial symptoms settled, and she was discharged home 2 days after her operation with normal bowel function.

Discussion

The incidence of trocar site hernia is estimated to be between 0.65% and 2.80% [1]. In a survey of the American Association of Gynecologic Laparoscopists, post-laparoscopy incisional hernias occur at an approximate incidence of 21 per 100,000 and are associated with significant morbidity [2]. The same survey revealed that 86.3% of herniae occurred in sites where the trocar diameter was 10 mm or more, and umbilical herniae were found in 75.70% as compared to lateral hernias in 23.70% [2]. In another retrospective study of 320 cases, the prevalence of trocar site herniation after laparoscopic fundoplication was minimal at 3% [3]. All herniae occurred at the midline supraumbilical port [3].

There are several factors implicating the etiology. They include large trocar size, incomplete closure of fascia at the trocar site, midline trocars, stretching of the port site for organ retrieval, the effect of a partial vacuum while port withdrawal, obesity, poor nutrition, and operation site infection [1, 4]. Reardon et al. [5] suggested in their paper that hernia may also be caused by repetitive motions in different directions during lengthy laparoscopic procedures. These motions may cause significant stretching of the port site, hence allowing a hernia to develop to a considerable size [5]. In the series by Mayol et al. [6], the incidence of port site hernia was higher in closed than in open (Hasson) technique.

There are very few similar reported cases. Tonouchi et al. [1] classified trocar site herniae into three main groups. The first group, where our case falls into, is early-onset hernia, which indicates dehiscence of anterior fascial plane and peritoneum [1]. The late-onset type develops several months after laparoscopy and contains the peritoneum as a hernia sac [1]. The special type indicates dehiscence of the whole abdominal wall [1].

Sirito et al. [7] described a similar complication after laparoscopic ovarian cystectomy; however, the hernia developed a year after the surgery and contained omentum.

Bourdel et al. [8]. reported a Richter's hernia, where only part of the bowel's wall is herniating with no complete obstruction, presenting through a 5-mm sheath incision after laparoscopic hysterectomy.

Our case describes this rare complication through a 5-mm lateral port, with complete bowel obstruction, in the absence of any of the recognized risk factors following a straightforward short surgical procedure, performed as an open laparoscopy with the sample retrieved through the 10-mm trocar. BMI was normal, with no significant health problems preoperatively. Therefore, would closing the 5-mm port site have prevented this serious complication from happening?

There is no satisfying answer for this question. Crist and Gadacaz suggested that fascial defects created by 5.5 mm do not require closing [9]. On the other hand, Tonouchi et al. [1] suggested that trocar site hernia may be reduced by closing the fascia in all port sites including lateral ones of 5 mm, and they advocated closing the fascial defect and peritoneum for 5-mm trocar defects if active manipulation has occurred during prolonged procedures. The evidence is clearly conflicting, and perhaps, more research needs to be done before a conclusion can be reached. However, after this particular case, we (the team involved in this case) will adapt closing the fascial defect for all ports of any size and location as a safer option with no significant delay in the operating time.

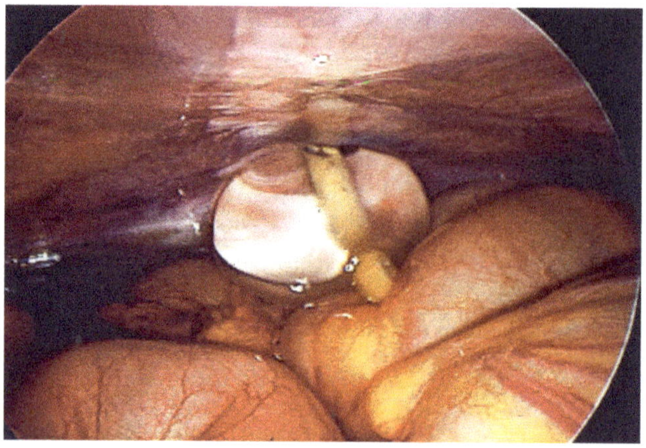

Fig. 4 Twenty minutes after reduction. Note the improved colour of the reduced bowel loop. A Foley catheter balloon was used to prevent gas leakage from abdominal cavity throughout the procedure

This case has highlighted a very important aspect of laparoscopic surgery: aftercare of patients and prompt recognition and management of postoperative complications. This patient was reviewed promptly by the same team who had performed the operation, and investigations were initiated in a timely way. A thorough review of the patient was performed, and the diagnosis was suspected from the start. This led to appropriate review by the surgical team. Radiology assistance was also readily available, though this all happened out of hours at night. She was treated laparoscopically as expertise was at hand and perhaps avoided an unnecessary laparotomy. She also did not require bowel resection, as the symptoms were seen without delay and theater was arranged for in time. We believe that units performing laparoscopic surgery should have adequate expertise and facilities to deal with potential complications albeit rare at any time, as this significantly alters the prognosis of those involved. Units should have a clear pathway for the referral of patients in the postoperative period for review in case of suspected complications.

Conflict of interest The corresponding author certifies that there is no actual or potential conflict of interest in relation to this article.

References

1. Tonouchi H, Ohmori Y, Kobayashi M, Kusunoki M (2004) Trocar site hernia. Arch Surg 139:1248–1256
2. Montz FJ, Holschneider CH, Munro MG (1994) Incisional hernia following laparoscopy: a survey of the American association of gynecologic laparoscopists. J Obstet Gynecol 84(5):881–884
3. Bowrey DJ, Blom D, Crookes PF, Bremner CG, Johansson JLM, Lord RV, Hagen JA, DeMeester SR, DeMeester TR, Peters JH (2001) Risk factors and the prevalence of trocar site herniation after laparoscopic fundoplication. Surg Endosc 15(7):663–666
4. Rao P, Ghosh K, Sudhan D (2008) Port site hernia: a rare complication of laparoscopy. Med J Armed Forces India 64:187–188
5. Reardon PR, Preciado A, Scarborough T, Matthews B, Marti JL (1999) Hernia at 5-mm laparoscopic port site presenting as early postoperative small bowel obstruction. J Laparoendosc Adv Surg Tech A 9(6):523–525
6. Mayol J, Garcia-Aguilar J, Ortiz-Oshiro E, De-Diego Carmona JA, Fernandez-Represa JA (1997) Risks of the minimal access approach for laparoscopic surgery: multivariate analysis of morbidity related to umbilical trocar insertion. World J Surg 21:529–533
7. Sirito R, Puppo A, Centurioni MG, Gustavino C (2005) Incisional hernia on the 5-mm trocar port site and subsequent wall endometriosis on the same site: a case report. Am J Obstet Gynecol 193(3 Pt 1):878–880
8. Bourdel N, Roman H, Lebouedec G, Lenglet Y, Accoceberry M, Canis M (2006) Richter's hernia occurring through a 5-mm laparoscopy sheath incision. Gynecol Surg 3:132–133
9. Crist DW, Gadacz TR (1993) Complications of laparoscopic surgery. Surg Clin North Am J 73:265–289

Risk assessment of the ergonomic aspects of laparoscopic theatre

A. Cutner · A. Stavroulis · N. Zolfaghari

Abstract An employer has a legal requirement to offer a safe working environment to its employees. The risks and hazards should be reduced as far as practicably possible, and the set-up should be as ergonomic as possible. Modern laparoscopic surgery carried out in an old-fashioned theatre without the advantages that an integrated operating room has to offer results in increased risk of injury to the staff. We have assessed the relative risks and determined reasons why modernisation is essential to the safety of the theatre team.

Keywords Laparoscopy · Integrated theatre · Ergonomics

Introduction

Operating rooms need to be fit for purpose. They are required to offer a safe environment for patients who undergo treatment and the staff who work within them. Previously, some aspects of the theatre environment were considered optional but are now the minimum acceptable standard. Examples of these include negative-pressure air conditioning [1], piped gas for anaesthetic machines [2] and laminar flow for orthopaedic joint surgery [3].

A hospital has a duty of care for the individuals responsible for surgery. The patient expectation is that the surgery will be carried out by skilled personnel in an appropriate environment.

There are certain expectations of the teams involved. Expectations of a surgeon include the following: to have the necessary skills to carry out the surgery that is planned [4], to work as a team to optimise outcome [5], to call for additional assistance where required and to forward plan this where possible. Expectations of the nursing staff are to have the correct nursing skills for the surgery, to prepare the theatre and equipment for the surgery to be carried out and to work with the surgeon to facilitate a good outcome [5].

Legally, employers must comply with relevant health and safety and employment legislation as well as the common law Duty of Care. Under the Management of Health and Safety at Work Regulations 1999, employers are responsible to complete a suitable and sufficient assessment of the risks to the health and safety that employees are exposed to whilst at work [6]. In addition, the same duty of care applies to anyone whose health and safety could be adversely affected by the employer's actions. The employer must identify risks and act upon these by instituting preventive and protective measures as far as reasonably practicable to protect the health of employees and others who may be affected.

Complying with the Duty of Care principle requires planning for the prevention of workplace-related illnesses and injuries. It is the employer's responsibilities to ensure that all reasonably practicable measures have been taken to identify workplace hazards and identify and apply preventative measures to control workplace risks against work-related illnesses and injuries.

Thus, there is a corporate responsibility to provide a facility that optimises surgical outcome and to provide an environment that does not place the patient or staff at an unacceptable level of risk of physical injury. This paper will address the risk assessment to staff performing advanced laparoscopic surgery in an unacceptable theatre environment. We acknowledge that our article is not applicable to all areas of surgery and merely addresses the laparoscopic environment.

A. Cutner · A. Stavroulis (✉) · N. Zolfaghari
Institute for Women's Health, UCLH NHS Foundation Trust, London, UK
e-mail: stavroulis@btinternet.com

What is ergonomics?

Ergonomics is "the scientific study of people at work, in terms of equipment design, workplace layout, the working environment, safety, productivity, and training". Ergonomics is based on anatomy, physiology, psychology and engineering, combined in a systems approach [7]. It is the study of designing equipment and devices that fit the human body, its movements and its cognitive abilities. In simple words, it is the science of best suiting the worker to his job.

With laparoscopic surgery, a man–machine environment has been brought into the operating room, which has created mental and physical challenges for the operating team. The science of ergonomics analyses these challenges and formulates guidelines for creating a work environment that is safe and comfortable for its operators whilst effective and efficient processes are maintained [8].

In the case of laparoscopic surgery, it is to make the setting and surroundings as favourable as reasonably practicable for the laparoscopic surgeon to do the surgery without awkward posture and with reasonable comfort [9].

What is a hazard and risk rating?

A hazard is a biological, chemical or physical agent that is reasonably likely to cause illness or injury in the absence of its control [10]. Risk is the likelihood that a specified undesired event will occur due to the realisation of a hazard by or during work activities or by the products and services created by work activities [11]. Risk in relation to occupational health and safety is defined as the likelihood that a person could be harmed by hazards in the workplace. The risk from the hazard should be determined by estimating the potential severity of harm and the likelihood that harm will occur.

Risk assessment is a tool to help an organisation or a department prevent accidents and ill health from occurring [12]. The requirement for risk assessment was first legally introduced in 1992 with the Management of Health and Safety at Work Regulations [13], even though the concept was contained within the Health and Safety at Work Act 1974 [14].

Risk rating selects or marks the values for consequences of hazards if they are not controlled (Table 1). The following risk matrix can be used to rate the risk [11]:

$$\text{Risk rating} = \text{Likelihood of the hazard causing harm} \times \text{Severity of the consequences.}$$

A risk rating of 16–25 (Table 2) demands immediate remedial action to remove the hazard in order to ensure patient care and safety, staff health and safety and to comply with relevant health and safety legislation [15].

Table 1 Risk rating matrix

Category	Harm (severity of the consequences)	Likelihood
1	Non-injury	Almost impossible
2	First aid	Unlikely
3	Fewer than 3 days off work	Possible
4	More than 3 days off work	Likely
5	Major injury	Almost certain

Comparison of risk between open and laparoscopic surgery

There are many differences between open and laparoscopic surgery. Open surgery has a high degree of freedom, and surgeons work in line with their visual axis. There is a three-dimensional direct vision and direct tactile feedback. There is no need for monitors, accessory equipment like gas insufflators or extra wiring. During laparoscopic surgery, there is two-dimensional vision and a loss of depth perception to some extent, as well as a fulcrum effect with tremor enhancement. There are only four degrees of freedom, and the major limitation is that the view is not under the control of the surgeon.

For open surgery, the level of vision is determined by the visual acuity of the operator, the size of the incision, retractors used and the quality of overhead lighting in the operating room. The surgeon works directly on the patient with the use of traditional instruments. In contrast, to perform the surgical procedure laparoscopically, the surgeon interacts with several technological applications and equipments and requires extra wires and cables.

The increased technological complexity and sometimes poorly adapted equipment for the laparoscopic theatre environment have increased the chances of the operating team, in general, and the surgeons, in particular, of being encouraged to adopt incorrect posture and consequently suffer from fatigue and discomfort during laparoscopic surgery and thus suffer from musculoskeletal injuries.

Laparoscopic surgery in a standard theatre environment

Performing laparoscopic surgery in a conventional operating room requires additional specialised equipment otherwise

Table 2 Action required according to risk rating score

Risk rating score	Action
1–4	No further action
5–9	Re-assess after next review
10–15	Action within 3 months
16–25	Immediate action

stored outside the theatre. Before the procedure, the theatre team must collect, prepare and connect the equipment, then take it away afterwards. These extra tasks pose a threat to efficiency and may lengthen turnover times. In addition, they increase the risk of physical injury to staff manoeuvring the equipment.

The average general operating theatre is not designed to house this equipment, leading to crowded workplaces, floors cluttered with tubing and wires, operative inefficiencies and safety problems for patients and staff [16]. The stack system is heavy to move and handle. Overall, there is an increased hazard and risk of physical harm.

The monitor is placed on top of a trolley with fixed height, and the trolley is placed wherever possible around the operating theatre. The fixed height of the trolley and its location within the operating theatre do not allow surgeons to adjust the height of the monitor in relation to their own height, and very often, surgeons are forced to adopt an awkward neck and back posture to view the operation on the monitor. Ergonomically, the best view for laparoscopy is with the monitor image at or within 25 optimal degrees below the horizontal plane of the eye. This leads to least neck strain [17, 18]. Other positions of the monitor will compromise surgical safety and result in repetitive strain injury to the surgeon. This will be exacerbated in long complex operations.

If there is one monitor and this is optimally placed for the surgeon, then the assistant who stands on the opposite side of the table is required to look over their shoulder for long periods of time. Besides neck pain, monitor positioning can be responsible for spondylosis [19].

In a non-integrated poorly designed theatre, the risk or likelihood of musculoskeletal injury during laparoscopic surgery to surgeons and their assistants and the risk of error in surgery are almost certain. The severity of the consequences or the injury to the surgeon, their assistant and to patients is quite high or major as musculoskeletal injury causes short-, medium- and long-term absenteeism amongst staff. Thus, the risk rating would be as follows:

$$\text{Risk rating}(25) = \text{Almost certain}(5) \times \text{Major}(5).$$

This risk rating is supported in the literature. In a recent publication, 85 % of laparoscopic surgeons reported suffering from work-related symptoms or injuries [20]. Much of the blame was placed on the piecemeal assembly of operating suites not designed for screen-based operations and on the co-opting of instrumentation from other specialties not intentionally designed for laparoscopic use [21, 22]. Guidelines have been introduced detailing proper positioning to minimize injuries, although implementation has been slow to non-existent [23].

Laparoscopic operations substantially increase the amount of equipment and the number of cables in the operating room. Such conditions create physical hazards for traffic in the operating theatre.

Laparoscopic surgery in an integrated theatre

The integrated theatre is a state-of-the-art system in which the laparoscopic equipment and multiple flat-screen monitors are permanently installed to be operational on demand inside the theatre. The equipment is installed in columns attached to a ceiling-mounted suspension system that facilitates versatile positioning away from the monitors. All the wiring is concealed inside the suspension system and led out through the ceiling. The laparoscopic equipment can be remotely controlled by the operating surgeon or by the circulating nurse using a touch panel at a control station. It links together, via an interface, all surgical equipment including the room and camera lights, gas insuflation and diathermy.

The Media Control provides settings that the individual surgeon can preselect, and with one button, the set-up takes place automatically. In addition, it can function as a tele-video conferencing system with transmission of images and can be used for telemedicine, telementoring and remote teaching.

It is easy to be used by all theatre staff and requires minimal training. Being boom-mounted is important as this is much safer for equipment and there are no trailing cables on the floor. It enables positioning of monitors where they are required, and it is easier for staff to move around and is important for health and safety as it minimises infection risk. Efficiency during the intraoperative period is significantly improved in the integrated theatre. The theatre nurses' tasks are relieved, which may reduce mental and physical workload and improve job satisfaction and patient safety [23]. The integrated theatre is designed to reduce theatre clutter and staff workload. It increases comfort, safety and efficiency, and it enhances the ergonomics and team performance [24–26].

Conclusion and discussion

Laparoscopic surgery provides patients with less painful surgery but is more demanding for the surgeon. The benefits for patients such as smaller incisions and shorter recovery periods are well established. However, the negative effect on surgeons and the team of repeatedly performing laparoscopic operations in an inappropriate environment is only just beginning to be appreciated.

The increased technological complexity and sometimes poorly adapted equipment have led to increased complaints of surgeon fatigue and discomfort during laparoscopic surgery. Better ergonomic integration and understanding ergonomics can not only make the life of the surgeon more comfortable in the operating room but also reduce physical strains on the surgeon [7]. In addition, the movement of heavy equipment around a theatre complex together with increased theatre clutter increases the hazards for all staff and adds to inefficiencies.

To comply with the legal requirements and to ensure health and safety of the operating team, the ergonomic integration and suitability of the laparoscopic operating room environment are essential. Future work on the benefits of performing surgery in an ergonomically sound environment might focus on its effect on staff interactions and teamwork.

Conflict of interest Alfred Cutner received funding for Storz for lectures and education purposes.

References

1. Chow TT, Kwan A, Lin Z, Bai W (2006) Conversion of operating theatre from positive to negative pressure environment. J Hosp Infect 64:371–378
2. Love-Jones S, Magee P (2007) Medical gases, their storage and delivery. Anaesth Intensive Care Med 8(1):2–6
3. Knobben BAS, van Horn JR, van der Mei HC, Busscher HJ (2006) Evaluation of measures to decrease intra-operative bacterial contamination in orthopaedic implant surgery. J Hosp Infect 62:174–180
4. The National Institute for Health and Clinical Excellence (2009) IPG283 Sacrocolpopexy using mesh for vaginal vault: guidance. http://www.nice.org.uk/nicemedia/live/11202/42864/42864.pdf. Accessed 29 Sep 2012
5. Mousquès J, Bourgueil Y, Le Fur P, Yilmaz E (2010) Effect of a French experiment of team work between general practitioners and nurses on efficacy and cost of type 2 diabetes patients care. Health Policy 98:131–143
6. The Health and Safety Executive (HSE). Employer's responsibilities. http://www.hse.gov.uk/workers/employers.htm. Accessed 29 Sep 2012
7. Supe AN, Kulkarni GV, Supe PA (2010) Ergonomics in laparoscopic surgery. J Minim Access Surg 6(2):31–36
8. Sanders MS, McCormick EJ (1993) Human factors in engineering and design, 7th edn. McGraw-Hill, New York
9. Kilbom A (1990) Measurement and assessment of dynamic work. In: Wilson EC Jr (ed) Evaluation of human work: a practical ergonomics methodology. Taylor and Francis, London, pp 641–661
10. National Advisory Committee on Microbiological Criteria for Foods (NACMCF) (1992) Hazard analysis and critical control point system. Int J Food Microbiol 16:1–23
11. The Health and Safety Executive (HSE) (2012) www.hse.gov.uk/quarries/education/powerpoint/topic5.ppt. Accessed 29 Sep 2012
12. The Health and Safety Executive (HSE) (2011) Five steps to risk assessment. http://www.hse.gov.uk/risk/fivesteps.htm. Accessed 29 Sep 2012
13. The National Archives (2012) The Management of Health and Safety at Work Regulations 1992. http://www.legislation.gov.uk/uksi/1992/2051/contents/made. Accessed 29 Sep 2012
14. The Health and Safety Executive (HSE) (2012) Health and Safety at Work etc. Act 1974. http://www.hse.gov.uk/legislation/hswa.htm. Accessed 29 Sep 2012
15. TUC (2008) Risk assessment. www.tuc.org.uk/extras/riskassessment.pdf. Accessed 29 Sep 2012
16. Alarcon A, Berguer R (1996) A comparison of operating room crowding between open and laparoscopic operations. Surg Endosc 10:916–919
17. Menozzi M, von Buol A, Krueger H, Miege C (1994) Direction of gaze and comfort: discovering the relation for the ergonomic optimization of visual tasks. Ophthalmic Physiol Opt 14:393–399
18. Hanna GB, Shimi SM, Cuschieri A (1998) Task performance in endoscopic surgery is influenced by location of the image display. Ann Surg 227:481–484
19. Kant IJ, de Jong LC, van Rijssen-Moll M, Borm PJ (1992) A survey of static and dynamic work postures of operating room staff. Int Arch Occup Environ Health 63:423–428
20. Park A, Lee G, Seagull FJ, Meenaghan N, Dexter D (2010) Patients benefit while surgeons suffer: an impending epidemic. J Am Coll Surg 210(3):306–313
21. Berguer R, Rab GT, Abu-Ghaida H, Alarcon A, Chung J (1997) A comparison of surgeons' posture during laparoscopic and open surgical procedures. Surg Endosc 11(2):139–142
22. Nguyen NT, Ho HS, Smith WD et al (2001) An ergonomic evaluation of surgeons' axial skeletal and upper extremity movements during laparoscopic and open surgery. Am J Surg 182 (6):720–724
23. van Det MJ, Meijerink WJHJ, Hoff C, Tottè ER, Pierie JPEN (2009) Optimal ergonomics for laparoscopic surgery in minimally invasive surgery suites: a review and guidelines. Surg Endosc 23:1279–1285
24. Herron DM, Gagner M, Kenyon TL, Swanstrom LL (2001) The minimally invasive surgical suite enters the 21st century: a discussion of critical design elements. Surg Endosc 15:415–422
25. Kenyon TA, Urbach DR, Speer JB, Waterman-Hukari B, Foraker GF, Hansen PD, Swanstrom LL (2001) Dedicated minimally invasive surgery suites increase operating room efficiency. Surg Endosc 15:1140–1143
26. van Det MJ, Meijerink WJHJ, Hoff C, Van Veelen MA, Pierie JPEN (2008) Ergonomic assessment of neck posture in the minimally invasive surgery suite during laparoscopic cholecystectomy. Surg Endosc 22:2421–2427

Permissions

The contributors of this book come from diverse backgrounds, making this book a truly international effort. This book will bring forth new frontiers with its revolutionizing research information and detailed analysis of the nascent developments around the world.

We would like to thank all the contributing authors for lending their expertise to make the book truly unique. They have played a crucial role in the development of this book. Without their invaluable contributions this book wouldn't have been possible. They have made vital efforts to compile up to date information on the varied aspects of this subject to make this book a valuable addition to the collection of many professionals and students.

This book was conceptualized with the vision of imparting up-to-date information and advanced data in this field. To ensure the same, a matchless editorial board was set up. Every individual on the board went through rigorous rounds of assessment to prove their worth. After which they invested a large part of their time researching and compiling the most relevant data for our readers.

The editorial board has been involved in producing this book since its inception. They have spent rigorous hours researching and exploring the diverse topics which have resulted in the successful publishing of this book. They have passed on their knowledge of decades through this book. To expedite this challenging task, the publisher supported the team at every step. A small team of assistant editors was also appointed to further simplify the editing procedure and attain best results for the readers.

Apart from the editorial board, the designing team has also invested a significant amount of their time in understanding the subject and creating the most relevant covers. They scrutinized every image to scout for the most suitable representation of the subject and create an appropriate cover for the book.

The publishing team has been an ardent support to the editorial, designing and production team. Their endless efforts to recruit the best for this project, has resulted in the accomplishment of this book. They are a veteran in the field of academics and their pool of knowledge is as vast as their experience in printing. Their expertise and guidance has proved useful at every step. Their uncompromising quality standards have made this book an exceptional effort. Their encouragement from time to time has been an inspiration for everyone.

The publisher and the editorial board hope that this book will prove to be a valuable piece of knowledge for researchers, students, practitioners and scholars across the globe.

List of Contributors

Liv Ahlborg
Division of Obstetrics and Gynecology, Södertälje Hospital, 152 86 Södertälje, Sweden

Leif Hedman
Department of Psychology, Umeå University, Umeå, Sweden

Lars Enochsson
Divisions of Surgery, Karolinska University Hospital, Stockholm, Sweden

Li Felländer-Tsai
Divisions of Orthopaedics, Karolinska University Hospital, Stockholm, Sweden

Carsten Rasmussen
Divisions of Obstetrics and Gynecology, Karolinska University Hospital, Stockholm, Sweden

A. Coosemans, R. Corona, K. Mailova and P. Koninckx
Department of Obstetrics and Gynecology, UZ Leuven, Campus Gasthuisberg, Leuven, Belgium

M. Praet
Department of Pathology, UZ Gent, Gent, Belgium

J. Verguts
Department of Obstetrics and Gynecology, University Hospital Leuven, Campus Gasthuisberg, Herestraat 49, 3000 Leuven, Belgium

Rasiah Bharathan
John Radcliffe Hospital, Headley Way, Oxford OX3 9DU, UK

Sarah Merritt
Department of Obstetrics & Gynaecology, St. Thomas' Hospital, Westminster Bridge Road, London SE1 7EH, UK

Hasib Ahmed
Department of Obstetrics & Gynaecology, Medway Maritime Hospital, Gillingham, Kent ME7 5NY, UK

R. P. G. ten Broek and H. van Goor
Department of Surgery, Radboud University Nijmegen Medical Centre, Nijmegen, The Netherlands

N. Kok-Krant, H. R. Verhoeve and E. A. Bakkum
Department of Gynaecology and Obstetrics, Onze Lieve Vrouwe Gasthuis, 1090 HM Amsterdam, The Netherlands

Johannes Ott, Agnes Jaeger-Lansky, Gunda Poschalko, Eleen Rothschedl and René Wenzl
Department of Gynecology and Obstetrics, Medical University of Vienna, Waehringer Guertel 18-20, 1090 Vienna, Austria

Regina Promberger
Department of Surgery, Medical University of Vienna Vienna, Austria

S. Sircar, G. J. Robson, J. A. Davis, J. K. Kennedy and F. Alexander-Sefre
Department of Gynaecological Oncology, Glasgow Royal Infirmary, Glasgow G4 0SF Scotland, UK

F. Alexander-Sefre
Ward 56B, Glasgow Royal Infirmary, Castle Street, Glasgow G4 0SF Scotland, UK

Kushal Chummun, Ray O'Sullivan and Walter Prendiville
National Clinical Skills Centre, Coombe Women and Infants, University Hospital, Dublin, Ireland

John P. Burke
Department of Surgery, Beaumont Hospital, Dublin, Ireland

Harald Krentel
CEGPA, Centro de Endoscopía Ginecológica Peruano Aleman, Lima, Peru
Städtisches Krankenhaus Eisenhüttenstadt, Gynecology and Obstetrics, Friedrich-Engels-Str. 39, 15890 Eisenhüttenstadt, Germany

Mercedes Almagro Ruiz
Hospital Eugenio Espejo, Quito, Ecuador

Ibrahim Alkatout, Liselotte Mettler, Walter Jonat, Christel Eckmann-Scholz and Thoralf Schollmeyer
Department of Gynecology and Obstetrics, University Hospitals Schleswig-Holstein, Campus Kiel, Arnold-Heller Strasse 3, House 24, 24105, Kiel, Germany

Martin Anlauf
Institute of Pathology, University Hospital Düsseldorf, 40225, Düsseldorf, Germany

Reitan Ribeiro and Monica Tessmann Zomer
Red Cross Hospital, Curitiba, Paraná, Brazil
Vita Batel Hospital, Curitiba, Paraná, Brazil Sugisawa Medical Center, Curitiba, Paraná, Brazil

William Kondo
Av. Getulio Vargas, 3163 ap 21, 80240-041 Curitiba, Paraná, Brazil
Red Cross Hospital, Curitiba, Paraná, Brazil
Vita Batel Hospital, Curitiba, Paraná, Brazil
Sugisawa Medical Center, Curitiba, Paraná, Brazil

Imaduldin Salah
College of Medicine, El Minya, Egypt

Jacques Donnez, Pascale Jadoul, Sébastien Colette, Mathieu Luyckx and Jean Squifflet
Pôle de Recherche en Gynécologie, Institut de Recherche Expérimentale et Clinique (IREC), Université Catholique de Louvain (UCL), 1200 Brussels, Belgium
Department of Gynecology, Cliniques Universitaires Saint-Luc, 1200 Brussels, Belgium

Olivier Donnez
Gynecology, CHU Mont-Godinne, Université Catholique de Louvain, 5530 Yvoir, Belgium

Jacques Donnez
Department of Gynecology, Université Catholique de Louvain, Cliniques Universitaires St Luc, Avenue Hippocrate 10, 1200 Brussels, Belgium

Y. Kaufman, L. Ostrovsky, O. Klein, I. Hirsh, R. Auslander and A. Lissak
Department of Obstetrics and Gynecology, The Lady Davis Carmel Medical Center, Technion Institute of Technology Medical School, 7 Michal Street, Haifa 34362, Israel

R. Pizov
Department of Anesthesiology and Critical Care, The Lady Davis Carmel Medical Center, Technion Institute of Technology Medical School, Haifa, Israel

Rakesh Sinha, Meenakshi Sundaram, Shweta Raje, Gayatri Rao, Manju Sinha and Rushindra Sinha
Gynaecological Endoscopy, Bombay Endoscopy Academy and Centre for Minimally Invasive Surgery (BEAMS), 674, 16th Cross Road Khar, West Mumbai, Mumbai, Maharashtra 400052, India

Mariëlla I. J. Withagen, Mark E. Vierhout and Kirsten B. Kluivers
Department of Obstetrics and Gynaecology, Radboud University Nijmegen Medical Centre, Nijmegen, The Netherlands

Alfredo L. Milani
Department of Obstetrics and Gynaecology, Reinier de Graaf Group, Delft, The Netherlands

Robin M. F. van der Weiden
Department of Obstetrics and Gynaecology, Sint Franciscus Gasthuis, 3045 PM, Rotterdam, The Netherlands

Benoit Rabischong, Demetrio Larraín, Michel Canis, Kris Jardon and Gerard Mage
Department of Obstetrics-Gynecology and Human Reproduction, CHU Estaing, 1 Place Lucie Aubrac, 63003 Clermont-Ferrand, France

Guillaume Le Bouëdec Christophe Pomel Jean-Louis Achard and Jacques Dauplat
Department of Gynecologic Oncology and Surgery, Jean Perrin Cancer Center, 58 rue Montalembert, 63011 Clermont-Ferrand, France

Fabrice Kwiatkowski
Department of Medical Research and Biostatistics, Jean Perrin Cancer Center, 58 rue Montalembert, 63011 Clermont-Ferrand, France

Guido H. H. Mannaerts
Department of Surgery, Sint Franciscus Gasthuis, Rotterdam, The Netherlands

Meenakshi Sundaram
674, 16th Cross Road, Behind Khar Gymkhana, Khar Pali, Khar (W), Mumbai 400 052, India

Haruhiko Kanasaki, Aki Oride, Kentaro Nakayama and Kohji Miyazaki
Department of Obstetrics and Gynecology, Shimane University School of Medicine, 89-1 Enya Cho, Izumo 693-8501 Shimane Prefecture, Japan

Anwar Moria, Nouf Aljaji, Louise Miner and Togas Tulandi
Department of Obstetrics and Gynecology, McGill University, Montreal, QC, Canada

Togas Tulandi
687 Pine Ave. West, Montreal, Quebec H3A 1A1, Canada

Henk W. R. Schreuder, Thyrza O. S. Pattij, Ronald P. Zweemer, and René H. M. Verheijen
Division of Woman and Baby, Department of Surgical and Oncological Gynecology, University Medical Centre Utrecht, Room F05-126, 3508 GA Utrecht, The Netherlands

Marchien W. van Baal
Department of Obstetrics and Gynaecology, Flevo Hospital, Almere, The Netherlands

Buket Taş
Erasmus Medical Centre Rotterdam, 's- Gravedijkwal 230 3015 CE Rotterdam, The Netherlands
Verboomstraat 30, 3082 JN Rotterdam, The Netherlands

Anders Meller Donatsky and Ismail Gögenur
Department of Surgery, University Hospital of Copenhagen, Herlev, Herlev Ringvej 75, 2730 Herlev, Denmark

Andreas Stavroulis, Alfred Cutner and Lih-Mei Liao
University London College Hospitals NHS Foundation Trust, 235 Euston Road, NW1 2BU London, UK

Haider Jan, Natasha Waters, Pat Haines and Andrew Kent
Royal Surrey County Hospital NHS Foundation Trust, Egerton Road, Guildford, Surrey GU2 7XX, UK

Martina Ribič-Pucelj, Branko Cvjetićanin and Vesna Šalamun
Department of Obstetrics and Gynecology, University Medical Centre Ljubljana, Šlajmerjeva 3, SI-1000 Ljubljana, Slovenia

Latchesar S. Tantchev, Grigor A. Gorchev, Slavcho T. Tomov, Zdravka V. Radionova and Angelika S. Velkova
Gynecologic Oncology Clinic, Medical University—Pleven, Georgi Kochev Str. 8a, 5800 Pleven, Bulgaria

Susan S. Khalil and Tamara N. Finger
Division of Minimally Invasive Surgery, Department of Obstetrics and Gynecology, St. Luke's-Roosevelt Medical Center, New York NY, USA

Patrick F. Vetere and Farr R. Nezhat
Division of Minimally Invasive Gynecologic Surgery, Department of Obstetrics and Gynecology, Winthrop University Hospital, Mineola NY, USA

Farr R. Nezhat
Division of Gynecologic, Oncology andMinimally Invasive Surgery, Department of Obstetrics and Gynecology, Columbia University, New York, NY 10019, USA
Department of Obstetrics and Gynecology, St. Luke's-Roosevelt Medical Center, 10th Floor, 1000 10th Avenue, New York, NY 10019, USA

Atef Darwish
Woman's Health University Center, Assiut University, Assiut, Egypt
Department of Obstetrics & Gynecology, Woman's Health University Hospital, 71111 Assiut, Egypt

Hans Brölmann
Department of Gynaecology, VU University Medical Centre, de Boelelaan 1117, 1181HVAmsterdam, The Netherlands

Vasilios Tanos
Department of Obstetrics and Gynaecology, Aretaeio Hospital, St George's Medical School, Nicosia University, Nicosia, Cyprus

Grigoris Grimbizis
Department of Obstetrics and Gynecology, Aristotle University of Thessaloniki, Thessaloniki, Greece

Thomas Ind
Department of Gynaecological Oncology, Royal Marsden Hospital, London, UK

Kevin Philips
Spire Hull and East Riding Hospital, London, UK

Thierry van den Bosch
Catholic University Leuven, Leuven, Belgium

Samir Sawalhe
Donauisar Klinikum Deggendorf-Dingolfing-Landau, Deggendorf, Germany

Lukas van den Haak and Frank-Willem Jansen
Leiden University Medical Centre, Leiden, The Netherlands

Johanna Pijnenborg
Elisabeth-twee steden Hospital, Tilburg, The Netherlands

Florin-Andrei Taran and Sara Brucker
Department for Women's Health, University Hospital Tuebingen, Eberhard Karls University, Tübingen, Germany

Arnaud Wattiez
IRCAD, Strassburg, France

Rudi Campo
Leuven Institute for Fertility and Embryology (LIFE), Leuven, Belgium

Peter O'Donovan
M.E.R.I.T. Centre, Bradford Royal Infirmary, Bristol, UK

Rudy Leon de Wilde
Pius Hospital, Oldenburg, Germany

Liliana Mereu, Luca Mencaglia, Alessandro Pontis and Giada Carri
Division of Gynecology, Centro Oncologico Fiorentino, Via Ragionieri 101, Sesto Fiorentino, Florence, Italy

Stefano Angioni and Alessandro Pontis
Division of Gynecology, Obstetrics and Pathophysiology of Human Reproduction, University of Cagliari, Cagliari, Italy

Giada Carri
Department of Obstetrics and Gynecology, Università Cattolica del Sacro Cuore, Roma, Italy

S. Tamburro, E. Nouhz and F. Calonaci
Department of Obstetrics & Gynecology, CH Thiers, Route du Fau, 63300 Thiers, France
Department Obstetrics and Gynecology, CHU Clermont Ferrand, CHU Estaing, 1 Place Lucie Aubrac, 63003 Clermont-Ferrand CEDEX 1, France

A. Wattiez
CHU Hôpital Hautepierre, Chirurgie gynécologique, 1 Avenue Molière, 67098 Strasbourg Cedex 2, France

Kate McIlwaine, M. Cameron, E. Readman, J. Manwaring and P. Maher
Department of Endosurgery, Mercy Hospital for Women, 163 Studley Rd.Heidelberg, VIC 3084, Australia

Hossam El-Din Shawki
Obstetrics and Gynecology Department, Faculty of Medicine, El Minia University, El Minia, Egypt

Juan Gilabert-Estelles
Department of Gynecology, University Hospital La Fe, Valencia, Spain
Unit of Gynecological Endoscopy, Hospital Casa de Salud, Av. Manuel Candela 41, 46010, 46009 Valencia, Spain

Juan Gilabert-Aguilar
Department of Gynecology, Hospital Arnau de Vilanova, Valencia, Spain
Unit of Gynecological Endoscopy, Hospital Casa de Salud, Av. Manuel Candela 41, 46010, 46009 Valencia, Spain

Sonia Chachan
Department of Gynaecology, Royal Surrey County Hospital, Guildford, Surrey GU2 7XX, UK

N. Waters and A. Kent
Department of Gynaecology, Institution: Minimal Access Therapy Training Unit, Post Graduate Medical School, University of Surrey, Manor Park, Guildford, Surrey GU2 7WG, UK

Revaz Botchorishvili, Fanny Desvignes and Gérard Mage
C.H.U. Clermont-Ferrand, Department of Gynecology and Obstetrics, Polyclinique de l'Hôtel Dieu, Clermont Ferrand, France

William Kondo
Boulevard Leon Malfreyt, 63058 Clermont-Ferrand CEDEX 1, France

A. Sayasneh, H. Nosib and H. Abdel-Rahman
Department of Obstetrics and Gynaecology, Hinchingbrooke Hospital, Huntingdon, UK

A. Cutner, A. Stavroulis and N. Zolfaghari
Institute for Women's Health, UCLH NHS Foundation Trust, London, UK

Index

www.ingramcontent.com/pod-product-compliance
Lightning Source LLC
LaVergne TN
LVHW081037210926
848485LV00004B/1042